6/07

04

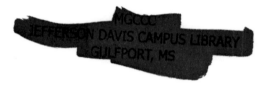

Psychiatric Disorders
in Pregnancy and the Postpartum

CURRENT CLINICAL PRACTICE

NEIL S. SKOLNIK, MD • SERIES EDITOR

Psychiatric Disorders
in Pregnancy
and the Postpartum

Principles and Treatment

Edited by

Victoria Hendrick, MD

Olive View–UCLA Medical Center
Sylmar, CA

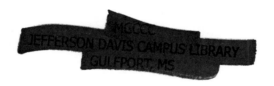

HUMANA PRESS ✳ TOTOWA, NEW JERSEY

© 2006 Humana Press Inc.
999 Riverview Drive, Suite 208
Totowa, New Jersey 07512

www.humanapress.com

Due diligence has been taken by the publishers, editors, and authors of this book to assure the accuracy of the information published and to describe generally accepted practices. The contributors herein have carefully checked to ensure that the drug selections and dosages set forth in this text are accurate and in accord with the standards accepted at the time of publication. Notwithstanding, as new research, changes in government regulations, and knowledge from clinical experience relating to drug therapy and drug reactions constantly occurs, the reader is advised to check the product information provided by the manufacturer of each drug for any change in dosages or for additional warnings and contraindications. This is of utmost importance when the recommended drug herein is a new or infrequently used drug. It is the responsibility of the treating physician to determine dosages and treatment strategies for individual patients. Further it is the responsibility of the health care provider to ascertain the Food and Drug Administration status of each drug or device used in their clinical practice. The publisher, editors, and authors are not responsible for errors or omissions or for any consequences from the application of the information presented in this book and make no warranty, express or implied, with respect to the contents in this publication.

This publication is printed on acid-free paper. ∞
ANSI Z39.48-1984 (American Standards Institute) Permanence of Paper for Printed Library Materials.

Production Editor: Robin B. Weisberg

Cover design by Patricia F. Cleary

For additional copies, pricing for bulk purchases, and/or information about other Humana titles, contact Humana at the above address or at any of the following numbers: Tel.: 973-256-1699; Fax: 973-256-8341; E-mail: orders@humanapr.com; or visit our Website: www.humanapress.com

Photocopy Authorization Policy:

Photocopy Authorization Policy: Authorization to photocopy items for internal or personal use, or the internal or personal use of specific clients is granted by Humana Press, provided that the base fee of US $30.00 per copy is paid directly to the Copyright Clearance Center (CCC), 222 Rosewood Dr., Danvers MA 01923. For those organizations that have been granted a photocopy license from the CCC, a separate system of payment has been arranged and is acceptable to the Humana Press. The fee code for users of the Transactional Reporting Service is 1-58829-486-2/06 $30.00.

Printed in the United States of America. 10 9 8 7 6 5 4 3 2 1

eISBN 1-59745-013-8

Library of Congress Cataloging-in-Publication Data

Psychiatric disorders in pregnancy and the postpartum : principles and treatment / edited by Victoria Hendrick.
    p. ; cm. -- (Current clinical practice)
  Includes bibliographical references and index.
  ISBN 1-58829-486-2 (alk. paper)
  1. Mental illness in pregnancy. 2. Pregnancy in mentally ill women. 3. Postpartum psychiatric disorders. 4. Mental illness in pregnancy--Treatment. 5. Postpartum psychiatric disorders--Treatment.
  [DNLM: 1. Mental Disorders--therapy--Pregnancy. 2. Postpartum Period--psychology.
3. Pregnancy Complications--therapy. WQ 240 P974 2006] I. Hendrick, Victoria C., 1963-
II. Series.
  RG588.P79 2006

  618.7'6--dc22

                                                                                          2005027758

Series Editor's Introduction

Psychiatric disorders during pregnancy and the postpartum period are common, underappreciated, and underdiagnosed maladies that affect many women at a time of their lives that they have long anticipated would be perhaps the happiest. These disorders rob both the woman and her child of the opportunity to enjoy and appreciate some of the most warm, comforting, special moments in each of their lives. Importantly, these disorders are entities that often respond to treatment, both with counseling and/or medications, and so it is therefore essential for primary care physicians— obstetrician/gynecologists, family physicians, internists, and pediatricians— to understand how to appropriately identify and be able to make decisions about treatment or referral. The results of physicians' interventions affect both mother and infant, as well as all members of their family.

Dr. Victoria Hendrick has done a wonderful service by organizing this evolving literature into one readable textbook, and in so doing has empowered primary care physicians to enable many women, at a time when they are feeling particularly fragile and vulnerable, to seek and find competent, compassionate care from their primary care physicians. For this, she deserves our thanks.

Neil Skolnik, MD
Professor of Family and Community Medicine
Temple University School of Medicine
Associate Director
Family Practice Residency
Abington Memorial Hospital

Preface

Women's risk for developing a psychiatric disorder is greatest during their reproductive years. Many women, therefore, are likely to require treatment for a psychiatric illness during pregnancy and breastfeeding. Contrary to common stereotype, pregnancy and the postpartum period are not times of relative quiescence of mental illnesses, but rather represent a time of high risk for illness exacerbation. Clinicians often feel apprehensive about treating pregnant and breastfeeding women since much of the information on safe psychiatric treatments is recent and has not been widely disseminated. Many of the studies on the use of psychiatric medications in pregnancy and lactation have been published only in the past five years. Furthermore, data can be difficult to interpret because of conflicting and inconclusive findings and a lack of awareness of the variety of issues that must be taken into account in choosing the treatment. These include the potential adverse effects on the child of untreated maternal psychiatric illnesses during pregnancy and the postpartum period, as well as the lesser known risks of prenatal medication exposure, such as neonatal toxicity and postnatal behavioral sequelae. Knowledge of the typical course of psychiatric illnesses during pregnancy and the postpartum is also necessary to make wise treatment decisions.

Psychiatric Disorders in Pregnancy and the Postpartum comprehensively reviews the treatment of psychiatric disorders in pregnancy and postpartum. Chapters focus on each of the major psychiatric illnesses, as well as on the potential impact of these illnesses on infants and children. The authors, all experts in the field of perinatal psychiatry, discuss a variety of treatments including medications, psychotherapy, parent education, and social skills training. *Psychiatric Disorders in Pregnancy and the Postpartum* will provide readers with the information necessary to make informed, careful decisions for the safest and most effective treatment of psychiatrically ill pregnant women and new mothers.

Victoria Hendrick, MD

Contents

ix

Contributors

JONATHAN S. ABRAMOWITZ, PhD • *OCD/Anxiety Disorders Program, Mayo Clinic, Rochester, MN*

LORI L. ALTSHULER, MD • *UCLA Mood Disorders Research Program, Department of Psychiatry, David Geffen School of Medicine at UCLA, Los Angeles, CA*

JENNIFER BALLEW, DO, PhD • *Clinical Neuroscience Training Program, Department of Psychiatry, Yale University School of Medicine, New Haven, CT*

MARY F. BRUNETTE, MD • *Dartmouth Medical School and the New Hampshire Dartmouth Psychiatric Research Center, Concord, NH*

ADRIENNE EINARSON, RN • *The Motherisk Program, Division of Clinical Pharmacology and Toxicology, The Hospital for Sick Children, Toronto, Ontario*

C. NEILL EPPERSON, MD • *Yale Behavioral Gynecology Program, Departments of Psychiatry and Obstetrics, Gynecology and Reproductive science, Yale University School of Medicine, New Haven, CT*

DEBRA L. FRANKO, PhD • *Department of Counseling and Applied Educational Psychology, Northeastern University and Harvard Eating Disorders Center, Boston, MA*

VICTORIA HENDRICK, MD • *Olive View–University of California, Los Angeles Medical Center, Sylmar, CA*

MONIQUE M. HERNANDEZ, MSW • *Psychiatry and Biobehavioral Sciences, David Geffen School of Medicine, University of California, Los Angeles, CA*

TERESA JACOBSEN, PhD • *School of Social Work, University of Illinois at Urbana-Champaign, Urbana, IL*

SANJOG KALRA, BSc • *Department of Pharmacology, University of Toronto and The Motherisk Program, Division of Clinical Pharmacology and Toxicology, The Hospital for Sick Children, Toronto, Ontario*

CAROL KIRIAKOS, MD • *Olive View–University of California Medical Center, Los Angeles and Sepulveda-Veterans Administration Medical Center, Los Angeles, CA*

KARIN LARSEN, PhD • *Department of Psychology, Mayo Clinic, Rochester, MN*

KAREN A. MIOTTO, MD • *Psychiatry and Biobehavioral Sciences, David Geffen School of Medicine, University of California, Los Angeles, CA*

KATHERINE M. MOORE, MD • *Department of Psychiatry, Mayo Clinic, Rochester, MN*

PHIVAN L. PHAM, BA • *Psychiatry and Biobehavioral Sciences, David Geffen School of Medicine, University of California, Los Angeles, CA*

MARY V. SEEMAN, MD • *Centre for Addiction and Mental Health, University of Toronto, Toronto, Ontario*

ELIZABETH SUTI, MFT • *UCLA Substance Abuse Service and Psychiatry and Biobehavioral Sciences, David Geffen School of Medicine, University of California, Los Angeles, CA*

1

General Considerations in Treating Psychiatric Disorders During Pregnancy and Following Delivery

Victoria Hendrick

Summary

Many pregnant women and new mothers require treatment for a psychiatric illness. The most common psychiatric illnesses among women of reproductive age involve depressive and anxiety disorders. More severe conditions, such as bipolar disorder or schizophrenia, also typically manifest their first symptoms during the reproductive years. In many cases, psychiatric treatment will include the use of a medication. This chapter reviews important considerations in providing psychiatric treatment during pregnancy and the postpartum period to maximize the safety and well-being of the mother and the child.

Key Words: Psychiatric disorder; pregnancy; postpartum; breast-feeding; women.

1. INTRODUCTION

Women are at the greatest risk of developing a psychiatric disorder between the ages of 18 and 45 yr *(1–3)*. Many women, therefore, may experience a psychiatric illness while they are pregnant or breast-feeding. The psychiatric disorders with the highest prevalence in women are depressive and anxiety disorders (Table 1). Women with histories of these disorders are at risk for relapse during pregnancy, particularly if they have experienced two or more relapses of the disorder *(4)*.

Ideally, women with a history of any recurrent psychiatric disorder should obtain a prepregnancy consultation to discuss the safest treatment

From: *Current Clinical Practice: Psychiatric Disorders in Pregnancy and the Postpartum: Principles and Treatment*
Edited by: V. Hendrick © Humana Press, Totowa, NJ

Table 1
Lifetime and 12-Mo Prevalence Rates
of Psychiatric Disorders in Women and Men

	Male		Female		Total	
	Lifetime	12 mo	Lifetime	12 mo	Lifetime	12 mo
Mood disorders						
Major depressive episode	12.7	7.7	21.3	12.9	17.1	10.3
Manic episode	1.6	1.4	1.7	1.3	1.6	1.3
Dysthymia	4.8	2.1	8.0	3.0	6.4	2.5
Any mood disorder	14.7	8.5	23.9	14.1	19.3	11.3
Anxiety disorders						
Panic disorder	2.0	1.3	5.0	3.2	3.5	2.3
Agoraphobia w/o panic disorder	3.5	1.7	7.0	3.8	5.3	2.8
Social phobia	11.1	6.6	15.5	9.1	13.3	7.9
Simple phobia	6.7	4.4	15.7	13.2	11.3	8.8
Generalized anxiety disorder	3.6	2.0	6.6	4.3	5.1	3.1
Any anxiety disorder	19.2	11.8	30.5	22.6	24.9	17.2
Substance use disorders						
Alcohol abuse w/o dependence	12.5	3.4	6.4	1.6	9.4	2.5
Alcohol dependence	20.1	10.7	8.2	3.7	14.1	7.2
Drug abuse w/o dependence	5.4	1.3	3.5	0.3	4.4	0.8
Drug dependence	9.2	3.8	5.9	1.9	7.5	2.8
Any substance abuse/dependence	35.4	16.1	17.9	6.6	26.6	11.3
Other disorders						
Antisocial personality	5.8	—	—	—	3.5	—
Nonaffective psychosis[a]	0.3	0.5	0.8	0.6	0.7	0.5
Any NCS disorder	48.7	27.7	47.3	31.2	48.0	29.5

[a] Nonaffective psychosis includes schizophrenia, schizophreniform disorder, delusional disorder, and atypical psychosis.
NCS, National Comorbidity Survey (7).

approach as they try to conceive and during the pregnancy. For women on psychiatric medications, the consultation should include a review of any previous attempts of medication discontinuation. If a patient has quickly relapsed after discontinuing a medication, she may need to remain on the medication while pregnant. However, if she has been able to remain well for at least several months while off the medication, she may be able to taper and discontinue the medication prior to attempting to conceive.

Women who are unlikely to conceive quickly (e.g., women in their mid- to late-30s or those with history of infertility in themselves or their partners) should consider remaining on the medication while trying to get pregnant. The medication can be discontinued once a pregnancy test is positive at approx 2 wk postconception. This approach produces minimal embryological exposure to the medication because the placental circulation is not established until 2–3 wk postconception (5). Certain medications should be tapered rather than stopped abruptly to minimize the likelihood of psychiatric relapse (e.g., mood stabilizers) and/or to avoid withdrawal symptoms (e.g., paroxetine, venlafaxine). Medications with antifolate properties, such as valproate and carbamazepine, should not be used for 6 wk postconception because they are linked with a substantial risk of neural tube defects (6).

Whether the discussion with the patient takes place prior to or following conception, it should review the following:

1. The available information on the risks of medication exposure during pregnancy and nursing.
2. The limitations of the data (e.g., small sample sizes, limited information on potential neurobehavioral sequelae of prenatal medication exposure, naturalistic designs that may not take into account confounding variables such as maternal use of nicotine, maternal health habits, etc.).
3. Treatment alternatives during pregnancy.
4. The patient's likelihood of a psychiatric relapse during pregnancy and the postpartum period.
5. Measures that may reduce likelihood of relapse (e.g., psychotherapy; couples counseling, attention to psychosocial stressors).
6. The general incidence of birth defects (approx 2–4%) regardless of prenatal medication exposure.

The clinician should ensure that the patient understands the information that has been presented to her. The risk–benefit discussion should continue over the course of the pregnancy and should be carefully documented. It is always best if the father is involved in this discussion.

Whenever possible, nonpharmacological interventions should take precedence over medications during pregnancy. Nonpharmacological interventions include individual and group psychotherapy, couple and family counseling, relaxation techniques, and attention to psychosocial

Table 2
FDA Use-in-Pregnancy Ratings

A	Controlled studies in women show no risk.
B	Animal studies show no risk, but there are no controlled studies in humans; or animal studies show adverse effect that has not been confirmed in human studies.
C	Animal studies show risk but there are no controlled studies in humans; or studies in animals and humans are not available.
D	There is evidence of risk in humans, but the drug may have benefits that outweigh the risk.
X	Risk outweighs any benefit.

stressors. However, if nonpharmacological interventions are inadequate or inappropriate for the patient's illness or if previous attempts at nonpharmacological interventions have been unsuccessful, medications may be necessary. Regardless of the treatment approach, the patient should be encouraged to obtain support from family and friends for infant care, to get as much sleep and rest as possible, and to reduce her other responsibilities. If possible, hiring a child-care assistant for even part of each day is extremely helpful.

Doses of psychiatric medications should be maintained at the minimum necessary. Monotherapy is always preferable to polytherapy. Whenever possible, the use of the medication should be minimized or avoided at least in the first trimester, particularly if pregnancy data on its safety are limited. Clinicians should base their choice of medication primarily on the latest research findings rather than on the Food and Drug Administration (FDA) Use-in-Pregnancy ratings (Table 2). The FDA Pregnancy Category B rating can be misleading: medications in this category are not necessarily safer to use in pregnancy than medications with Pregnancy Category C labeling because they may have been placed in this category if animal studies show no fetal risk while there are as yet no human data. Category C-labeled medications for which human data show low risk may be preferable to Category B-labeled medications for which there are no human data.

In prescribing psychiatric medications to pregnant women, it is important to keep in mind that many medications exacerbate the common physiological experiences of pregnancy. For example, medications with anticholinergic effects (e.g., tricyclic antidepressants, certain antipsychotic agents) are likely to worsen constipation. Also, several psychiatric medications worsen the orthostatic hypotension and/or fatigue common in pregnancy (Table 3).

In addition to attending to the risks of medication use in pregnancy, clinicians should emphasize the importance of avoiding nicotine, alcohol, and illicit drugs and of obtaining good nutrition. Education about proper dietary habits and weight management can be helpful for chronically mentally ill women who often follow poor diets (8). Women with schizophrenia are at high risk for obesity, a risk factor for neural tube defects (9).

2. UNINTENDED PREGNANCY

More than 50% of pregnancies in the United States are unplanned (10), and many women become pregnant while taking medications. Clinicians working with chronically mentally ill women should keep in mind their relatively high incidence of unprotected sex and inadequate use of contraception (11). For women who do not wish to conceive, it is wise to provide education about methods of contraception and to inquire about recent missed menstrual periods. Adequate contraception has become particularly important following the widespread use of the "atypical" antipsychotic medications (e.g., olanzapine, quetiapine) that, unlike the older antipsychotic agents, do not raise prolactin levels and therefore do not interfere with women's ability to conceive.

3. EFFECT OF PREGNANCY ON DRUG METABOLISM

Physiological changes in pregnancy can affect serum concentrations of psychiatric medications (Table 4). Some of these changes may increase or decrease the dose necessary for some medications. The blood level of nortriptyline, a tricyclic antidepressant, has been found to drop below the therapeutic range as women reach the fifth month of pregnancy (12). Certain hepatic enzymes in the cytochrome P450 system are induced by high levels of estradiol and progesterone during pregnancy (13–16). These include 3A4, which breaks down quetiapine and clozapine, and 2D6, which metabolizes risperidone. Cytochrome 1A2, on the other hand, becomes less active during pregnancy (17). Because 1A2 is the main metabolizing enzyme for olanzapine, blood levels of this medication may increase during pregnancy.

Wide interindividual variations exist in the degree of medication clearance present during pregnancy (18). For medications that must remain within a specific therapeutic window (e.g., lithium, tricyclic antidepressants, antiepileptic drugs), it is advisable to increase the monitoring frequency of blood levels of medications. Although the optimal frequency

Table 3
FDA Use-in-Pregnancy Ratings for Specific Medications

Medication	FDA Use-in-Pregnancy Rating
Anxiolytics and sedatives	
Alprazolam (Xanax)	D
Buspirone (Buspar)	B
Clonazepam (Klonopin)	D
Diazepam (Valium)	D
Flurazepam (Dalmane)	X
Lorazepam (Ativan)	D
Temazepam (Restoril)	X
Zolpidem (Ambien)	B
Antidepressants	
Amitriptyline (Elavil, Endep)	D
Bupropion (Wellbutrin)	B
Citalopram (Celexa, Lexapro)	C
Clomipramine (Anafranil)	C
Desipramine (Norpramin, Pertofrane)	C
Doxepin (Adapin, Sinequan)	C
Fluoxetine (Prozac, Sarafem)	C
Fluvoxamine (Luvox)	C
Imipramine (Tofranil)	D
Mirtazapine (Remeron)	C
Nefazodone (Serzone)	C
Nortriptyline (Aventyl, Pamelor)	D
Paroxetine (Paxil)	C
Sertraline (Zoloft)	C
Trazodone (Desyrel)	C
Venlafaxine (Effexor)	C
Mood stabilizers	
Lithium (Lithobid, Eskalith)	D
Valproate (Depakote, Depakene)	D
Carbamazepine (Tegretol)	D
Gabapentin (Neurontin)	C
Lamotrigine (Lamictal)	C
Oxcarbazepine (Trileptal)	C
Antipsychotics	
Aripiprazole (Abilify)	C
Clozapine (Clozaril)	B
Fluphenazine (Prolixin)	C
Haloperidol (Haldol)	C
Olanzapine (Zyprexa)	C

Table 3 *(Continued)*

Medication	FDA Use-in-Pregnancy Rating
Risperidone (Risperdal)	C
Quetiapine (Seroquel)	C
Trifluoperazine (Stelazine)	C
Ziprasidone (Geodon)	C
Stimulants	
Dextroamphetamine (Adderall, Dexedrine)	C
Methylphenidate (Ritalin)	C
Anticholinergic agents	
Diphenhydramine (Benadryl)	B
Hydroxyzine (Atarax)	C
Trihexyphenidyl (Artane)	C
Antihypertensive agents	
Propanolol (Inderal)	C
Clonidine (Catapres)	C
Hormone supplements	
Levothyroxine	A
Oral contraceptives	X
Analgesics	
Acetaminophen (Tylenol)	B
Ibuprofen (Motrin)	B
Naproxen (Naprosyn)	B
Sumatriptan (Imitrex)	C

of monitoring has not been established, a wise rule would be to check medication blood levels at least monthly during the second and third trimesters of pregnancy. If a medication dosage is increased during pregnancy, it should probably be reduced following delivery to avoid the possibility of toxicity in the mother following the birth.

4. PSYCHIATRIC MEDICATION USE NEAR TERM

Some medications may produce toxicity or withdrawal effects in the newborn. These include the selective serotonin reuptake inhibitors (e.g., fluoxetine, paroxetine), which have been linked with neonatal jitteriness, respiratory distress, and hypoglycemia *(19,20)*, and benzodiazepines (e.g., clonazepam, diazepam, lorazepam), which can produce excessive

Table 4
Effects of Pregnancy on Medication Concentrations

Physiological changes in pregnancy	Effect on medication concentrations
Increase in hepatic metabolism	Increased medication clearance
Increase in renal clearance	Increased medication clearance
Increase in volume of distribution	Reduction in blood levels of medications
Decrease in protein binding	Increase in free fraction of protein-bound medications (e.g., valproate, carbamazepine)
Slowed gastrointestinal transit time	Increase in gastrointestinal absorption of medications.

sedation or withdrawal-like symptoms in the newborn *(21)*. Depending on the stability of the mother's condition during pregnancy, it may be advisable to taper the dose of the psychiatric medication 2–4 wk before the estimated delivery date to minimize the risk of neonatal withdrawal symptoms. Following the birth, the original medication dose should be resumed to minimize the possibility of a relapse of the mother's psychiatric illness in the postpartum period.

5. POSTPARTUM

The weeks following delivery are a time of vulnerability to psychiatric disorders for many women *(22)*. Mood and anxiety disorders are particularly likely to recur or worsen during these weeks. These conditions not only cause significant distress to the mother but can disrupt family life and, if prolonged, can negatively impact the child's emotional and social development *(23)*. Clinicians should encourage patients to identify family members or friends who can help with child-care responsibilities if the mother experiences a relapse of psychiatric illness in the postpartum. Women with severe mental illnesses may be deficient in parenting skills and need a referral to a parenting education class.

Women with a history of psychiatric disorder may benefit from the prophylactic use of psychiatric medication begun the day of delivery. However, data on this approach are limited and inconsistent *(24)*.

Certain side effects can be especially problematic to new mothers. For example, several psychiatric medications produce significant sedation and can therefore impair a new mother's ability to attend adequately to her infant. Weight gain is another common side effect, and women who are trying to lose the weight they gained during pregnancy may be hesitant to take medications with such an effect. New mothers may be looking forward to the end of the pregnancy to resume their pregravid intimate relationships with their partners and may prefer to avoid medications that impair sexual functioning, a widespread side effect of many antidepressants.

Many new mothers begin contraception following the birth of a child, and clinicians should consider the potential impact of hormonal contraceptives on psychiatric medications. Estrogen-containing hormonal contraceptives inhibit CYP3A4 and may therefore reduce clearance for medications that are metabolized by this enzyme, including diazepam and imipramine (25,26). On the other hand, estrogen-containing hormonal contraceptives can induce hepatic conjugative enzymes and may therefore increase the metabolism of medications that are conjugated before elimination by the kidney, such as lamotrigine (27).

Conversely, hormonal contraceptives can be rendered ineffective by the concomitant use of medications that increase their metabolism, including carbamazepine, oxcarbazepine, topiramate, modafinil, and St. John's wort (28). Women should be encouraged to use a high-potency oral contraceptive (i.e., containing at least 50 µg/d of estradiol) or an alternative method of contraception while taking these medications.

An additional consideration in evaluating new mothers with histories of psychiatric disorders is the possibility of premenstrual relapse of psychiatric symptoms. Once a new mother's menstrual cycles resume, she may experience an exacerbation or relapse of symptoms in the days prior to onset of menses. If this premenstrual relapse occurs repeatedly and the patient is taking a psychiatric medication, an increase of medication dose by 50% from midcycle to onset of menses may help.

6. USE OF PSYCHIATRIC MEDICATIONS DURING BREAST-FEEDING

The decision to use psychiatric medications in new mothers should take into consideration whether the patient will be breast-feeding. If so, it is best to prescribe a medication for which safety data exist in breast-feeding and to use the lowest effective dose. Before the mother begins the medication, the infant's behavior and sleep and feeding patterns should be established. Changes in these patterns may reflect a side effect of the medication in the infant.

For medications that lack safety data in breast-feeding, the medication's pharmacokinetic parameters can provide useful information about its likely passage into breast milk. High protein-binding and short half-lives are associated with lower concentrations of the medication in milk and therefore less infant exposure. The medication's potency is another consideration: for example, fluoxetine has approximately one-sixth and one-fifteenth the serotonergic potency of sertraline and paroxetine, respectively. Therefore, a serum concentration of 100 ng/mL of fluoxetine is approximately equivalent in potency to a serum concentration of 6.7 ng/mL of paroxetine. Additional factors that influence the nursing infant's exposure to medication include the presence of active metabolites and timing of the mother's dose. For example, breast milk concentrations of sertraline and fluoxetine peak approx 6–10 h after the mother takes the medication *(29,30)*.

Clinicians and/or patients who want more data on the infant's level of medication exposure can obtain an infant serum concentration of medication. No cut-off has been established for a safe serum level of medication in infants, but an undetectable level provides reassurance. The infant's serum concentration of medication should be obtained after the medication levels are likely to be at steady state (i.e., at least five medication half-lives). Levels of the medication's metabolites, if any, should also be obtained.

In prescribing psychiatric medications to nursing mothers, it is important to consider the infant's age: an older infant has a greater capacity to metabolize medications than a newborn. Supplementation with bottle-feeding will reduce the infant's exposure to the drug.

7. CONCLUSION

Clinicians who work with pregnant and postpartum women are likely to encounter patients requiring treatment for psychiatric conditions. Whenever possible, these patients should be treated with nonpharmacological approaches. If psychopharmacological treatment is necessary, the choice of medication should be guided primarily by its safety data during pregnancy and breast-feeding and by the patient's psychiatric history. In deciding on the course of treatment, the clinician and patient should engage in a careful risk–benefit discussion before any medication is initiated. These risks and benefits may change over the course of treatment and should therefore be reexamined periodically. Medication dosage requirements may vary during pregnancy and should be adjusted as necessary. Women with mood and anxiety disorders require close monitoring following delivery as they are at risk of experiencing a postpartum relapse or exacerbation of the illness. Many medications lack safety data in breast-feeding, but general estimates of the infant's likely exposure can be made from the medication's pharmacokinetic parameters and from blood levels of medication in the infant. Women who initiate hormonal contraception following delivery should avoid psychiatric medications that diminish the contraceptive's efficacy.

REFERENCES

1. Weissman, M. M. and Jensen, P. (2002) What research suggests for depressed women with children. J. Clin. Psychiatry 63, 641–647.
2. Stevens, J. R. (2002) Schizophrenia: reproductive hormones and the brain. Am. J. Psychiatry 159, 713–719.
3. Suppes, T., Dennehy, E. B., and Gibbons, E. W. (2000) The longitudinal course of bipolar disorder. J. Clin. Psychiatry 61 Suppl 9, 23–30.
4. Altshuler, L. L., Hendrick, V., and Cohen L. (1998) Course of mood and anxiety disorders during pregnancy and the postpartum period. J. Clin. Psychiatry 59, 29–33.
5. Creasy, R. K. and Resnik, R. (1994) Maternal-Fetal Medicine: Principles and Practice, 3rd ed. Philadelphia, WB Saunders, pp. 96–97.
6. Hernandez-Diaz, S., Werler, M. M., Walker, A. M., et al. (2000) Folic acid antagonists during pregnancy and the risk of birth defects. N. Engl. J. Med. 343, 1608–1614.
7. Kessler, R. C., McGonagle, K. A., Zhao, S., et al. (1994) Lifetime and 12-month prevalence of DSM-III-R psychiatric disorders in the United States: results from the National Comorbidity Survey. Arch. Gen. Psychiatry 51, 8–19.
8. Tardieu, S., Micallef, J., Gentile, S., et al. (2003) Weight gain profiles of new antipsychotics: public health consequences. Obes. Rev. 4,129–138.
9. Koren, G, Cohn, T., Chitayat D., et al. (2002) Use of atypical antipsychotics during pregnancy and the risk of neural tube defects in infants. Am. J. Psychiatry 159, 136–137.
10. Moos, M. K. (2003) Unintended pregnancies: a call for nursing action. MCN Am. J. Matern. Child Nurs. 28, 24–30.
11. Coverdale, J., Aruffo, J., and Grunebaum, H. (1992) Developing family planning services for female chronic mentally ill outpatients. Hosp. Commun. Psychiatry 43, 475–478.
12. Altshuler, L. L. and Hendrick, V. (1996) Pregnancy and psychotropic medication: changes in blood levels. J. Clin. Psychopharmacol. 16, 78–80.
13. Schwartz, J. B. (2003) The influence of sex on pharmacokinetics. Clin. Pharmacokinet. 42, 107–121.
14. Meibohm, B., Beierle, I., and Derendorf, H. (2002) How important are gender differences in pharmacokinetics? Clin. Pharmacokinet. 41, 329–342.
15. Hagg, S., Spigset, O., and Dahlqvist, R. (2001) Influence of gender and oral contraceptives on CYP2D6 and CYP2C19 activity in healthy volunteers. Br. J. Clin. Pharmacol. 51, 169–173.
16. Wadelius, M., Darj, E., Frenne, G., et al (1997) Induction of CYP2D6 in pregnancy. Clin. Pharmacol. Ther. 62, 400–407.
17. Zaigler, M., Rietbrock, S., Szymanski, J., et al (2000) Variation of CYP1A2-dependent caffeine metabolism during menstrual cycle in healthy women. Int. J. Clin. Pharmacol. Ther. 38, 235–244.

18. McCune, J. S., Lindley, C., Decker, J. L., et al (2001) Lack of gender differences and large intrasubject variability in cytochrome P450 activity measured by phenotyping with dextromethorphan. J Clin. Pharmacol. 41, 723–731

19. Costei, A. M., Kozer, E., Ho, T., et al. (2002) Perinatal outcome following third trimester exposure to paroxetine. Arch. Pediatr. Adolesc. Med. 156, 1129–1132

20. Cohen, L. S., Heller, V. L., Bailey, J. W., et al. (2000) Birth outcomes following prenatal exposure to fluoxetine. Biol. Psychiatry 48, 996–1000.

21. Swortfiguer, D., Cissoko, H., Giraudeau, B., et al (2005) Neonatal consequences of benzodiazepines used during the last month of pregnancy. Arch. Pediatr. [Epub ahead of print]

22. Miller, L. J. (2002) Postpartum depression. JAMA 287:762–765.

23. Grace, S. L., Evindar, A., and Stewart D. E. (2003) The effect of postpartum depression on child cognitive development and behavior: a review and critical analysis of the literature. Arch. Women Ment. Health 6, 263–274.

24. Howard, L., Hoffbrand, S., Henshaw, C., et al. (2005) Antidepressant prevention of postnatal depression. Cochrane Database Syst. Rev. 2, CD004363.

25. Abernathy, D. R., Greenblatt, D. R., Divoll M., et al. (1982) Impairment of diazepam metabolism by low-dose estrogen-containing oral-contraceptive steroids. N. Engl. J. Med. 306, 791–792.

26. Abernathy, D. R., Greenblatt, D. J., and Shader, R. I. (1984) Imipramine disposition in users of oral contraceptive steroids. Clin. Pharmacol. Ther. 35, 792–797.

27. Sabers, A., Buchholt, J. M., Uldall, P., and Hansen, E. L. (2001) Lamotrigine plasma levels reduced by oral contraceptives. Epilepsy Res. 47, 151–154.

28. Doose, D. R., Wang, S. S., Padmanabhan, M., et al. (2003) Effect of topiramate or carbamazepine on the pharmacokinetics of an oral contraceptive containing norethindrone and ethinyl estradiol in healthy obese and nonobese female subjects. Epilepsia 44, 540–549.

29. Hendrick, V., Stowe Z. N., Altshuler, L. L., et al.(2001) Fluoxetine and norfluoxetine concentrations in nursing infants and breast milk. Biol. Psychiatry 50, 775–782.

30. Stowe, Z. N., Owens, M. J., Landry, J. C., et al. (1997) Sertraline and desmethylsertraline in human breast milk and nursing infants. Am. J. Psychiatry 154, 1255–1260.

2

Prevalence, Clinical Course, and Management of Depression During Pregnancy

Sanjog Kalra and Adrienne Einarson

Summary

Depression has been identified by the World Health Organization as a major cause of morbidity in the 21st century. As women between 25 and 44 yr represent the population at highest risk for depression, a substantial number are likely to become pregnant while suffering from this illness. In this chapter, we summarize the prevalence and clinical course of depression during pregnancy. We also document evidence-based information regarding the safety and efficacy of both pharmacological and nonpharmacological treatments of prenatal depression. In addition, we discuss other issues surrounding the treatment of depression, such as abrupt discontinuation syndrome, poor neonatal adaptability, and an increase in the rate of spontaneous abortions, associated with the use of certain antidepressant drugs. Of equal importance, we also review the emerging literature on the potential adverse effects of untreated depression during pregnancy.

Depression is an important issue that must be addressed when women become pregnant. A variety of pharmacological and nonpharmacological treatment options are available, the vast majority of which appear to be relatively safe. Women suffering from depression during pregnancy must be treated individually, and the benefits and/or risks of treatment or nontreatment should be weighed carefully using evidence-based information. This approach will ensure the best possible outcomes for the mothers and their babies.

Key Words: Depression; pregnancy; risks; prevalence; course; treatment; safety.

1. INTRODUCTION

Depression has been identified by the World Health Organization as a major cause of morbidity in the 21st century *(1)*. The Global Burden

From: *Current Clinical Practice: Psychiatric Disorders in Pregnancy and the Postpartum: Principles and Treatment*
Edited by: V. Hendrick © Humana Press, Totowa, NJ

of Disease study *(2)* states that major depression will become the second leading worldwide cause of disease burden by 2020. In the United States alone, the prevalence of depression has been estimated by the National Institutes of Health at between 5 *(3)* and 10.3% *(4)*.

Major depressive disorder (MDD) is threefold more common in women than in men *(5)*. Furthermore, the prevalence of depression is highest in women between the ages of 25 and 44 *(6)*. Therefore, a large group of women are likely to experience depression during their childbearing years. Recent studies document the incidence of depression during pregnancy in about 30% of all patients in the United States *(7)*. Women who have been depressed prior to pregnancy appear to be at an elevated risk for depressive episodes during subsequent pregnancies *(8)*.

2. PREVALENCE

Studies focusing on the prevalence of depression during pregnancy have recently increased, with 21 studies published in the last 9 yr in contrast to only 9 studies published between 1985 and 1995 *(9)*.

2.1. Current Prevalence Data

Although wide variations exist in estimates of the prevalence of depression in pregnancy *(10,11)*, recent evidence suggests that the prevalence of depression during the first trimester of pregnancy is approx 7.4% *(12)*. During the second trimester, prevalence of the disease rises to 12.8%, and remains virtually unchanged at 12% in the third trimester *(12)*. It is critical to note, however, that many women choose not to participate in prenatal care until well into the second trimester. Therefore, the low prevalence of depression observed during the first trimester may simply be the result of depressed women not seeking prenatal care during that period *(12)*. Also of note is the fact that postpartum depression in some patients is known to begin prenatally and increase dramatically in severity during the postpartum period *(1)*.

2.2. Tools Used to Detect the Presence
of Depressive Symptoms in Pregnancy

Much of the recent epidemiological data on depression has been obtained via the use of lay-administered self-report questionnaires, some of which have been validated for use in pregnant women. The items contained in the questionnaires are based on those contained in previously validated instruments and the diagnostic criteria for MDD set forth by the fourth edition of the *Diagnostic and Statistical Manual of Mental Disorders* (DSM-IV) *(13)*. These lay-administered tools facilitate data collection from a variety of patient groups. Furthermore, they reveal the presence of depressive symptoms without the need for time-consuming, costly analyses by mental health professionals. Specific details regarding four of the most commonly used self-report inventories are outlined here.

2.2.1. BECK DEPRESSION INVENTORY

The Beck Depression Inventory (BDI), first introduced in 1961, was revised and re-released in 1978 as a brief 10-min, self-administered questionnaire capable of detecting the presence of depressive symptoms in both female and male psychiatric patients. The BDI consists of 21 questions regarding various aspects of mood, including but not limited to sadness, suicidal ideation, loss of weight, and social withdrawal *(14,14a)*. The BDI has been validated for use in pregnant women via comparison against the National Institute of Mental Health Diagnostic Interview Schedule III *(15)*. It should be noted, however, that responses to items on the BDI referring to physical disturbances (loss of sleep, fatigability) are often positive in nondepressed obstetric patients because of the changing physical demands of pregnancy. This fact should be kept in mind when using the BDI to assess the severity of depression in these patients *(12,16)*. The cutoff score denoting the presence of depressive symptoms is 16 or more.

2.2.2. EDINBURGH POSTNATAL DEPRESSION SCALE

The Edinburgh Postnatal Depression Scale (EPDS), first published in the *British Journal of Psychiatry* in 1987 *(16)*, is also validated for use in pregnant populations *(17)*. This 10-question inventory specifies that it should not be used as a diagnostic tool, and all results should be confirmed by a careful clinical assessment. Women who score above the cutoff of 12 are likely to be suffering from a depressive illness. The EPDS has a sensitivity of 0.50 and a specificity of 0.90 for the detection of depressive symptoms during pregnancy *(18)*. It detects only mood-related signs of depressive symptoms in order to avoid false-positives owing to erroneous detection of physiological symptoms consistent with depression as well as normal pregnancy *(12)*.

2.2.3. PRIMARY CARE EVALUATION OF MENTAL DISORDERS PATIENT HEALTH QUESTIONNAIRE

Validated in 3000 obstetric patients via comparison with telephone-psychologist assessments, the Primary Care Evaluation of Mental Disorders Patient Health Questionnaire (PRIME-MD, PHQ) is considered an accurate instrument for the detection of recent psychosocial stressors and functional impairment due to mood disorders in pregnant populations *(19)*. The original PRIME-MD was a clinician-administered inventory but was adapted to a patient self-administered questionnaire, with a sensitivity of 0.70 and a specificity of 0.95 *(20)*. Scores of 5–9 are indicative of mild depression, 10–14 of moderate depression requiring psychotherapeutic intervention, and 15 or higher of severe depression requiring immediate pharmacotherapy and likely hospitalization *(21)*.

2.2.4. CENTER FOR EPIDEMIOLOGICAL STUDY DEPRESSION SCALE

The Center for Epidemiological Study Depression Scale (CES-D), developed by the National Institutes of Health in 1970, has been used extensively in psychiatric research *(22)*. Although not yet validated for use in pregnant populations, the CES-D is one of the most common instruments used by first-line clinicians and researchers to detect the presence and prevalence of depressive symptoms, both in the general population and in pregnancy. In the general population it has a sensitivity of 1.0 and a specificity of 0.88 for the detection of major depression (1 mo prevalence) when using the cutoff score of 16 or higher to denote the presence of depressive symptoms *(23)*.

2.2.5. VARIABILITY IN STUDY DATA

It should be noted that studies have been conducted in patients at varying stages of pregnancy. Such variation exists both within and between many of the studies recently conducted on the epidemiology of depression during gestation. Moreover, the type and severity of depressive symptoms between and even within relapse episodes can change. Such changes in symptomatology may have an impact on the accuracy of the results obtained from these studies.

Additionally, one must note the effect of socioeconomic status (SES) on the prevalence of depression and the responses to the self-report questionnaires used in these studies. A negative correlation has been shown between the prevalence of depression and SES *(24,25)*.

3. CLINICAL COURSE

MDD is a highly complex disorder with a variable clinical course. The clinical presentation of the disorder is characterized by one or more major depressive episodes (MDEs), defined by the DSM-IV as 2 or more weeks of depressed mood, anhedonia, and/or loss of interest with any five of the following symptoms: difficulties in concentration, fatigue, feelings of worthlessness or guilt, insomnia or hypersomnia, thoughts of death, suicidal ideation, weight change, and psychomotor difficulties (agitation or retardation) *(13)*. It is important to note, however, that many of the somatic symptoms cited by the DSM-IV as integral to the diagnosis of depression are also highly common during pregnancy, especially insomnia, weight change, and fatigue. A clinical assessment for depression in any obstetric patient should therefore focus more on the cognitive aspects of depression (feelings of guilt, worthlessness; anhedonia) rather than the physical symptoms.

3.1. Risk Factors

Numerous risk factors have been identified for prenatal depression. Those most commonly observed are previous depressive illness, lack of social support, negative life events in the preceding pregnancy *(26)*, negative attitudes toward pregnancy, unplanned or first pregnancy, physical discomfort (e.g., nausea), and previous stillbirth *(27,28)*. Additionally, poor prenatal care, poor marriage dynamics, remarriage, and substance abuse/dependency have also been identified as risk factors for depression in pregnancy *(29–31)*.

The single most significant predictor of postpartum depression (PPD) is prenatal depression *(32–35)*. A meta-analysis by Beck and colleagues *(33,36)* revealed a comprehensive list of predictors of PPD, including prenatal depression, child-care stress, life stress, lack of social support, prenatal anxiety, maternal relationship dissatisfaction (e.g., marital problems), history of previous depression, difficult or unpredictable infant temperament, maternity blues (tearfulness, anxiety, irritability, and labile mood in the first 10 d postdelivery) *(37)*, low self-esteem, and low SES *(33,38)*. PPD begins during the later stages of pregnancy in 25% of patients *(39)*.

As mentioned earlier, peak prevalence of depression in females occurs during the childbearing years, between ages 25 and 44 *(6)*. An apparent clustering of depression occurs between ages 20 and 30 *(9,40,41)*. MDD in obstetric patients is characterized by one or more MDEs (6–12 mo in length if left untreated) *(9,40)*.

Fifty percent of patients treated for MDD experience full remission of their symptoms *(42)*. However, 85% of recovered patients relapse to a subsequent MDE within 15 yr of treatment *(42)*, and a large proportion of these patients remain chronically depressed *(43,44)*.

Symptoms of prenatal depression, which can occur at any time during pregnancy, can vary in intensity, duration, and type. To date, however, there has not been a clearly established pattern of symptom progression or change in antenatal depression *(45)* because investigations on the topic have yielded conflicting results. One study that examined mood in a group of depressed pregnant patients during the first trimester noted improvements in mood over the second and third trimesters of pregnancy *(46)*, whereas the results of a second prospective study showed depressive symptoms to be at their height in the third trimester (34–38 wk) *(47)*. Further study in this area is ongoing.

4. RISKS OF UNTREATED DEPRESSION DURING PREGNANCY

Many pregnant, depressed women experience an amplification of physical symptoms during pregnancy, including increased heart rate, loss of appetite, stomach pain, headaches, and sexual dysfunction *(48)*, during both the period leading up to and during MDEs. However, the risks of untreated depression go well beyond the somatic symptoms cited previously. Past studies suggest that the most notable adverse pregnancy outcomes associated with antenatal depression include increases in spontaneous preterm delivery *(49,50)*, low birthweight (LBW), and small-for-gestational age infants *(9)*. There are, however, a number of intermediate risks associated with inadequate treatment of depression during pregnancy, all of which are also associated with both short- and long-term deleterious maternal and neonatal health effects *(9)*. These risks are summarized below.

4.1. Functional Impairment

Recent research suggests that women who are either depressed or are experiencing severe anxiety during the first trimester of their pregnancies exhibit some degree of functional impairment *(51)*. This impairment may take the form of reduced work productivity, continuous and/or prolonged absence from work *(52)*, and increased health care utilization *(53)*. In cases where the depressed woman is the only working member of a family, such an impairment could also have negative consequences on her family; her family's financial status, for example, would likely decline.

4.2. Substandard Maternal Nutrition and Increased Maternal Weight Loss

As loss of appetite is often associated with depression, untreated depression during pregnancy may result in substandard maternal nutrition and lower-than-normal maternal weight gain. Studies have shown that intrauterine growth retardation (IUGR) and low neonatal birthweights have been linked to inadequate maternal nutrition and/or low maternal weight gain *(54)*. The Centers for Disease Control have classified LBW as the second leading cause of neonatal morbidity and mortality *(55)*.

4.3. Substance Abuse

Although a causal relationship between depression and substance abuse has not been clearly elucidated, the connection between depression and substance abuse (especially smoking and alcohol use) is of note. Depression during pregnancy is significantly associated with prenatal substance abuse. Finnish studies have found substance abuse to be co-morbid with depression in 6.4% of women *(56)*. Also, in a recent US study of 186 pregnant women, 8% were found to have both psychiatric illnesses and substance abuse disorders *(57)*. More critically, a study of 1014 women of low SES showed depressive symptoms (as per CES-D scores ≥16) to be significantly associated with smoking, as well as alcohol and cocaine use *(57a)*. Alcohol consumption, smoking, and street drug use have been clearly associated with neonatal morbidity and mortality when used or consumed in even small to moderate amounts during pregnancy *(9)*.

4.4. Pregnancy-Induced Hypertension

Pregnancy-induced hypertension (PIH) is considered a serious complication during pregnancy *(9)*, and pre-eclampsia, a form of PIH, has been associated with depression during pregnancy *(58)*. Some of the symptoms associated with severe pre-eclampsia are hypertension, proteinuria, with associated edema in the last half of pregnancy, headaches, visual disturbances, and upper abdominal pain *(9,59,60)*. Although the etiology of this condition is as yet uncharacterized, investigators have hypothesized that altered elimination of vasoactive hormones as a result of depression may increase the risk for PIH *(58,61)*. A recent Finnish study found a 2.5-fold increase in the risk of pre-eclampsia in pregnant women suffering from depression *(61)*.

4.5. Inadequate Prenatal Care

The lack of motivation and self-esteem associated with depression during pregnancy may lead to inadequate prenatal care because depressed women are known not to seek out prenatal care until well into their pregnancies *(62)*. Previous studies have found that women with psychiatric disorders attend fewer than 50% of prenatal care appointments *(62)*. A cohort study of almost 10.6 million births found a relative risk (RR) of 2.8 for preterm birth in Caucasian women with inadequate prenatal care compared to women with prenatal care throughout their pregnancies *(63)*. Additionally, these researchers additionally found an

RR of 3.3 for fetal death and an RR of 1.7 for postnatal death in women lacking prenatal care throughout their pregnancies *(64,65)*. Upon adjustment for the presence of various maternal high-risk conditions, the RRs for fetal and postnatal deaths remained elevated at 4.3 and 1.6, respectively, in women without any high-risk conditions and without prenatal care *(64,65)*. Furthermore, the study identified a negative relationship between the number of prenatal care visits and the risks for both fetal and postnatal deaths. These findings clearly underscore the potential dangers of inadequate prenatal care.

4.6. Postpartum Depression

Perhaps one of the most notable consequences of untreated antenatal depression is the subsequent increase in risk for PPD. Although a number of recent studies have examined the incidence of PPD in women with antenatal depression, the most notable evidence comes from studies using Beck's Postpartum Depression Predictors Inventory (BPDPI) *(38)*. A recent meta-analysis of 26 studies using BPDPI showed prenatal depression to be an extremely strong predictor of PPD *(33)*.

4.7. Poor Neonatal Behavioral Development

Recent investigations have shown that infants born to depressed mothers tend to exhibit excessive crying, lower orientation scores, inferior excitability, and few expressions of interest shortly after birth, indicating the possibility of neurodevelopmental consequences of maternal depression in the newborn *(66,67)*.

Altered levels of cortisol, norepinephrine, and dopamine have been detected in babies of depressed mothers *(9)*. Moreover, in depressed pregnant women, levels of cortisol and norepinephrine have been elevated and levels of dopamine have been reduced during the third trimester of pregnancy. Furthermore, these altered levels have been found to significantly predict similar alternations in the levels of these substances in neonates *(67)*. These findings lend support to the hypothesis that biological imbalances associated with depression in the mother may affect fetal mood development and hormone distribution, especially given that cortisol, dopamine, and norepinephrine are known to cross the placenta (to varying degrees) *(68)*. Mother–baby interactions are also known to suffer in women with depressed mood *(69)*.

5. TREATMENT OF DEPRESSION DURING PREGNANCY

A number of options for the treatment of depression during pregnancy are available. Interpersonal psychotherapy (IPT) has been shown to be effective in the treatment of women diagnosed with prenatal depression *(9)*. Studies have also noted the efficacy of electroconvulsive therapy (ECT) in the treatment of severely depressed and suicidal pregnant patients *(70,71)*. Most notably, an increase in the use of pharmacotherapy for the treatment of depression during pregnancy has been noted in several studies *(72)*.

The selection of a treatment modality for depression in pregnant patients is generally a function of the severity of the disorder and its associated symptoms. The clinical management of depression during pregnancy should occur on a case-by-case basis. The decision-making process should center on informed decision making by the patient, with the assistance of her health care provider *(73)*.

5.1. Nonpharmacological Treatment Options

5.1.1. INTERPERSONAL PSYCHOTHERAPY

Two major studies involving the use of IPT for pregnant, depressed women were undertaken by the same investigator *(74,75)*. Both investigations found IPT to be an effective therapy for antepartum depression *(74,75)*. It should be noted, however, that no investigations have compared IPT to antidepressant treatment. Although data on the efficacy of IPT for prenatal depression are not as extensive as those for antidepressants, it is a reasonable treatment option for patients who wish to avoid the use of medications or who experience antidepressant-refractory illness.

5.1.2. ELECTROCONVULSIVE THERAPY

Data from several investigations now exist that attest to the safety of ECT in pregnancy. Recent reviews on the subject *(70,71)* suggest that ECT is both safe and efficacious for the treatment of severe and/or anti-depressant-refractory forms of MDD. A recent review cites 300 case reports regarding the use of ECT in pregnancy over the past half century. Among the cited reports, only four cases of premature labor were described, and premature membrane rupture did not occur in any case *(76)*. Given the reports of its relative safety and efficacy, some clinicians may wish to consider ECT as an alternative to antidepressant therapy *(76)*.

5.2. Pharmacological Treatment Options

The baseline incidence of congenital malformations in the general population is approx 1–3% *(77–79)*. The greatest potential for drug-related physical teratogenesis occurs in the first 12 wk of pregnancy, because the majority of organogenesis occurs within this period. It should be noted, however, that studies are required in all trimesters to clearly establish a given drug's safety in pregnant patients. A summary of the safety of the pharmacological treatments discussed here can be found in Table 1.

5.2.1. TRICYCLIC ANTIDEPRESSANTS AND SAFETY IN PREGNANCY

Imipramine, the first of the tricyclic antidepressants (TCAs), was introduced in 1958 *(80)*. Since then, more than 10 other TCAs have been designed, produced, and marketed. These agents achieve their anti-depressant effects principally via inhibition of central norepinephrine reuptake and, to a lesser extent, serotonin reuptake *(80)*. Although TCAs have been widely prescribed, their use has declined over the past 20 yr, likely due to the advent of medications with fewer adverse effects. In the early 1970s, a case report of a child born with bilateral amelia following *in utero* TCA exposure *(81)* caused widespread fear that TCAs were teratogenic. Since then, 3 prospective and more than 10 retrospective studies have become available regarding the safety of TCA use in the first trimester of pregnancy *(82–88)*. The individual and pooled results of these studies suggest that TCA use in pregnancy is not associated with an increase in the risk of congenital malformations above the baseline.

It should be noted that transient withdrawal symptoms have been noted following TCA exposure in late gestation, including irritability, rapid breathing, and urinary retention *(89)*.

5.2.2. SELECTIVE SEROTONIN REUPTAKE INHIBITORS

Selective serotonin reuptake inhibitors (SSRI) antidepressants, although relatively new, are the most widely prescribed antidepressants in the world today *(90)*. The advent of these agents highlighted the role that serotonin or 5-hydroxytryptamine plays in the pathophysiology of mental illness.

SSRIs show remarkable selectivity for the serotonergic system over the noradrenergic or cholinergic systems and, as such, have much wider therapeutic windows and more favorable tolerability profiles compared with earlier antidepressant medications *(91,92)*.

5.2.2.1. Fluoxetine (Prozac). Of all the SSRIs currently prescribed in pregnancy, fluoxetine is the best studied. Fluoxetine has been demon-strated to cross the placenta in both animal *(93)* and human studies *(94,95)*. Fluoxetine was shown to cross the placenta in larger amounts than all other SSRIs, with the exception of citalopram *(95)*.

Five recent prospective studies *(83,96–98a)* and four retrospective studies have examined the safety of fluoxetine use in pregnancy *(82,99–101)*. In these nine studies, more than 1700 pregnancies exposed to fluoxetine at vary-

Table 1
Summary of Antidepressants in Pregnancy

Class	Drugs studied	Safety in pregnancy
Tricyclic antidepressants	Clomipramine, amitriptyline, imipramine, doxepin, dothiepin, trimipramine, nortriptyline, lofepramine, desipramine, maprotiline, protriptyline	As a group, considered relatively safe to use in pregnancy; however, associated with maternal toxicities and neonatal withdrawal
Selective serotonin reuptake inhibitors	Fluoxetine, paroxetine, citalopram, sertraline, fluvoxamine	All except fluvoxamine are well studied and considered relatively safe for use in pregnancy; however, have been associated with perinatal complications including jitteriness, respiratory distress, hypoglycemia
Monoamine oxidase inhibitors	Tranylcypromine, phenelzine; no others studied	Not recommended for use in pregnancy because of paucity of data and possible toxicities
Others	Venlafaxine, bupropion, trazodone, nefazodone, mirtazapine, St. John's wort (SJW)	Based on one prospective comparative study on each drug, venlafaxine bupropion, trazodone, and nefazodone appear to be relatively safe in pregnancy; data on mirtazapine and SJW limited

ing stages (1418 prospectively, 289 retrospectively) were examined. None of these studies showed an increase in the rate of major malformations—physical deformities that are life-threatening, require major surgery, or are associated with serious cosmetic or functional effects (102) —above the 1–3% baseline risk that exists in the general population. Moreover, all but two of these studies (83,97) showed no statistically significant increases in the risk for spontaneous abortion, LBW or major neonatal health complications following exposure to fluoxetine in early or late pregnancy or throughout gestation *(82,83,96–101)*. It should be noted that the vast majority of the 1280 prospectively followed pregnancies were compared with matched controls, and no differences in the rates of major malformations between the two groups were seen.

Chambers and colleagues prospectively examined 228 pregnant women taking fluoxetine throughout gestation and compared their outcomes with those of 254 prospectively identified comparator women exposed to known nonteratogens. In this investigation, the incidence of major malformations in the fluoxetine-exposed group (5.5%) was no different from that observed in the nonteratogen-exposed comparator group (4%) The rate of spontaneous abortions also did not differ significantly between the fluoxetine exposed and comparator groups (10.5 vs 9.1%, respectively). This study did, however, find a significant increase in the rate of three or more minor anomalies, LBW and length, preterm delivery, and admission to special care nurseries in infants whose mothers were exposed to fluoxetine in the third trimester *(97)*. The study also observed an increase in poor neonatal adaptation, characterized by transitory jitteriness, respiratory difficulty, and cyanosis upon feeding in infants exposed to fluoxetine in late gestation (*see* Section 5.3.1. for a brief discussion of poor neonatal adaptation). Confidence in the results obtained from this study *(97)* is limited by several methodological issues, including a lack of control for the effects of the underlying depressive illness. Additionally, maternal age in the fluoxetine-exposed group was higher than in the control group, a factor known to affect birthweight *(103)*. Furthermore, a large proportion of the women in the fluoxetine-exposed group were also exposed to nicotine and other psychoactive medications.

In a study by Pastuszak et al. *(83)*, 128 gravid women taking a mean daily dose of 25.8 mg of fluoxetine during the first trimester were followed and compared with two matched control groups (each of 74 patients) exposed to either TCAs or known nonteratogens. The investigators found no differences in the rates of major malformations between any of the comparison groups, but they did find a slightly increased risk of spontaneous abortions in the fluoxetine- and TCA-exposed groups (13.5 and 12.2%, respectively) vs the nonteratogen comparator group (6.8%). These increases, however, did not reach statistical significance. Moreover, as is the case in the study by Chambers et al. *(97)*, it is unclear whether the higher incidence of spontaneous abortions observed in both the fluoxetine- and TCA-exposed groups was the result of the effects of the medications, the underlying maternal depression, or other factors.

Another prospective study by Hendrick et al. found an increase in LBW in the infants of mothers exposed to high-dose fluoxetine (40–80 mg/d) throughout gestation, despite comparable maternal weight gain across all experimental groups *(98a)*. Women exposed to nicotine, alcohol, or recreational drugs were excluded, thereby removing these as potential confounding factors. It should be noted, however, that this study had no matched comparator group.

A significant concern associated with psychoactive medication use during pregnancy is the potential for long-term neurodevelopmental abnormalities, including cognitive and language impairment and behavioral teratogenesis. A study by Nulman et al. assessed global IQ, language development, temperament, mood, arousability, activity-level distractibility, and behavior in the children of 80 mothers exposed to TCAs and 55 mothers exposed to fluoxetine during pregnancy *(104)*. Assessment of IQ and language development occurred between 16 and 86 mo of postnatal age. These investigators found no differences in any parameter examined between the TCA-exposed, fluoxetine-exposed, and non-antidepressant-exposed groups.

5.2.2.2. Paroxetine (Paxil). The use of paroxetine during pregnancy has also been the subject of recent study. Paroxetine has been shown to cross the placenta in detectable amounts in a recent human placental kinetics study *(95)*.

Currently, data on paroxetine use in pregnancy are somewhat limited. To date, published data on 305 exposures to paroxetine at varying stages in pregnancy (274 prospectively followed and 31 retrospectively evaluated) *(82,99,101,105,106)* are available. None of these studies has shown an increase in the risk of major malformations compared with the general population or a matched comparator group *(105,106)*. Additionally, these studies have found no evidence linking paroxetine use at any time in pregnancy to an increase in spontaneous abortions or other major neonatal health complications. One of these studies did report evidence of poor neonatal adaptation in infants whose mothers used paroxetine in the third trimester *(106)*.

Recently, an unpublished retrospective, cohort study (supplemented by a nested case–control study) examined the effects of antenatal exposure to various antidepressants, including paroxetine (studied only via *post hoc*, secondary analyses) on pregnancy outcome. This study, conducted by GlaxoSmithKlein (GSK) utilized medical records taken from two large medical databases, containing medication (and pharmacy dispensing) records from more than 25 health insurance providers *(106a)*. The results of *post hoc* analyses from this study showed an adjusted odds ratio of 1.84 (95% CI 1.16–2.91) for congenital malformations associated with paroxetine exposure during the first trimester. The adjusted odds ratio increased to 2.20 (95% CI 1.34–3.63) following the exclusion of data from women exposed to other antidepressants or known teratogens during the study period. The results of this investigation suggested an overall risk of 4% for the development of major malformations following paroxetine exposure in the first trimester (an increase of 1% over the baseline risk) *(106b)*.

The adjusted odds ratio for cardiovascular defects following first-trimester exposure to paroxetine was found to be 2.26 (95% CI 1.17–4.33). The odds ratio diminished to 2.08 (95% CI 1.03–4.23) following the exclusion of data from women exposed to other antidepressants and/or known cardiovascular teratogens during the study period. These data represent an overall risk of 2% for cardiovascular defects (a twofold increase over the 1% baseline risk for cardiovascular defects in the general population) associated with first-trimester paroxetine exposure *(106a,106b)*. The results of this study have recently prompted the US Food and Drug Administration (FDA) to label paroxetine as a "Category D" (demonstrated risk to the fetus) drug.

Although the data from this large epidemiological study are among the first that suggest teratogenicity following paroxetine use during pregnancy, confidence in the results obtained is limited by several methodological issues. Briefly, both the retrospective nature of the study design and the use of *post hoc* analyses to obtain the adjusted odds ratios for cardiovascular malformations and congenital malformations decrease the grade of evidence ascribable to the results obtained. The lack of a matched control group and the limited medical/clinical data (including information on disease severity) available from the insurance databases used further limits the interpretation of the results obtained *(106c)*. Finally, and perhaps most troublingly, much of the data used in the GSK study was based on pharmacy dispensing records for the various antidepressants studies and thus, did not provided any information on how many of the patients prescribed paroxetine actually consumed their medications regularly and at the doses prescribed (i.e., the degree of paroxetine exposure).

Overall, the data available regarding paroxetine use during pregnancy are conflicting. Although the results of the unpublished GSK study just cited do suggest some degree of caution regarding antenatal paroxetine use, the overall risks of general and/or cardiac malformations in children whose mothers were exposed to paroxetine during the first trimester are only modestly above the risks for these negative pregnancy outcomes in the general population. In general, the available data regarding antenatal paroxetine safety, the potential health risks of untreated depression during pregnancy, and individual patient responsiveness to paroxetine should all be carefully considered when making decisions regarding the commencement, modification and particularly the cessation of paroxetine use during pregnancy.

5.2.2.3. Citalopram (Celexa, Lexapro). Limited data are available on the use of citalopram during pregnancy. Citalopram has been shown to cross the human placenta in detectable amounts and to a greater degree than all other SSRI antidepressants *(95)*, with the exception of fluvoxamine, whose placental kinetics have yet to be clearly established.

Ericson et al. recently reported the outcome of 375 prospectively followed exposures to citalopram in early pregnancy, of which 364 were exposures to citalopram alone with the remainder being exposures to citalopram in combination with another SSRI or TCA antidepressant *(99)*. The investigators found no statistically significant increases in the incidence of major malformations compared to that expected in the general population. An association between the use of citalopram (and other SSRIs) early in pregnancy and an increase in preterm delivery was noted. This increase, however, was thought by the investigators to be a consequence of the underlying maternal disease.

A second prospective, comparison study followed 11 mothers exposed to citalopram throughout gestation. Pregnancy outcome as well as neurodevelopment was evaluated up to 1 yr of age. No major or minor malformations were detected as part of this study. Additionally, all infants were neurodevelopmentally normal at 1 yr of age *(107)*.

Most recently, The Motherisk Program prospectively followed 106 women exposed to citalopram during their pregnancies (98 in first trimester and 48 throughout gestation) *(107a)*. Their preliminary results documented 92 (86.6%) live births, 11 (10.3%) spontaneous abortions, 2 (1.9%) therapeutic abortions, 1 (0.9%) stillbirth, and 3 (3.2%) major malformations in the citalopram-exposed group. Upon comparison with two matched comparator groups, each consisting of 106 women exposed to other antidepressants or known nonteratogens (respectively), no statistically significant differences in the rates of major malformations, spontaneous abortions, elective terminations, or stillbirths were found between any of the comparison groups.

At present the pregnancy data are on citalopram and not on its isomer, *S*-citalopram (Lexapro).

5.2.2.4. Sertraline (Zoloft). Sertraline has been shown to cross the human placenta in significantly smaller amounts than other SSRI antidepressants *(95,107b)*.

Published literature on 213 pregnancies exposed to sertraline (181 prospectively followed and 32 retrospectively evaluated) is available. A prospective controlled cohort study by The Motherisk Program *(105)* followed 147 women exposed to sertraline in the first trimester of pregnancy. Of the women exposed, 127 (86%) gave birth to live infants, 12 (9%) experienced spontaneous abortions, and 7 (5%) chose to undergo therapeutic abortions. Among the 127 live births, 4 (3.2%) malformations were observed. There were no statistically significant differences among the observed rates of spontaneous abortions, elective abortions, major malformations, or stillbirths between the SSRI-exposed and matched comparator groups *(105)*.

A second study prospectively followed 32 pregnancies exposed only to sertraline in early pregnancy and 2 other pregnancies exposed to sertraline and other SSRI agents at similar stages of gestation. The rate of major malformations seen in infants of sertraline-exposed women was not statistically different than that observed in the general population *(99)*.

5.2.2.5. Fluvoxamine (Luvox). Very limited data are available regarding the use of fluvoxamine in pregnancy. In a multicenter, prospective, cohort-comparator study by The Motherisk Program *(105)*, 26 women exposed to fluvoxamine in the first trimester of pregnancy were followed. Of the 26 women exposed, 22 (88%) gave birth to live infants. Two of the remaining four women had spontaneous abortions, and two women therapeutically aborted their pregnancies. In the group of live births, three (12%) major malformations were observed. Given the small sample size of this study, these data are not definitive regarding fluvoxamine use in pregnancy.

Additionally, 66 women who took fluvoxamine early in their pregnancies were retrospectively examined by the European Network of Teratology Information Services. This group observed 49 live births with 1 malformation among them, 9 therapeutic abortions (of which 1 was of a malformed fetus), 6 spontaneous abortions, and 2 stillbirths. Although no control group was available for comparison in this study, the rates of live births, spontaneous abortions, and malformations was similar to that expected in the general population.

5.2.3. Other Antidepressants

5.2.3.1. Venlafaxine (Effexor). Venlafaxine, a phenethylamine bicyclic derivative, is chemically unrelated to all other antidepressants *(108)*. Venlafaxine achieves its therapeutic effects via inhibition of both serotonin and norepinephrine reuptake. It has no significant affinity for central acetylcholine or histamine receptors—hence its mild adverse effects profile *(109)*.

To date, only one study evaluating the safety of venlafaxine use in pregnancy exists. In this multicenter study from Motherisk *(108)*, 150 women exposed to venlafaxine in the first trimester of pregnancy (35 of whom took the drug throughout pregnancy) were followed. Of the 150 women, 125 gave birth to live infants, 18 had spontaneous abortions, and 7 had therapeutic abortions. Two major malformations were observed among the 125 live births. The outcomes of these pregnancies were compared to those of two matched-comparator groups, each consisting of 150 women, exposed exclusively to SSRI antidepressants or nonteratogens, respectively. No statistically significant differences in the rates of major malformations, therapeutic abortions, mean gestational ages, or mean birthweights were observed between the exposed and comparator groups. It should be noted that the incidence of spontaneous abortions in the venlafaxine- and antidepressant-exposed groups (12 and 10.7%, respectively) was higher than that in the nonteratogenic comparator group (7.3%). This difference between the groups, however, was not statistically significant.

5.2.3.2. Bupropion (Wellbutrin). Bupropion, an amino ketone compound, is marketed both as an antidepressant and as an aid for smoking cessation. The antidepressant mechanism of bupropion is presently not well understood but is thought to involve both central noradrenergic and dopaminergic pathways *(110)*. Data on the outcomes of 226 pregnancies exposed to bupropion are available from the manufacturer. The outcomes of these pregnancies suggest no increase in the rate of major malformations resulting from exposure to bupropion during pregnancy *(111)*. Recently, a study completed by The Motherisk Program followed 136 women exposed to bupropion in the first trimester or throughout gestation and compared their pregnancy outcomes to those of two comparator groups exposed to other antidepressants (57 women) or known nonteratogens (126 women). Among the 136 exposed pregnancies, there were 105 live births, 20 spontaneous abortions, 10 therapeutic abortions, 1 stillbirth, 1 neonatal death, and no malformations observed. Upon comparison with the matched control groups, no statistically significant differences in the rates of major malformations, stillbirths, neonatal deaths, or major neonatal health complications were detected *(112)*.

This study examined the safety of bupropion during pregnancy in women using it as an antidepressant and/or as smoking-cessation aid. Upon comparison of the pregnancies exposed to bupropion for either indication with matched nonteratogen-exposed comparators, the incidence of spontaneous abortions was significantly higher in the bupropion-exposed group (14.7%) than in the control group (4.5%) ($p < 0.009$) *(112)*.

Interestingly, however, when the incidence of spontaneous abortions in women using bupropion as an antidepressant only (15.4%) was compared with that of women using other antidepressants and nonteratogens (12.3 and 6.7%, respectively), no statistically significant difference between the groups was detected ($p < 0.18$) *(112)*. Nicotine has been shown by several groups to increase the risk of spontaneous abortions *(113–118)*. Accordingly, this study *(112)* attempted to account for the effects of nicotine by matching the nonteratogen-exposed control group with the bupropion group for smoking status and number of cigarettes smoked per day *(112)*. No association between the increase of spontaneous abortions and smoking status was noted in this study. In actuality, there was no difference in the rates of spontaneous abortions among the depressed and smoking women (15.4 vs 16.2%). However, the number of smokers in this study was small ($N = 37$), and further study with a larger sample size is indicated.

5.2.3.3. Trazodone and Nefazodone (Desyrel, Serzone). Trazodone and nefazodone, both of which are phenylpiperazine antidepressants, exert their therapeutic effects via inhibition of central serotonin and norepinephrine reuptake. Nefazodone has reduced affinity for cholinergic and α-adrenergic receptors and is therefore less sedative than trazodone *(109)*.

Presently, one multicenter prospective comparison study evaluating the safety of trazodone and nefazodone during pregnancy is available *(119)*. This study followed 147 women exposed to either drug in the first trimester (52 of whom continued either drug throughout pregnancy) and compared them with two comparison groups, consisting of 147 women each, exposed to other antidepressants or nonteratogens, respectively. Upon completion of the study, there were 121 (82.4%) live births, 20 (13.6%) spontaneous abortions, and 6 (4%) therapeutic abortions. Of the 121 live births, 2 (1.6%) were found to have major malformations. There was no difference in the incidence of major malformations between the drug-exposed and comparison groups. It should be noted, however, that fewer spontaneous abortions were observed in the nonteratogen-exposed control group (8.1%) than in either the trazodone/nefazodone (13.6%) or the antidepressant-exposed group (11.5%). Although the differences in the rate of spontaneous abortions between the groups were not statistically significant, they mirror similar increases seen in studies with other antidepressants (discussed earlier).

5.2.3.4. Mirtazapine (Remeron). Mirtazapine, introduced in the United States in the late 1990s, is a new antidepressant that augments noradrenergic and serotonergic transmission *(111)*. To date, there have been no prospective controlled studies evaluating the safety of mirtazapine during pregnancy. A Turkish group recently followed the pregnancies of two women exposed to this drug in early and mid- first trimester *(120)*. Both pregnancies resulted in the birth of healthy infants (40 and 39 wk gestation, respectively), one of whom had mild hyperbilirubinemia and mild gastroesophageal reflux that resolved without treatment.

5.2.3.5. Saint John's Wort. Saint John's Wort (SJW) (*Hypericum perforatum*) is the most common herbal therapy for depression in use today *(121)*. The active ingredient, thought to be hypericin, is capable of antidepressant effects via inhibition of serotonin, norepinephrine, and dopamine reuptake *(122,123)*.

SJW is generally considered safer than most currently prescribed antidepressant medications *(124–127)* probably because "natural" or herbal products are considered inherently safer than pharmaceuticals by the general population *(128)*. To date, only two cases regarding obstetric self-medication with SJW have been published *(129)*. Of these cases, follow-up data on only one is available. The woman in this case took SJW from 24 wk gestation until term and gave birth to a normal, healthy child.

5.2.3.6. Monoamine Oxidase Inhibitors. The use of monoamine oxidase inhibitors (MAOIs) in pregnancy has not been well studied, mainly because they are used infrequently as drugs of "last resort" *(130)*. In animal studies, the use of MAOIs in pregnancy has been shown to cause fetal growth retardation *(131,132)*. Human data concerning MAOI safety during pregnancy is limited. A published case series associated MAOI use in pregnancy with an increased incidence of major malformations *(85)*. Specific details concerning the exposures or malformations, however, were unavailable.

Given the discouraging data available, its potential interactions with medications such as terbutaline (hypertensive crisis) *(76)*, and the availability of other more studied antidepressants, MAOI use during pregnancy should be avoided.

5.3. Reported Adverse Outcomes

5.3.1. POOR NEONATAL ADAPTABILITY

The use of SSRI agents in late gestation has been associated with poor neonatal adaptability, a transient period of jitteriness, difficulty breathing, and some difficulty feeling *(106,133,134)*. As such, infants born to mothers exposed to SSRIs near term should be carefully monitored. These adverse effects are, however, transient, self-limiting generally require no treatment, and appear to have no long-lasting effects on the infants.

5.3.2. Increase in Spontaneous Abortions

Of note, some of the previously mentioned studies reported an increased rate of spontaneous abortions in the antidepressant-exposed groups compared with the nonteratogen-exposed groups. This difference was statistically significant in three of these studies (two on fluoxetine and one on bupropion) *(83,97,112)*. Although the observed rates of spontaneous abortions in any of the antidepressant-exposed groups have not exceeded the reported 10–20% baseline rate in the general population *(82)*, this finding requires further study.

5.3.3. Abrupt Discontinuation Syndrome

Given that at least 50% of pregnancies are unplanned *(102,135)*, many women first become aware of their pregnancies well into the first trimester. These women may abruptly discontinue taking all medications, including antidepressants, in attempts to minimize drug exposure to their fetuses. Einarson and colleagues interviewed 36 pregnant women 1 mo after they received counseling regarding the safety of antidepressant use in pregnancy *(136)*. They found that 34 of these women discontinued their medication abruptly (28 on the advice of their health care providers). Of these women, 26 (70.3%) reported deteriorating physical and psychological health. Eleven of these women reported suicidal ideation, and 4 were hospitalized.

Abrupt discontinuation of certain antidepressants may be associated with a "discontinuation syndrome," characterized by any or all of the following: nausea and vomiting, diarrhea, diaphoresis, hot or cold flashes, tremors, excess lacrimation, syncope, anxiety, panic attacks, low energy, fatigue, and mood swings *(136)*. Most critically, sudden discontinuation of antidepressants has been associated with relapse of the underlying psychiatric condition *(137)*. In the case of antenatal depression, this is of particular concern given the deleterious health effects associated with untreated depression during pregnancy.

5.3.4. Persistent Pulmonary Hypertension in the Newborn

At press time, a newly released case–control study reported a significantly elevated risk of persistent pulmonary hypertension in the newborn (PPHN) in infants exposed to SSRIs following the 20th week of gestation. Although the absolute risk of PPHN in SSRI-exposed infants was relatively low (~ 1 in 100), it was six times higher than that of control group infants. The study findings raise an important concern and should be reviewed carefully during risk–benefit discussions regarding treatment of depression during pregnancy. Children exposed to SSRIs prior to the 20th week of gestation, or to non-SSRIs at any time of pregnancy, were not found to be at an increased risk for PPHN *(138)*.

5.3.5. DIRECTIONS FOR FUTURE STUDY

Despite recent evidence supporting the safety of antidepressant use in pregnancy *(82,83,96–101,105–108,112,119,121)*, several questions remain unanswered.

The sample size in the vast majority of studies assessing the safety of these medications in pregnancy is statistically small. Most studies *(108,112,119)* have only an 80% power to detect a fourfold increase in the risk of major malformations ($\alpha = 0.05$). Almost 800 cases in each treatment group would be required to detect a twofold increased risk, and thousands of cases would be required to detect rare defects.

At present, only one study has assessed the long-term neurodevelopment (i.e., global IQ score, language and behavioral development, and cognitive abilities) of children exposed to antidepressants (fluoxetine and TCAs) *in utero (104)*. Therefore, the long-term effects of *in utero* exposure to these medications (except for fluoxetine) remain poorly characterized. It should be noted that this is an area of active research.

6. CONCLUSION

In this chapter we have reviewed some of the key issues surrounding prenatal depression, including its prevalence, course, and treatment options. Depression during pregnancy is an important issue that cannot be ignored given its high prevalence in general and obstetric populations. It has become apparent, according to data from recent studies, that deleterious effects are associated with untreated depression during pregnancy. Women should not be denied treatment simply because they are pregnant, as there appears to be a relatively safe arsenal of both pharmacological and nonpharmacological treatments available. Women should be given evidence-based information concerning treatment options. Such information would allow them and their health care providers to make appropriate decisions that will ensure the best possible outcomes for themselves and their babies.

REFERENCES

1. Buist, A. (2000) Managing depression in pregnancy. Aust Fam Physician 29(7), 663–667.
2. Murray, C. J. and Lopez, A. D. (1996) Evidence-based health policy lessons from the Global Burden of Disease Study. Science 274, 740–743.
3. Regier, D. A., Narrow, W. E., Rae D. S., et al. (1993) The de facto US mental and addictive disorders health system. Arch Gen Psychiatry 50, 85-94.
4. Kessler, R. C., McGonagie, K. A., Zhao, S., et al. (1994) Lifetime and 12-month prevalence of DSM-III-R psychiatric disorders in the United States: results from the National Comorbidity Survey. Arch Gen Psychiatry 51, 8–19.
5. Weissman, M. M., Bland, R., Joyce, P. R., et al. (1993) Sex differences in rates of depression: cross-national perspectives. J. Affect. Disord. 29, 77–84.

6. Burke, K. C., Burke, J. D., Rae, D. S., et al. (1991) Comparing age at onset of major depression and other psychiatric disorders by birth cohorts in five US community populations. Arch Gen Psychiatry 48, 789–795.
7. Kendell, R. E., Wainwright, S., Hailey, A., et al. (1976) The influence of childbirth on psychiatric morbidity. Psychol Med. 6, 297–302.
8. Kumar, R., and Robson, M. (1984) A prospective study of emotional disorders in childbearing women. Br. J. Psychiatry 144, 35–47.
9. Bennett, H. A., Einarson, A., Taddio, A., et al. (2004) Depression during pregnancy: overview of clinical factors. Clin. Drug Invest. 24, 157–179.
10. Affonso, D. D., Lovett, S. Paul, N., et al. (1990) A standardized interview that differentiates pregnancy and postpartum symptoms from perinatal clinical depression. Birth 17, 121–130.
11. McKee, M. D., Cunningham, D., Jankowski, K. R., et al. (2001) Health-related functional status in pregnancy: relationship to depression and social support in a multi-ethnic population. Obstet. Gynecol. 97, 988–993.
12. Bennett, H. A., Einarson, A., Taddio, A., et al. (2004) Prevalence of depression during pregnancy: systematic review. Obstet. Gynecol. 103, 698–709.
13. American Psychiatric Association. (1994) Diagnostic and Statistical Manual of Mental Disorders. Washington, DC: American Psychiatric Association.
14. Beck, A. T. (1961) An inventory for measuring depression. Arch. Gen. Psychiatry 4, 53–61.
14a. Beck, A. T., Rush, H. A., Shaw, B. F., and Emery, G. (1979) Cognitive Therapy of Depression. New York: Guilford Press.
15. Holcomb, W. L., Stone, L. S., Lustman, P. J., et al. (1996) Screening for depression in pregnancy: characteristics of the Beck Depression Inventory. Obstet. Gynecol. 88, 1021–1025.
16. Salamero, M., Marcos, T., Gutierrez, F., et al. (1994) Factorial study of the BDI in pregnant women. Psychol. Med. 24, 1031–1035.
17. Cox, J. L., Holden, J. M., and Sagovsky, R. (1987) Detection of postnatal depression: development of the Edinburgh Postnatal Depression Scale. Br. J. Psychiatry 150, 782–786.
18. Murray, D. and Cox, J. L. (1990) Screening for depression during pregnancy with the Edinburgh depression scale (EPDS). J. Reprod. Infant Psychol. 8, 99–107.
19. Spitzer, R. L., Williams, J. B., Kroenke, K., et al. (2000) Validity and utility of the PRIME-MD patient health questionnaire in assessment of 3000 obstetric-gynecology study. Am. J. Obstet Gynecol. 183, 759–769.
20. Spitzer, R. L., Kroenke, K., Williams J. B. W., and the Patient Health Questionnaire Primary Care Study Group. (1999) Validation and utility of a self-report version of PRIME-MD: The PHQ Primary Care Study. JAMA 282, 737–744.
21. Pfizer Inc. (1999) PRIME-MD: Patient Health Questionnaire (PHQ). Available from http://providers.ipro.org/dox/AMI_Depression/DOC/Patient_Health_Question.doc. Accessed June 2004.
22. Radloff, L. S. (1977) The CES-D scale: a self-report depression scale for research in the general population. Appl. Psychol. Measure. 1, 385–401.
23. Radloff, L. S. and Locke, B. Z. (1986) The community mental health assessment survey and the CES-D scale. In: Weissman, M. M., Myers, J. K., and Ross, C. E., eds. Community Surveys of Psychiatric Disorders. Surveys in Psychosocial Epidemiology 4, 177–189.
24. Lorant, V., Deliege, D., Eaton, W., et al. (2003) Socioeconomic inequalities in depression: a meta-analysis. Am. J. Epidemiol. 157, 98–112.

25. Boyd, R. C., Pearson, J. L., and Blehar, M. C. (2002) Prevention and treatment of depression in pregnancy and the postpartum period: summary of a maternal depression roundtable: a UA perspective. Arch. Women Ment. Health 4, 79–82.
26. Collins, N. L., Dunkel-Schetter, C., Lobel, M., et al. (1993) Social supporting pregnancy: psychosocial correlates of birth outcomes and postpartum depression. J. Pers. Soc. Psychol. 6, 1243–1258.
27. Burger, J., Horwitz, S. M., Forsyth, B. W., et al. (1993) Psychological sequelae of medical complications during pregnancy. Pediatrics 91, 566–571.
28. Hughes, P., Turnton, P., and Evans, C. (1999) Stillbirth as a risk factor for depression and anxiety in the subsequent pregnancy: cohort study. Br. Med. J. 318, 1721–1724.
29. Kitamura, T., Sugawara, M., Sugawara, K., et al. (1996) Psychosocial study of depression in early pregnancy. Br. J. Psychiatry 168, 732–738.
30. Johanson, R., Chapman, G., Murray, D., et al. (2000) The North Staffordshire Maternity Hospital prospective study of pregnancy-associated depression. J. Psychosom. Obstet. Gynecol. 21, 93–97.
31. Mäki, P. (2003) Parental Separation at Birth and Maternal Depressed Mood in Pregnancy: Associations with Schizophrenia and Criminality in the Offspring. Oulu, Finland: Oulu University Press.
32. Steiner, M. and Tam, W. Y. K. (1999) Postpartum depression in relation to other psychiatric disorders. In: Miller, L.J. ed. Postpartum Mood Disorders. Washington, DC: American Psychiatric Press, pp. 47–63.
33. Beck, C. T. (2002) Revision of the postpartum depression predictors inventory. J Obstet Gynecol Neonatal Nurs 31, 394–402.
34. Miller, L. J. (2002) Postpartum depression. JAMA 287, 762–765.
35. O'Hara, M. W. and Swain, A. M. (1996) Rates and risk of postpartum depression-a meta-analysis. Int. Rev. Psychiatry 8, 37–54.
36. Beck, C. T. (2001) Predictors of postpartum depression: an update. Nurs. Res. 50, 275–285.
37. Hendrick, V. and Altshuler, L. (2002) Management of major depression. Am. J. Psychiatry 159, 1667–1673.
38. Beck, C. T. (1998) A checklist to identify women at risk for developing postpartum depression. J. Obstet. Gynecol. Neonatal Nurs. 27, 39–46.
39. Evans, J., Heron, J., Francomb, H., et al. (2001) Cohort study of depressed mood during pregnancy and after childbirth. Br. Med. J. 323, 257–260.
40. Weissman, M. M., Bland, R. C., Canino, G. J., et al. (1996) Cross-national epidemiology of major depression and bipolar depression. JAMA 276, 293–299.
41. Eaton, W. W., Anthony, J. C., Gallo, J., et al. (1997) Natural history of diagnostic Interview Schedule/DSM-IV major depression: the Baltimore Epidemiologic Catchment Area follow-up. Arch. Gen. Psychiatry 54, 993–999.
42. Parikh, S. V. and Lam, R. W. (2001) Clinical guidelines for the treatment of depressive disorder: 1. definitions, prevalence, and health burden. Can. J. Psychiatry 46, 13–20S.
43. Thornicroft, G. and Sartorius N. (1993) The course and outcome of depression in different cultures: 10-year follow-up of the WHO collaborative study on the assessment of depressive disorders. Psychol. Med. 23, 1023–1032.
44. Keller, M. B. (1982) Recovery in major depressive disorder: analysis with the life table and regression models. Arch. Gen. Psychiatry 39, 905–910.
45. Altshuler, L. L., Hendrick, V., and Cohen, L. S. (1998) Course of mood and anxiety disorders during pregnancy and the postpartum period. J. Clin. Psychiatry 59(Suppl. 2), 29–33.

46. Kumar, R. and Robson, M. K. (1984) A prospective study of emotional disorders in childbearing women. Br. J. Psychiatry 144, 35–47.

47. O'Hara, M. W., Zekoski, E. M., Philipps, L. H., et al. (1990) Controlled prospective study of postpartum mood disorders: comparison of childbearing and nonchildbearing women. J. Abnorm. Psychol. 1, 3–15.

48. Kelly, R. H., Russo, J., and Katon, W. (2001) Somatic complaints among pregnant women cared for in obstetrics: normal pregnancy or depressive and anxiety symptom amplification revisited? Gen. Hosp. Psychiatry 23, 107–113.

49. Kelly, R. H., Russo, J., Holt, V. L., et al. (2002) Psychiatric and substance use disorders as risk factors for low birth weight and preterm delivery. Obstet. Gynecol. 100, 297–304.

50. Orr, S. T., James, S. A. and Blackmore Prince, C. (2002) Maternal prenatal depressive symptoms and spontaneous preterm births among African-American women in Baltimore, Maryland. Am. J. Epidemiol. 156, 797–802.

51. Birndorf, C. A., Madden, A., Portera, L., et al. (2001) Psychiatric symptoms, functional impairment, and receptivity toward mental health treatment among obstetrical patients. Int. J. Psychiatry Med. 31, 355–365.

52. Bixo, M., Sundstrom-Poromaa, I., Bjorn, I., et al. (2001) Patients with psychiatric disorders in gynecologic practice. Am. J. Obstet. Gynecol. 185, 396–402.

53. Simon, G., VonKorff, M., and Barlow, W. (1995) Health care costs of primary care patients with recognized depression. Arch. Gen. Psychiatry 52, 850–856.

54. Committee to Study the Prevention of Low Birthweight. (1998) Etiology and Risk Factors. Washington, DC: National Academic Press.

55. Children's Dental Health Project (2003) Periodontal disease association with poor birth outcomes: state of the science and policy implications. Available from http://www.cdhp.org/downloads/Publications/Policy/ PTLBW.pdf. Accessed June 2004.

56. Pajulo, M., Savonlahti, E., Sourander, A., et al. (2001) Antenatal depression, substance dependency and social support. J. Affect. Disord. 65, 9–17.

57. Kelly, R. H., Zatzick, D. F., and Anders, T. F. (2001) The detection and treatment of psychiatric disorders and substance use among pregnant women cared for in obstetrics. Am. J. Psychiatry 158, 213–219.

57a. Zuckerman, B., Amaro, H., Bauchner, H., et al. (1989) Depressive symptoms during pregnancy: relationship to poor health behaviours. Am. J. Obstet. Gynecol. 160, 1107–1111.

58. Paarlberg, K. M., Vingerhoets, J. J., Passchier, J., et al. (1995) Psychosocial factors and pregnancy outcome: a review with emphasis on methodological issues. J. Psychosom. Res. 39, 563–595.

59. National High Blood Pressure Education Working Group. (1990) National High Blood Pressure Education Working Group report on high blood pressure in pregnancy. Am. J. Obstet. Gynecol. 163, 1689–1712.

60. Brooks, M.B. (2004) Pregnancy, pre-eclampsia. Available from http://www.emedicine.com/emerg/topic480.htm. Accessed June 2004.

61. Kurki, T., Hilesmaa, V., Raitasalo, R., et al. (2000) Depression and anxiety in early pregnancy and risk for pre-eclampsia. Obstet. Gynecol. 95, 487–490.

62. Kelly, R. H., Danielsen, B., Golding, J., et al. (1999) Adequacy of prenatal care among women with psychiatric diagnoses giving birth in California in 1994 and 1995. Psychiatr. Serv. 50, 1584–1590.

63. Vintzileos, A., Anath, C. V., Smulian, C. V., et al. (2002) The impact of prenatal care in the United States on preterm births in the presence and absence of antenatal high-risk conditions. Am. J. Obstet. Gynecol. 187, 1254–1257.

64. Vintzileos, A., Smulian, C. V., Scorza, W. E., et al. (2002) The impact of prenatal care on postnatal deaths in the presence and absence of antenatal high-risk conditions. Am. J. Obstet. Gynecol. 187, 1258–1262.
65. Vintzileos, A. M., Ananth, C. V., Smulian, J. C., et al. (2002) Prenatal care and black-white fetal death disparity in the United States: heterogeneity by high-risk conditions. Obstet. Gynecol. 99, 483–489.
66. Lundy, B. and Field, T. (1996) Newborns of mothers with depressive symptoms are less expressive. Infant Behav. Dev. 19, 419–424.
67. Lundy, B., Jones, N. A., Field, T., et al. (1999) Prenatal depression effects on neonates. Infant Behav. Dev. 22, 119–129.
68. Gitau, R., Cameron, A., Fisk, N. M., et al. (1998) Fetal exposure to maternal cortisol. Lancet 352, 707–708.
69. Murray, L. (1992) The impact of postnatal depression on infant development. J. Child Psychol. 33, 543–561.
70. Ferrill, M. J., Kehoc, W. A., and Jacisin, J. J. (1992) ECT during pregnancy: physiologic and pharmacologic considerations. Convuls. Ther. 8, 186–200.
71. Miller, L. J. (1994) Use of electroconvulsive therapy during pregnancy. Hosp. Commun. Psychiatry 45, 444–450.
72. Olfson, M., Marcus, S. C., Druss, B., et al. (2002) National trends in the outpatient treatment of depression. JAMA 287, 203–209.
73. Wisner, K. L., Zarin, D. A., Holmboe, E. S., et al. (2000) Risk-benefit decision making for treatment of depression during pregnancy. Am. J. Psychiatry 157, 1933–1940.
74. Spinelli, M.G. (1997) Interpersonal psychotherapy for depressed antepartum women: a pilot study. Am. J. Psychiatry 154, 1028–1030.
75. Spinelli, M. G. and Endicott, J. (2003) Controlled trial of interpersonal psychotherapy versus parenting education program for depressed women. Am. J. Psychiatry 160, 555–562.
76. Cohen, L. S., Nonacs, R., Viguera, A. C., et al. (2004) Diagnosis and treatment of depression during pregnancy. CNS Spectr. 9, 206–216.
77. Portnoi, G., Chng, L. A., Karimi-Tabesh, L., et al. (2003) Prospective comparative study of the safety and effectiveness of ginger for the treatment of nausea and vomiting in pregnancy. Am. J. Obstet. Gynecol. 189, 1374–1377.
78. Einarson, A., Phillips, E., Mawji, F., et al. (1998) A prospective controlled multicentre study of clarithromycin in pregnancy. Am. J. Perinatol. 15, 523–525.
79. Fabro, S. E. (1987) Clinical Obstetrics. New York: John Wiley.
80. Baldessarini, R. J. (2001) Drugs and the treatment of psychiatric disorders: depression and anxiety disorders. In: Hardman, J. G., Limbird, L. E., Goodman Gilman, A., eds. The Pharmacological Basis of Therapeutics, 10th ed. New York: McGraw-Hill, pp. 447–483.
81. McBride, W. G. (1972) Limb deformities associated with iminodibenzyl hydrochloride [letter]. Med. J. Aust. 1, 492.
82. McElhatton, P. R., Garbis, H. M., Eléphant, E., et al. (1996) The outcome of pregnancy in 689 women exposed to therapeutic doses of antidepressants. A collaborative study of the European network of teratology information services (ENTIS). Reprod. Toxicol. 10, 286–294.
83. Pastuszak, A., Schick-Bschetto, B., Zuber, C., et al. (1993) Pregnancy outcome following first-trimester exposure to fluoxetine (Prozac). JAMA 269(17), 2246–2248.
84. Morrow, A. W. (1972) Imipramine and congenital abnormalities [letter]. NZ Med. J. 75, 228–229.

85. Heinonen, O. P., Slone, D. and Shapiro, S. (1977) Birth Defects and Drugs in Pregnancy. Littleton, MA: Publishing Services Group.
86. Misri, S. and Sivertz, K. (1991) Tricyclic drugs in pregnancy and lactation: a preliminary report. Int. J. Psychiatry Med. 21, 157–171
87. Altshuler, L. L., Cohen, L., Szuba, M. P., et al. (1996) Pharmacologic management of psychiatric illness during pregnancy: dilemmas and guidelines. Am. J. Psychiatry 153, 592–606.
88. Briggs, G. G., Freeman, R. K., and Yaffe, S. J. (2002) Drugs in Pregnancy and Lactation, 6th ed. Philidelphia: Lippincott Williams and Wilkins.
89. Shearer, W. T., Schreiner, R. L., and Marshall, R. E. (1972) Urinary retention in a neonate secondary to maternal ingestion of nortriptyline. J. Pediatr. 81, 570–572.
90. Petersen, T., Dording, C., Neault, N.B., et al. (2002) A survey of prescribing practices in the treatment of depression. Prog. Neuropsychopharmacol. Biol. Psychiatry 26, 177–187.
91. Preskorn, S. H. and Fast, G. A. (1991) Therapeutic drug monitoring for antidepressants: efficacy, safety and cost effectiveness. J. Clin. Psychiatry 52(Suppl.), 23–33.
92. Preskorn, S. H. and Burke, M. (1992) Somatic therapy for major depressive disorder: selection of an antidepressant. J. Clin. Psychiatry 53(Suppl. 1), 5–18.
93. Pohland, R. C., Byrd, T. K., Hamilton, M., et al. (1989) Placental transfer and fetal distribution of fluoxetine in the rat. Toxicol. Appl. Pharmacol. 98, 198–205.
94. Heikkine, T., Ekblad, U., and Laine, K. (2002) Transplacental transfer of citalopram, fluoxetine and their primary demethylated metabolites in isolated perfused human placenta. Br J Obstet Gynaecol 109, 1003–1008.
95. Hendrick, V., Stowe, Z. N., Altshuler, L. L., et al. (2003) Placental passage of antidepressant medications. Am. J. Psychiatry 160, 993–996.
96. Goldstein, D. J. (1995) Effects of third trimester fluoxetine exposure on the newborn. J. Clin. Psychopharmacol. 15, 417–420.
97. Chambers, C. D., Johnson, K. A., Dick, L. M., et al. (1996) Birth outcomes in pregnancy women taking fluoxetine. N. Engl. J. Med. 335, 1010–1015.
98. Goldstein, D. J., Corbin, L. A., and Sundell, K. L. (1997) Effects of first-trimester fluoxetine exposure on the newborn. Obstet. Gynecol. 89, 713–718.
98a. Hendrick, V., Smith, L. M., Suri, R., et al. (2003) Birth outcomes following prenatal exposure to antidepressant medications. Am. J. Obstet. Gynecol. 188, 812–815.
99. Ericson, A., Källén, B., and Wiholm, B. E. (1999) Delivery outcome after the use of antidepressants in early pregnancy. Eur. J. Clin. Pharmacol. 55, 503–508.
100. Cohen, L. S., Heller, V. L., Bailey, J. W., et al. (2000) Birth outcomes following prenatal exposure to fluoxetine. Biol. Psychiatry 48, 996–1000.
101. Simon, G. E., Cunnignham, M. L., and Davis, R. L. (2002) Outcomes of prenatal antidepressant exposure. Am. J. Psychiatry 159, 2055–2061.
102. Koren, G., Pastuzak, A., and Ito, S. (1998) Drugs in pregnancy. N. Engl. J. Med. 338, 1128–1137.
103. Robert, E. (1996) Treating depression in pregnancy [editorial]. N. Engl. J. Med. 335, 1056–1058.
104. Nulman, I., Rovet, J., Stewart, D. E., et al. (1997) Neurodevelopment of children exposed in utero to antidepressant drugs. N. Engl. J. Med. 336, 258–262.
105. Kulin, N. A., Pastuszak, A., Sage, S. R., et al. (1998) Pregnancy outcome following maternal use of the new selective serotonin reuptake inhibitors. A prospective controlled multicenter study. JAMA 279, 609–610.

106. Costei, A. M., Kozer, E., Ho, T., et al. (2002) Perinatal outcome following third trimester exposure to paroxetine. Arch. Pediatr. Adolesc. Med. 156, 1129–1132.

106a. GlaxoSmithKline study EPIP083. GSK medicine:bupropion and paroxetine. Epidemiology study: preliminary report on bupropion in pregnancy and the occurrence of cardiovascular and major congenital malformation. Available: http://ctr.gsk.co.uk/summary/paroxetine/epip083.pdf (accessed 2006 Jan 26).

106b. Health Canada Endorsed Important Safety Information on Paxil (paroxetine). Available: http://www.hc-sc.gc.ca/dhp-mps/medeff/advisories-avis/prof/paxil_4_hpc-cps_e.html (accessed 2006 Jan 26).

106c. Williams, M. and Wooltorton, E. (2005) Paroxetine (Paxil) and congenital malformations. CMAJ, 173(11), 1320–1321.

107. Heikkinen, T., Ekblad, U., Kero, P., et al. (2002) Citalopram in pregnancy and lactation. Clin. Pharmacol. Ther. 72, 184–191.

107a. Sivojelezova, A., Shuhaiber, S., Sarkissian, L., et al. (2003) Citalopram use in pregnancy: evaluation of fetal risk [abstract]. Ottawa, ON: Canadian Society of Clinical Pharmacology.

107b. Hostetter, A., Ritchie, J. C., and Stowe, Z. N. (2000) Amniotic fluid and umbilical cord blood concentrations of antidepressants in three women. Biol. Psychiatry 48, 1032–1034.

108. Einarson, F., Fatoye, B., Sarkar, M., et al. (2001) Pregnancy outcome following gestational exposure to venlafaxine: a multicenter prospective controlled study. Am. J. Psychiatry 158, 1728–1730.

109. Ward, H. E. (1997) The newer antidepressants. IM Intern. Med. 18, 65–76.

110. Ascher, J. A., Cole, J. O., Colin, J. N., et al. (1995) Bupropion: a review of its mechanism of antidepressant activity. J. Clin. Psychiatry 56, 395–401.

111. Einarson, A. and Koren, G. (2004) New antidepressants in pregnancy. Can. Fam. Physician 50, 227–229.

112. Chan, B. F., Koren, G., Fayez, I., et al. (2005) Pregnancy outcome of women exposed to bupropion during pregnancy: a prospective comparative study. Am. J Obstet. Gynecol. 192, 932–936.

113. Lambers, D. S. and Clark, K. E. (1996) The maternal and fetal physiologic effects of nicotine. Semin. Perinatol. 20(2), 115–126.

114. Benowitz, N. L. (1991) Nicotine replacement therapy during pregnancy. JAMA 266(22), 3174–3177.

115. O'Campo, P., Davis, M., and Gielen, A. (1995) Smoking cessation interventions for pregnant women: review and future directions. Semin. Perinatol. 19(4), 229–225.

116. Stillman, R. J., Rosenberg, M. J., and Sachs, B. P. (1986) Smoking and reproduction. Fertil. Steril. 46(4), 545–566.

117. Werler, M., Pober, B., and Holmes, L. (1985) Smoking and pregnancy. Teratology 32, 473–481.

118. Abel, E. L. (1980) Smoking during pregnancy: a review of effects on growth and development of offspring. Hum. Biol. 52(4), 593–625.

119. Einarson, A., Bonari, L., Voyer-Lavigne, S., et al. (2003) A multicentre prospective controlled study to determine the safety of Trazodone and Nefazodone use during pregnancy. Can. J. Psychiatry 48, 106–110.

120. Kesim, M., Yaris, F., Kadioglu, M., et al. (2002) Mirtazepine use in two pregnant women: Is it safe? Teratology 66, 204.

121. Goldman, R. D. and Koren, G. (2003) Taking St. John's wort during pregnancy. Can. Fam. Physician 49, 29–30.

122. Muller, W. E., Singer, A., and Wonnemann, M. (1998) Hyperforin represents the neurotransmitter reuptake inhibiting constituent of Hypericum extract. Pharmacopsychiatry 31(Suppl. 1), 16–21.

123. Nathan, P. (1999) The experimental and clinical pharmacology of St John's wort (*Hypericum perforatum*). Mol. Psychiatry 4, 333–338.
124. Linde, K. and Mulrow, C. D. (2000) St John's wort for depression. Cochrane Database Syst. Rev. CD000448.
125. Woelk, H., Bukard, G., and Grunwald, J. (1994) Benefits and risks of the Hypericum extract LI 160: drug monitoring study with 3250 patients. J. Geriatr. Psychiatry Neurol. 7(Suppl. 1), S34–38.
126. Schrader, E., Meier, B., and Brattstrom, A. (1998) Hypericum treatment of mild-moderate depression in a placebo-controlled study. Hum. Psychopharmacol. 13, 163–169.
127. Einarson, A., Lawrimore, T., Brand, P., et al. (2000) Attitudes and practices of physicians and naturopaths toward herbal products, including use during pregnancy and lactation. Can. J. Clin. Pharmacol. 7, 45–49.
128. O'Hara, M. A., Keifer, D., Farrell, K., et al. (1998) A review of 12 commonly used medicinal herbs. Arch. Fam. Med. 7, 523–535.
129. Grush, L. R., Nierenberg, A., Keefe, B., et al. (1998) St John's wort during pregnancy. JAMA 280, 1566.
130. Einarson, A. (2003) Abrupt discontinuation of psychotropic drugs during pregnancy. Mental Fitness. 2:26, 35-39.
131. Compendium of Drug Therapy. (The Obstetrician and Gynecologist's) (1984) New York: Biomedical Information Corp.
132. Poulson, E.and Robson, J. M. (1964) Effect of phenelzine and some related compounds on pregnancy. J. Endocrinol. 30, 205-215.
133. Castiel--Levinson, R., Merlob, P., Linder, N., and Sirota, L., and Klinger, G. (2006) Neonatal abstinence syndrome after in utero exposure to selective serotonin reuptake inhibitors in term infants. Arch. Pediatr. Adoles. Med. 160, 170–173.
134. Nordeng, H., Lindemann, R., Perminov, K.V, et al. (2001) Neonatal withdrawal syndrome after *in utero* exposure to selective serotonin reuptake inhibitors. Acta Pædiatr. 90, 228–291.
135. Better news on populations. (1993) Lancet 339, 1600.
136. Einarson, A., Selby, P., and Koren, G. (2001) Abrupt discontinuation of psychotropic drugs during pregnancy: fear of teratogenic risk and impact of counseling. J. Psychiatry Neurosci. 26, 44–48.
137. Rosabaum, Z. J. (1997) Clinical management of antidepressant discontinuation. J. Clin. Psych. 58(Suppl. 7), 37–40.
138. Chambers, C. D., Hernandez-Diaz, S., van Marter, L. J., Werler, M. M., Louik, C., Jones, K. L., and Mitchell, A. A. (2006)) Selective serotonin reuptake inhibitors and risk of persistent pulmonary hypertension of the newborn. NEJM 354, 579–587.

3

Postpartum Depression

A Common Complication of Childbirth

C. Neill Epperson and Jennifer Ballew

Summary

Postpartum depression (PPD) or, simply, postpartum are the most commonly used lay terms for describing major depressive disorder occurring in the postnatal period. Whether the disorder occurs *de novo*, is a relapse of a previous depressive episode, or has its origin in the antepartum period, depression after childbirth is associated with significant maternal and infant morbidity and, in worst cases, mortality. With most epidemiological studies demonstrating a prevalence of 10–13%, PPD is one of the most common complications of childbirth *(1,2)*. Yet, the pathogenesis, natural history, and treatment of the disorder have been shrouded in mystery and myth as society and science has imbued motherhood with a cloak of sanctity that cuts both ways. Attempts to protect mothers and their offspring from unnecessary intrusions or potential harm have unwittingly limited detection of PPD in the clinical setting and the investigation of its pathogenesis and treatment in the scientific arena.

Thus, PPD continues to be a major public health problem, with more than 400,000 women in the United States alone suffering each year from this potentially devastating disease. The overarching purpose of this chapter is to review the studies that provide the most rigorous and up-to-date findings regarding the detection, pathogenesis, and treatment of depression occurring in the postnatal period. In doing so, this chapter will enable the primary care provider to become more comfortable in assessing postpartum women and treating those who, in many cases, would otherwise go without care.

Key Words: Postpartum; depression; children; treatment, breast-feeding.

From: *Current Clinical Practice: Psychiatric Disorders in Pregnancy and the Postpartum: Principles and Treatment*
Edited by: V. Hendrick © Humana Press, Totowa, NJ

1. DETECTION:
THE FIRST STEP TO SYMPTOM RESOLUTION

1.1. The "Mental Health-Friendly" Environment

The creation of a clinical environment, including the physical space as well as the medical and office staff, that explicitly and implicitly includes mental health as a vital part of a healthy lifestyle is key to enabling women to divulge their concerns regarding their mood, thought processes, and behaviors during pregnancy and the postnatal period. Prominently displaying educational materials about anxiety and depression during pregnancy and the puerperium along with information about other common pregnancy-related issues helps to destigmatize mental disorders. Directly inquiring about symptoms of depression and anxiety at every pre- and postnatal appointment sends the unequivocal message that the clinician values the patient as an individual with specific needs and concerns.

Engaging the services of a local wellness expert to provide in-office workshops on activities to promote mental well-being during pregnancy and beyond or a mental health professional to lead groups discussing the adjustments required of motherhood, clearly indicates the practice's commitment to and investment in its patients' mental health. Each of these can be accomplished with relatively little financial or time commitment on the part of busy primary care providers. With increasing numbers of mental health care providers requesting fee-for-service, it is crucial that the primary care practice invests in prevention services and provides in-house counseling for those who require immediate psychiatric assessment. Otherwise, valuable nursing and staff time is consumed trying to find a mental health care provider who can see the patient during a postpartum crisis.

1.2. Routine Screening for Mental Illness
in Pregnant and Postpartum Women

For clinicians who wish to institute routine screening for postnatal depression, there are two excellent patient-rated instruments to aid in the detection of depression in postpartum women. The Edinburgh Postnatal Depression Scale (EPDS; 3) is a 10-item instrument that requires the woman to rate herself on a scale of 0 (*no, not at all*) to 3 (*yes, all of the time*) on questions such as "I have been able to laugh and see the funny side of things," "I have blamed myself unnecessarily when things go wrong," and "I have felt sad or miserable." The instrument is easily tallied, and a score of 12.5 or more has been shown to indicate the presence of a probable case of postpartum depression (PPD) in studies of women attending primary care clinics *(4–6)*. A more recently developed instrument, the Postpartum Depression Screening Scale (PDSS) *(7,8)*, is tailored to assess symptoms specific to new mothers and has excellent sensitivity and specificity to detect PPD. The PDSS has 35 items compared with the 10 questions in the EPDS, but is written at a third-grade level and can be completed by most people within 5–10 min. A PDSS score of 35–59 indicates normal adjustment after delivery, a score of 60–79 indicates "minor" PPD (i.e., likely requires formal psychiatric evaluation), and a score of 80–175 is a positive screen for major PPD, in which case the patient should be referred for mental health evaluation as soon as possible.

To assess for the presence of other psychiatric disorders in addition to depression, the clinician can administer the Primary Care Evaluation of Mental Disorders patient health questionnaire (PRIME-MD; Pfizer Inc., New York). When used to assess the prevalence of psychiatric disorders in a study of 2747 women attending seven obstetrics/gynecological (OB/GYN) practices, investigators found a prevalence of 19% for any psychiatric diagnosis in those women who were pregnant or postpartum *(9,10)*. This was similar to the rate of psychiatric disorders in the entire group and suggests that general screening for mental illness should occur in all OB/GYN patients.

1.3. The Differential Diagnosis

Once a postpartum woman has been identified as suffering from a mood disturbance, determining the nature, timing of onset, duration, and severity of the symptoms is essential to making a correct diagnosis (Table 1). The differential diagnosis ranges from normal adjustment and the baby blues to anxiety disorders, PPD, postpartum psychosis, and/or bipolar disorder.

In addition, organic causes such as thyroid dysfunction must be ruled out. Approximately 5% of all postpartum women *(11)* and 50% of the 10% of women who have thyroid peroxidase antibodies during early gestation develop thyroid dysfunction during the first 9 mo after delivery *(12,13)*. One-third of these women will develop permanent hypothyroidism *(14)*, and findings from several studies suggest that women who are thyroid peroxidase antibody-positive during early gestation are at increased risk of PPD regardless of postpartum thyroid function *(15–18)*.

As noted in Table 1, the baby blues are so common (26–85% of postpartum women) that they are considered to be part of the normal reaction to childbearing *(19–21)*. This syndrome, characterized by

Table 1

Characteristics of the Baby Blues, Postpartum Depression (PPD), and Postpartum Psychosis: Sorting Through the Differential Diagnosis

Characteristics	Baby blues	PPD	Postpartum psychosis
Prevalence	40–60%	10–15%	0.2%
Timing			
Peaks 3–4 d postpartum	√		
Onset within 6 mo postpartum		√	
Onset within 2–4 wk postpartum			√
Duration			
hours to a few days	√		
>2 wk to months		√	
>4 d to months			√
Symptoms			
Feeling overwhelmed	√	√	
Anxiety	√	√	
Mood lability	√	√	√
Depressed mood	√	√	
Decreased interest or pleasure		√	
Inappropriate guilt		√	
Appetite/weight change		√	
Obsessions		√	
Irritability	√	√	
Decreased libido [a]		√	
Difficulty sleeping but tired	√	√	
Suicidal/infanticidal thoughts		√	√
Agitation		√	√
Decreased need for sleep			√
Unusual thoughts or behaviors			√
Hallucinations			√
Hypersexuality			√
Hyperactivity			√
Confusion/disorientation			√

[a] Symptom included in the DSM-IV criteria for major depressive disorders.

dysphoric mood, tearfulness, irritability, emotional lability, anxiety, and sleep disturbance, peaks around 3–4 d postpartum and resolves within hours to a few days. Although the baby blues are self-limited in duration, the more severe the symptoms during this time period, the more likely the woman is to meet criteria for major depressive disorder (MDD) at

6 wk postpartum *(22,23)*. Given the frequency of the baby blues, all pregnant women should be informed about the potential for mood symptoms during the first week after delivery and encouraged to contact their health care provider if the symptoms last longer than a few days or are so severe that they limit their ability to function.

PPD, although also quite common (10–15% of postpartum women), results in distress and impairment in function that can linger well into the first postnatal year if not treated *(24)*. The diagnosis of PPD is made using the fourth edition of the *Diagnostic and Statistical Manual of Mental Disorders* (DSM-IV) criteria for MDD. If the symptoms occur within the first 4 wk after delivery, an additional specifier, "with postpartum onset," may be added to the MDD diagnosis. Although the symptoms of PPD can overlap with those of the baby blues and postpartum psychosis, a clinical presentation that is dominated by decreased need for sleep, agitation, heightened activity or rapid speech, bizarre or unusual behavior, is frequently indicative of postpartum psychosis. This disorder is most often similar to the mania of bipolar affective disorder (BPAD). The portion of women with psychosis in the postnatal period who will not have ongoing BPAD is not clear, but one can suspect that those postpartum psychotic women with no previous psychiatric history may have a "pure puerperal psychosis," which is time-limited with treatment. Psychosis can be subtle when commingled with depression, and thus, questions regarding unusual thoughts or experiences should be queried regardless of whether the patient is behaving "normally" during the office visit.

Although the DSM-IV does not provide distinct diagnostic nomenclature for PPD and psychosis, studies have found several differences in the clinical presentation of depression and psychosis occurring in the puerperium vs that occurring at other times. Postpartum psychoses are more frequently accompanied by a confused and disorganized clinical picture *(25,26)*, which can wax and wane. Symptoms of postpartum psychosis can include thought disorganization, bizarre behavior, lack of insight, delusions of reference, persecution, jealousy, grandiosity, suspiciousness, impaired sensorium/orientation, and self-neglect *(25)*.

Although the intensity of obsessions and compulsions do not differ between women with puerperal and nonpuerperal depression, aggressive obsessions regarding the infant are more common in women who present with depression after delivery *(27)*. Thus, unless other obsessions or compulsions are present, the diagnosis of co-morbid obsessive-compulsive disorder is usually not appropriate in the context of PPD. Women with PPD often have violent thoughts that they will drown or stab the baby or

Table 2
Examples of Questions to Use in the Primary Care Setting to Probe
for Psychiatric Disorders in Postpartum Women

Symptoms	Probe
General well-being	"Motherhood can be quite an adjustment. How has it been going for you?"
Depressed mood	"Have you been feeling down or more sad recently?"
Anxious mood	"Do you find that you are feeling more tense and on edge than usual?" "Are you worrying about even small things?"
Obsessions/worries	"Many moms have frequent concerns about their baby's health and well-being. Are there certain worries or thoughts about your baby or other things that keep bothering you even when you try to stop thinking about them?"
Psychosis	"Have you or your family members noticed that you don't seem to be your usual self lately?" "Have you been experiencing any unusual thoughts or feelings?"
Infanticidal or suicidal thoughts	"It can be hard to be a new mother, and sometimes infants can be very frustrating. Have you been so frustrated with [infant's name] that you have had thoughts or feelings of hurting him/her?"
	"Sometimes people feel so bad or upset that they don't feel like living anymore. Have you had these kinds of feelings recently?"

throw the baby down the stairs. When there are no signs of psychosis and the mother reports that these thoughts are highly distressing, it is usually not necessary to make a referral for emergency inpatient care. In the presence of psychosis and/or suicidal ideation, these thoughts are often not as upsetting to patients because the motivation for contemplating killing one's children can be altruistic or an extension of a suicide plan (28). The psychotic or suicidal mother's tentative hold on reality makes her at high risk for infanticidal behavior (28,29), and thus inpatient hospitalization with initiation of pharmacotherapy is the standard of care.

The prevalence of infanticidal thinking in women with PPD, with or without psychosis, is quite high. A study of severely psychiatrically ill and hospitalized women in India found that 43% reported infanticidal ideas, whereas 36% reported infanticidal behavior *(29)*. This high percentage is not surprising given that hospitalization could have occurred as a result of the presence of such thoughts. However, a study conducted in the United States found that 41% of depressed mothers with children younger than 3 yr reported having thoughts of harming their infants compared with 7% of the mothers in the control group *(30)*. Therefore, complete screening for PPD or postpartum psychosis must include thoughts about harming the infant and/or children in addition to thoughts of suicide.

1.4. Who Is at Risk for Postpartum Mood Disturbances?

Of women who present with PPD, 20–30% have had a previous episode of MDD *(31)*. Other risk factors include a personal history of severe premenstrual dysphoria *(32)*, family history of mood disorder *(2)*, marital discord *(33–35)*, lack or inadequacy of a confiding relationship *(36,37)*, and the number of stressful life events in the previous year *(35,38)*. Regarding perinatal events, pregnancy loss is associated with posttraumatic symptoms and depression *(39)*, but, in general, studies of the impact of obstetrical complications on postpartum mood have been mixed *(33,34,37,40,41)*. There is no consistent evidence that the choice to breast- or bottle-feed has any significant impact on mood in the first weeks after delivery *(19,22,42)*.

2. BIOLOGICAL UNDERPINNINGS OF POSTPARTUM MOOD DISORDERS

"Why me? Why now?" are questions commonly asked by women suffering from postpartum mental illness, particularly those who have never previously experienced a serious psychiatric disturbance. Although according to the DSM-IV, PPD is not diagnostically distinct from MDD that is not childbirth-related *(24)*, the hormonal milieu of pregnancy and the puerperium is so unique that investigators have focused on these hormonal changes as key factors in the pathogenesis of PPD. Several recent and thorough reviews of the relationship between PPD and endocrine function have been published *(18,43)*. Tables 3–6 provide an overview of the findings from studies focused primarily on the relationship between ovarian, adrenal, and thyroid hormones and postpartum mood disorders.

Although no clear relationship between one particular hormone and PPD emerges, the most compelling investigations of the pathogenesis of

Table 3
Estrogen in the Pathogenesis of Postpartum Depression (PPD)

Study (reference)	Findings	Implications
Weik, 1991 (45)	Growth hormone response to apomorphine was accentuated in at-risk women who became symptomatic during the postpartum	Estradiol may enhance postsynaptic dopamine receptor sensitivity, increasing risk for postpartum psychosis or mood instability
O'Hara, 1990 (19)	In 182 women followed prospectively, the baby blues was associated with higher free estriol levels in the third trimester and greater drop in levels within the first day postpartum	Lends support to theory that estrogen withdrawal may precipitate the baby blues
Ahokas, 1999 (46), 2000 (47), 2001 (48)	Twelve women with postpartum psychosis and low serum estradiol levels were successfully treated with estradiol; 23 women with PPD and low serum estradiol improved as treatment with estradiol increased serum estradiol to follicular phase levels	PPD and psychosis in hypogonadal postpartum women may be responsive to treatment with estradiol; supports notion that hypogonadism contributes to symptom onset

PPD emphasize the importance of the individual's sensitivity to pregnancy-related hormonal changes *(44,45)*. By focusing on women who have demonstrated vulnerability to mood changes during the puerperium by having experienced PPD with a previous pregnancy, Bloch and colleagues overcame several of the shortcomings of previous studies. Women were studied outside of the postpartum period when manipulation of hormone levels would not interfere with breast-feeding nor exacerbate PPD at a time when recovery is crucial for both the mother and child. Administration of supraphysiological levels of estrogen and progesterone to mimic a pregnancy allowed the investigators to compare mood responses in those at high risk of depressive symptoms (history of PPD group) with those who are at low risk (no history of PPD), while at the same time controlling the hormonal milieu in each subject such that serum estradiol and progesterone levels were not significantly different between groups. Those women with a previous history of PPD experienced a significant worsening of their mood during the hormone administration and withdrawal phases of the study, with five out of the eight women becoming clinically depressed again. In contrast, women without a history of PPD did not experience a change in mood during the study. The potential mood-altering effects of the progesterone metabolite allopregnanolone, which is a potent γ-aminobutyric acid type A receptor agonist that has been implicated in the pathogenesis of premenstrual and postpartum mood changes *(49,65,66)*, was not evaluated in this investigation using the pseudopregnancy paradigm.

Alternatively, another group focused on at-risk women immediately in the puerperium to determine whether their response to a neuroendocrine challenge could predict the likelihood of them experiencing mood instability *(69)*. Women with a history of BPAD or schizoaffective disorder who experienced an illness relapse during the puerperium had an exaggerated growth hormone response on postpartum day 3 (prior to onset of mood instability) to an injection of apomorphine, an agent that stimulates postsynaptic dopamine receptors in the median eminence of the hypothalamus. The authors propose that the estrogen-induced alterations in dopaminergic function during pregnancy lead to hypersensitivity of postsynaptic dopamine receptors after delivery and thus contribute to mood changes in at-risk women *(67–71)*.

Finally, the vast majority of parturient women (93%) have blunted hypothalamic–pituitary–adrenal (HPA) axis function for weeks if not months following childbirth *(72)*, secondary to profound increases in corticotropin-releasing hormone and cortisol during pregnancy. Although it is not clear whether women who develop the baby blues and PPD have

Table 4

Progesterone in the Pathogenesis of Postpartum Depression (PPD)

Study (reference)	Findings	Implications
Ross, 2004 (49)	Plasma progesterone and 5-α-dihydroprogesterone (5-α-DHP) were higher in women with PPD than controls; levels of progesterone in pregnancy were lower in women who subsequently developed PPD; scores on the Edinburgh Postnatal Depression Scale correlated with plasma levels of 5-α-DHP and allopregnanolone.	Reduction in progesterone metabolism to 5-α-DHP and subsequently to allopregnanolone may precipitate PPD.
Lawrie, 1998 (50)	Administration of progestogen in postpartum was associated with more depression at 6 wk postpartum than placebo; estradiol and progesterone levels were lower in the progestogen group	Synthetic progestogens may worsen postpartum mood; they are not associated with increases in serum progesterone levels.
O'Hara, 1991 (31)	No significant association was found between free progesterone levels in plasma and PPD	No evidence that total or free progesterone levels are associated with PPD
Bulter, 1986 (51)	No significant association was found between total progesterone levels in plasma and PPD	No evidence that total or free progesterone levels are associated with PPD

Ballinger, 1982 (52)	No significant association was found between total progesterone levels in plasma and PPD	No evidence that total or free progesterone levels are associated with PPD
Heidrich, 1994 (53)	No significant association was found between total progesterone levels in plasma and PPD	No evidence that total or free progesterone levels are associated with PPD
Harris, 1989 (54)	Depressed breast-feeding women had lower salivary progesterone levels than nondepressed breast-feeding women; the opposite was true for bottle-feeders.	Breast-feeding alters progesterone levels secondary to suppressing menstrual cyclicity and thus could have confounded findings.
Harris, 1994 (55)	($N = 120$) Association between progesterone levels and PPD in early postpartum period (days 2–10), but none by d 35 postpartum	Modest association between maternal mood and salivary progesterone concentration in early postpartum period
Nott, 1976 (56)	($N = 27$) Weak association between magnitude of the change in progesterone levels and PPD	Little indication of association between progesterone and PPD

Table 5

The Hypothalamic–Pituitary–Adrenal Axis in the Pathogenesis of Postpartum Depression (PPD) or Psychosis

Study (reference)	Findings	Implications
Singh, 1986 (57)	No association between cortisol levels and postpartum psychosis	No evidence that cortisol levels or degree of suppression by dexamethasone is involved in postpartum psychosis
O'Hara, 1991 (31)	93% of postpartum women were dexamethasone nonsuppressors (DNSs)	Pregnancy-related elevations in corticotropin-releasing factor and cortisol render most women as DNSs, thus associations with the blues cannot be ruled out
Harris, 1996 (58)	Evening cortisol levels were lower in the 7 (out of 120) women who developed PPD	Dysregulation of the hypothalamic–pituitary–adrenal (HPA) axis may be involved in PPD
Magiakou, 1996 (59)	Adrenocorticotrophic hormone (ACTH) response to corticotropin-releasing hormone was blunted to a greater degree in women with baby blues or PPD than healthy postpartum women.	No evidence that cortisol levels or degree of suppression by dexamethasone is involved in postpartum psychosis
Bloch, 1999 (44)	Women with history of PPD had greater cortisol response to supraphysiological levels of estradiol and progesterone	Pregnancy-related alterations in HPA axis function continue into the postpartum and may contribute to mood symptoms in vulnerable individuals

Table 6

Thyroid Hormones and β-Endorphins in the Pathogenesis of Postpartum Depression (PPD) or Psychosis

Study (reference)	Findings	Implications
Stewart, 1988 (60)	No difference in thyroid hormone levels or antibodies in 30 women with postpartum psychosis vs controls	No evidence that thyroid hormones or the presence of thyroid antibodies is associated with postpartum psychosis
Bokhari, 1998 (61)	Case report of a postpartum woman with psychosis that coincided with postpartum thyroiditis and resolved as she became euthymic	Limited to one report
Kuijpen, 2001 (17)	Thyroperoxidase antibodies associated with PPD at 12 wk gestation, 4 and 12 wk postpartum ($N = 291$)	Small but significant fraction of PPD cases associated with thyroid dysfunction
Smith, 1990 (62)	Greater drop in serum β-endorphin levels from delivery to postnatal day 2 found in those with mood symptoms	Relationship between PPD and β-endorphin cannot be elucidated by the Smith and Glover studies
Glover, 1994 (63)	No association observed between serum β-endorphin levels and mood on postpartum day 3	
Harris, 2002 (64)	Randomized placebo-controlled trial of thyroxine in the prevention of PPD in thyroid antibody-positive women; thyroxine administration did not reduce the occurrence of PPD	Does not support the use of thyroid supplementation in the treatment of PPD

a longer period of HPA axis dysregulation than those who are asymptomatic *(73)*, this alteration in neuroendocrine function may be sufficient to unmask mood disturbance in vulnerable individuals. No association between cortisol and cortisol suppression to dexamethasone has been shown for puerperal psychosis *(57)*.

In summary, no specific aspect of the hormonal milieu of pregnancy or the puerperium has been implicated, without contradiction, in the pathogenesis of postpartum mood disorders. However, many studies have been limited to peripheral measures of neuroendocrine function and thus lack the power of neuroimaging techniques to hone in on alterations in central nervous system function in symptomatic women. With this said, several studies of the treatment of PPD and psychosis provide additional support for the importance of estrogen fluctuations and postpartum hypogonadism in the pathogenesis of postpartum mental illness.

3. TREATMENT OF POSTPARTUM MOOD DISORDERS

3.1. Incorporating the Biopsychosocial Model of Treatment

It is important to take into consideration the psychosocial as well as the biological contributions to mental disorders in any patient presenting with depression or psychosis. This is particularly true when women present in the puerperium. At no other time in a woman's life is she required to navigate a developmental transition that is potentially wrought with challenging psychodynamic issues, and changes in interpersonal relationships, all in the context of sleep deprivation and profound hormonal and physiological adjustments. Thus, treatment must address potential situational and interpersonal factors as well as target the specific symptoms.

3.2. Management of the Breast-Feeding Patient

Given that 62% of women breast-feed for at least the first 6 wk after delivery *(74)*, informed consent regarding the risks and benefits of exposing the newborn to a psychotropic agent and/or maternal mental illness must be discussed and documented. The benefits of breast-feeding, even in developed countries, are extensive and include convenience and cost savings in addition to the health advantages offered to the infant and enhanced emotional security via parental bonding. The American Academy of Pediatrics recommends exclusive breast-feeding during the first 6 mo of life to promote "optimal" growth and development *(75)*. Extensive research provides compelling evidence that human milk feeding reduces the risk of respiratory *(76)* and urinary tract infections *(77)*, otitis media *(78)*, bacteremia and bacterial meningitis *(79)*, allergic diseases *(80)*, sudden infant death syndome *(81)*, and insulin-dependent diabetes mellitus *(82)*. Exclusive breast-feeding may enhance neurodevelopment *(83–85)*.

Several other groups have published comprehensive reviews focusing on the use of psychotropic medications during nursing *(18,86–93)*. A frequently updated source for clinicians prescribing all classes of medications is *Drugs in Pregnancy and Lactation: A Reference Guide to Fetal and Neonatal Risk (94)*.

Regarding breast-fed babies, it is useful to keep in mind that older children will be better able to fully and efficiently metabolize drugs than newborns. Likewise, preterm infants or babies with impaired liver or kidney function will have more difficulty effectively metabolizing medications. Children who are exclusively breast-fed are likely to be exposed to higher amounts of drugs than those who are not breast-fed or who receive supplemental formula feedings.

The importance of continued breast-feeding to the mother must be balanced with her anxiety regarding infant exposure to a particular agent, and the disruption in sleep that is particularly profound in nursing mothers. The practice of pumping and then discarding breast milk either in the morning after a bedtime dose of a sleep aid or when the medication is expected to peak in breast milk can limit the degree of infant exposure to medications. However, the studies indicating the point at which the drug peaks in breast milk are restricted to sertraline, paroxetine *(95,96)*, and fluoxetine *(97)*. Some women may find that pumping is either impractical because of other responsibilities or raises their anxiety level about the infant's medication exposure. Finally, many mothers who are highly committed to breast-feeding but find full-time breast-feeding too onerous may enjoy the option of partial breast-feeding, particularly once breast-feeding has been well established.

Table 7 summarizes the breast-feeding safety profile of antidepressants most frequently used to treat depression. The relatively extensive literature focusing on selective serotonin reuptake inhibitors (SSRIs) in nursing indicates that most infants can continue to nurse when their mothers are prescribed these agents without risk of adverse events. Significantly less is known about the safety of venlafaxine or bupropion in nursing infants. Although the older antidepressants such as the tricyclics are not included in Table 7, they appear to be relatively safe for use during nursing *(98)*. However, these agents pose more side effects for the mother and are no longer considered to be first-line treatments for depression *(99–115)*.

Table 7
Studies of Selective Serotonin Reuptake Inhibitors (SSRIs) in Breast-feeding

Study (reference)	Sample size	Maternal dose	Infant serum concentration	Comments
Sertraline (Zoloft)				
Stowe et al., 2003 (178)	N = 26	25–200 mg	Sertraline: ND to 3 ng/mL; Desmethylsertraline: ND to 10 ng/mL	MWAD: ~5.4%, during lactation
Epperson et al., 2001 (179)	N = 14	25–200 mg	Sertraline: ND Desmethylsertraline: ND	Infants experienced little to no blockade of platelet serotonin reuptake
Hendrick et al., 2001 (97)	N = 30	25–200 mg	Sertraline:< 1–8 ng/mL; Desmethylsertraline: < 1–12 ng/mL	No adverse effects reported
Dodd et al., 2000 (97a)	N = 10	50–150 mg	Sertraline levels were below the detection limit of 2 ng/mL in all infants	No adverse effects reported
Birnbaum et al., 1999 (169)	N = 3	50–100 mg	Sertraline: < 5 ng/mL; Desmethylsertraline: < 5 ng/mL	No adverse effects reported

56

Study	N	Dose	Levels	Comments
Wisner et al., 1998 (180)	N = 9	50–200 mg	Sertraline: ND to 3 ng/mL Desmethylsertraline: ND to 6 ng/mL 1 and 2 infants had unusually high sertraline and desmethylsertraline levels, respectively	No adverse effects were reported
Kristensen et al., 1998 (181)	N = 8	1.05 mg/kg/day	Sertraline: ND Desmethylsertraline: ND	MWAD: ~0.2–1.32%; no adverse effects reported
Stowe et al., 1997 (95)	N = 11	25–150 mg	Sertraline: ND to 3 ng/mL; Desmethylsertraline: ND to 10 ng/mL	No adverse effects reported; very low infant blood levels
Mammen et al., 1997 (182)	N = 3	50–100 mg	Sertraline: < 2.0 ng/mL; Desmethylsertraline: < 2.0 ng/mL	Benign neonatal sleep myoclonus reported in one infant, resolved by 6 months
Altshuler et al., 1995 (183)	N = 1	100 mg	Sertraline: ND; Desmethylsertraline: ND	No adverse effects reported; mother was also taking nortriptyline
Fluoxetene (Prozac)				
Suri et al., 2002 (184)	N = 10	Mean dose 34 ± 12.8 mg	Fluoxetine: ND-84 ng/mL; Norfluoxetine: ND-39 ng/mL	Using several methods of calculation of infant exposure, maximum infant dose over an entire year of nursing would appear to equal approx 120 mg

(continued)

Table 7 *(Continued)*

Study (reference)	Sample size	Maternal dose	Infant serum concentration	Comments
Hendrick et al., 2001 (97)	N = 19	10–60 mg	Fluoxetine: < 1–84 ng/mL; Norfluoxetine: < 1–265 ng/mL	No adverse effects reported; infants of mothers taking < 20 mg/day likely to have very low blood levels
Birnbaum et al., 1999 (169)	N = 13	20–80 mg	Fluoxetine: ND-82 ng/mL; Norfluoxetine: ND-250 ng/mL	No adverse effects reported; detectable concentrations of fluoxetine and/or norfluoxetine were noted in 78% of exposed infants; all but three infants were exposed *in utero* as well as during lactation; one infant also exposed to a TCA, another to clonazepam, and another to clonazepam and valproic acid
Chambers et al., 1999 (116)	N = 26	20–40 mg	n/a	Evidence of reduced growth curves in fluoxetine-exposed infants; no behavioral effects reported; retrospective cohort study design
Kristensen et al., 1999 (185)	N = 14	0.51 mg/kg/day	Fluoxetine: 20–252 ng/L; Norfluoxetine: 17–187 ng/L	MWAD: average was 6.81% (range 2.15 to 12%); colic was reported in two infants
Yoshida et al., 1998 (186)	N = 4	20–40 mg	Fluoxetine: ND; Norfluoxetine: ND	MWAD: 3–10%; no adverse effects reported

ND, nondetectable; MWAD, maternal weight-adjusted dose; n/a, not applicable.

Study	N	Dose	Infant level	Comments
Brent et al., 1998 (117)	N = 1	20 mg	Fluoxetine: 61 ng/mL; Norfluoxetine: 57 ng/mL	Transient seizure-like activity and one episode peripheral cyanosis reported by mother (all unwitnessed by medical personnel); mother was also taking carbamazepine and buspirone
Taddio et al., 1996 (187)	N = 10	0.39 mg/kg/day	Infant daily dose estimated to be 0.65 mg	MWAD: 10.8%; no adverse effects reported
Lester et al., 1993 (188)	N = 1	20 mg	Fluoxetine: 340 ng/mL; Norfluoxetine: 208 ng/mL	High infant drug levels correlated with symptoms of colic
Burch et al., 1992 (189)	N = 1	20 mg	n/a	No adverse effects reported
Paroxetine (Paxil)				
Merlob et al., 2004 (190)	N = 27	20 mg	n/a	Irritability reported in one infant; prospective cohort study design
Hendrick et al., 2000 (191)	N = 16	5–30 mg	ND	No adverse effects reported
Stowe et al., 2000 (96)	N = 16	Avg= 23.1 mg	< 2.0 ng/mL	No adverse effects reported
Begg et al., 1999 (192)	N = 10	10–30 mg	ND	MWAD: 1.3%; no adverse effects reported
Ohman et al., 1999 (193)	N = 6	20–40 mg	n/a	MWAD: 0.7–2.9%; no adverse effects reported

(continued)

59

Table 7 (Continued)

Study (reference)	Sample size	Maternal dose	Infant serum concentration	Comments
Misri et al., 1999 (194)	N = 24	10–40 mg	< 2.0 ng/mL	MWAD: 1.1%; no adverse effects reported
Birnbaum et al., 1999 (169)	N = 2	30 mg	< 20 ng/mL	No adverse effects reported; one infant exposed in utero and during lactation, the other exclusively during lactation but also exposed to clonazepam in utero and during lactation
Spigset et al., 1996 (195)	N = 1	20 mg	n/a	No adverse effects reported
Citalopram (Celexa)				
Lee et al., 2004 (196)	N = 31	10–60 mg	n/a	Prospective cohort study; one report of decreased sleep and restlessness in infant after citalopram use initiated
Heikkinen et al., 2002 (197)	N = 11	20–40 mg	Citalopram: ~3.3 mg/mL; Desmethylcitalopram: ~2.8 mg/mL at 2 months old	MWAD: 0.2–0.3% during lactation
Schmidt et al., 2000 (198)	N = 1	40 mg	Citalopram: 12.7 ng/mL	MWAD: 5.4% during lactation; sleep disturbance in infant, improved with decrease to 20 mg daily

Reference	N	Dose	Drug levels	Effects
Rampono et al., 2000 (199)	N = 7	20–40 mg	Citalopram: < 2.3 mg/mL; Desmethylcitalopram: < 2.2 mg/mL	MWAD: 4.4–5.1% during lactation
Jensen et al., 1997 (200)	N = 1	20 mg	Citalopram: 7 nM; Desmethylcitalopram: < 10 nM	MWAD: ~5%, during lactation; no adverse effects reported
Spigset et al., 1997 (201)	N = 3	20–40 mg	n/a	MWAD: 0.7–5.9% during lactation; single-dose citalopram; no adverse effects reported
Fluvoxamine (Luvox)				
Kristensen et al., 2002 (202)	N = 2	50–150 mg	n/a	MWAD: 0.8–1.38%; no adverse effects reported
Hendrick et al., 2001 (97)	N = 50	100–150 mg	ND	No adverse effects reported
Piontek et al., 2001 (203)	N = 2	50–300 mg	ND	No adverse effects reported up to 3 years after exposure
Yoshida et al., 1997 (204)	N = 1	100 mg	n/a	No adverse effects reported
Wright et al., 1991 (205)	N = 1	200 mg	n/a	No adverse effects reported

(continued)

Table 7 (Continued)

Study (reference)	Sample size	Maternal dose	Infant serum concentration	Comments
Bupropion (Wellbutrin)				
Briggs et al., 1993 (206)	N = 1	300 mg	ND	No adverse effects reported
Baab et al., 2002 (206a)	N = 2	75 mg/bid 150 mg/d	Below limit of detection	No adverse effects reported.
Chaudron et al., 2004 (206b)	N = 1	150 mg (SR)	Drug blood level not obtained. Infant was not febrile during seizure, which was witnessed by the mother. The description of the behavior was consistent with seizures of a 6 mo infant	6 mo infant had seizure after exposure to two doses. Infant evaluated in pediatric seizure clinic, laboratory test and EEG unremarkable.
Venlafaxine (Effexor)				
Hendrick et al., 2001 (206c)	N = 2	75 mg, 150 mg	Limit of detection was 10 ng/mL. Parent drug not detectable. Metabolite O-desmethylvenlafaxine was 16 ng/mL in one infant and 12 ng/mL in the other	Metabolite is measurable in infants. No adverse effects were reported.
Ilett et al., 2002 (207)	N = 6	225–300 mg	5 mg/L in one infant; ND in five other infants	MWAD: 5.5–7.3%; no adverse effects reported

Of the SSRIs, fluoxetine is the most extensively studied in breast-fed infants, and the findings remain more controversial. Higher infant serum concentrations of fluoxetine and its metabolites are found in some breast-fed infants compared with those exposed to other SSRIs (Table 7). One retrospective study *(116)* found significantly reduced growth curves in children exposed to fluoxetine through breast milk, and there is one case report of transient seizure activity possibly associated with maternal fluoxetine use *(117)*. The clinical significance of this latter report is questionable because the seizures were never confirmed by a medical professional. Although the majority of studies focusing on the use of fluoxetine during breast-feeding suggest that there are no apparent adverse effects, long-term developmental and behavioral effects of fluoxetine or any other SSRI exposure via lactation have not been investigated.

Benzodiazepines *(118–128)*, mood stabilizers *(129–158)*, and antipsychotic medications *(159–168)* are all used frequently in the treatment of postpartum psychiatric disorders, despite the lack of thorough, well-controlled studies in this population. In general, short-term, low-dose use of benzodiazepines is considered fairly safe during lactation. No long-term adverse effects have been reported in exclusively breast-fed children whose mothers were taking benzodiazepines on a regular basis *(169)*, but there have been a few case reports of transient sedation in breast-fed infants, which improved on cessation of breast-feeding *(170,171)*. The shorter-acting benzodiapines (alprazolam, lorazepam) are favored over those with longer half-lives (clonazepam, diazepam). Two small studies have suggested that the nonbenzodiazepine hypnotics zolpidem and zalepron are safe in nursing *(172,173)*

Of the mood stabilizers, lithium has been the most extensively studied in breast-feeding mother–infant pairs. Unfortunately, lithium has been linked to several serious adverse effects in nursing infants, including hypotonia, hypothermia, cyanosis, and electrocardiogram abnormalities *(174)* and is therefore not recommended in nursing. If lithium absolutely must be used in a woman who insists on breast-feeding, infant lithium levels are indicated. Valproic acid and carbamazepine are both considered reasonably safe to use while nursing, although careful monitoring for infant hepatotoxicity is recommended *(174,175)*. The inevitable sleep deprivation that goes along with breast-feeding may pose additional problems for women with bipolar disorder, further emphasizing the need for a low threshold for cessation of breast-feeding in these patients.

The literature regarding the use of antipsychotic agents during lactation is particularly scarce, making it difficult to recommend breast-feeding by women who require these medications. One group has reported that breast-fed infants of mothers taking haloperidol and chlorpromazine simultaneously were slow in meeting developmental milestones *(176)*. Clozapine, being highly lipophilic, has been shown to accumulate in high concentrations in breast milk and has been associated with sedation, autonomic instability, and agranulocytosis in a handful of case reports *(175)*. There is one published case report of perinatal cardiomegaly in an infant whose mother was taking olanzapine throughout pregnancy and breast-fed until postpartum day 7, but because jaundice and sedation persisted after bottle-feeding was initiated, the authors suggest there was no relationship to olanzapine in this case *(177)*. The other atypical antipsychotics have not been associated with adverse outcomes during lactation, but as mentioned, the data are limited.

3.3. Treatment Studies: The Few and Far Between

Given the evolving evidence that maternal mood disorders negatively impact child development *(208–213)*, aggressive treatment, and even prophylaxis, of postpartum disorders is warranted. As discussed earlier, the signs and symptoms of PPD occur across a broad spectrum, and thus individual treatment plans should be tailored to the needs of the individual patient. Depression caused by general medical causes (i.e., thyroid dysfunction, anemia, and nutritional deficits) should always be ruled out with a thorough medical history, physical exam, and appropriate lab tests.

As stated earlier, the treatment of PPD is currently based on standards for nonpuerperal depression because there are no double-blind, placebo-controlled studies of antidepressants in the treatment of MDD with postpartum onset. There is some reluctance on the part of researchers to conduct these studies, in part because of the ethical considerations of withholding treatment in subjects who would receive a placebo. However, differences in treatment response to medication cannot be ruled out without such studies. Although there is a relatively high spontaneous remission rate in women with milder symptoms who present early in the puerperium *(214)*, moderate to severe depression that has been present for a number of months is unlikely to remit without psychotherapy or pharmacological interventions *(215)*.

3.3.1. RANDOMIZED CONTROLLED CLINICAL TRIALS

Although relatively few well-controlled studies have focused on the treatment of PPD specifically, one study found that women with mild depression who were enrolled within the first couple of months of childbirth responded to treatment with fluoxetine with or without the addition of a cognitive behavioral-type therapy *(214)*. Additionally, six sessions of this type of psychotherapy were equally effective in reducing depressive symptoms. Findings from this study suggest that women with milder PDD can be successfully treated with medication or psychotherapy alone, but there is no evidence of synergism when used together.

Alternatively, in a study of women with more severe cases of PPD with longer duration (mean of 8 mo) a 12-wk course of interpersonal psychotherapy was effective in reducing depression, but women in the comparison group who were on the waiting list during the 12 wk experienced no significant improvement in their symptoms despite being involved in study-related mood assessments during this time *(215)*. Thus, depression that is well established is unlikely to spontaneously remit, and interpersonal therapy appears to be quite an effective nonpharmacological intervention.

Because of the dramatic hormonal shifts associated with pregnancy and childbirth and the known association between gonadal steroid hormones and mood *(216)*, the role of estrogen in the treatment of PPD has been questioned. Women with a history of PPD appear to be more sensitive to the mood-altering effects of high levels and withdrawal of sex steroids *(44)*. Therefore, the only other pharmacological intervention that has been studied in a double-blind, placebo-controlled fashion found transdermal administration of estrogen effective in decreasing depressive symptoms for up to 6 mo *(217)*. These findings were intriguing as the hormone appeared to distinguish itself from placebo within the first 2 wk of treatment. However, the results of the study were difficult to interpret because half of the women were being treated with traditional antidepressants at the same time that they underwent randomization to estrogen or placebo. The lack of clarity regarding whether estrogen alone or estrogen plus an antidepressant is more effective than placebo in treating PPD has limited most clinicians' enthusiasm for using estrogen as a mainstay of treatment for PPD. In addition, there are theoretical concerns that using estrogen early in the puerperium could increase the risk of thromboembolic events because the postnatal period is a time of relative hypercoagulability.

3.3.2. NONRANDOMIZED INTERVENTIONS

Sertraline at doses of 50–150 mg/d were found to significantly reduce Hamilton Depression Rating Scale Scores in a group of 21 women with PPD of moderate severity *(218)*. An open-label study of women with PPD and documented estradiol deficiency indicated that physiological sublingual doses of 17-β estradiol may be an effective treatment, with onset of response within the first week of administration *(48)*. Progesterone, in contrast, has not been shown to be beneficial in PPD *(219)*, and, in fact, long-acting norethisterone enanthate given within 48 h of delivery has been associated with an increased risk of developing PPD *(50)*.

Although no controlled studies have been conducted in PPD for obvious reasons, electroconvulsive therapy (ECT) is known to be a safe, rapid, and effective treatment for nonpuerperal depression. At least one study *(220)* has shown ECT to be effective in treating severe cases of PPD and is particularly recommended for women experiencing active suicidal ideation.

A number of other nonpharmacological options for treating PPD have been investigated with some modicum of success. Most communities have organized support groups composed of women who are currently experiencing this disorder and who can help each other feel less socially ostracized, learn coping skills, and provide an emotionally supportive environment *(221)*. Family education and marital counseling may also be considered for some couples, especially given the known correlation between PPD and stressful life events and marital discord *(36,37)*. Home visits by a midwife or doula may also be beneficial to vulnerable families *(222)* and can add to the mother's sense of social support and alleviate some of the strain of caretaking experienced by other family members.

Patients should additionally be encouraged to take time for themselves, to rest and relax, and to not hesitate to ask friends and family for help as needed. As with other forms of depression, exercise, proper nutrition, and adequate sleep will all contribute to symptom alleviation. Case reports have indicated that bright light therapy *(223)* and even massage *(224)* may be feasible, nonpharmacological treatments for PPD.

3.4. Prevention Strategies

PPD offers the rare opportunity in psychiatry to predict both the onset and duration of the disorder. Thus, it is particularly relevant to consider prevention of this illness and to screen all pregnant women for risk factors. Randomized controlled studies have demonstrated that antenatal *(225)* and postnatal *(226)* group therapy interventions have successfully decreased the incidence of PPD in women at risk. Notably, at least one controlled trial has shown that supportive counseling of mothers with PPD provided by nonspecialists was equally effective in protecting the maternal–child relationship, as was counseling provided by mental health specialists *(227)*.

Women with a history of previous PPD may benefit from prophylactic administration of sertraline *(228)*, but treatment with nortriptyline has not been proven more effective than placebo *(229)*. It has also been shown that women with increased consumption of omega-3 fatty acids, in particular docosahexaenoic acid (DHA), are less likely to develop PPD compared with women with low DHA intakes *(230)*.

3.5. Treating Postpartum Psychosis

As of mid-2005 there is no consensus regarding which medications are most effective in treating postpartum psychosis *(231)*. Because postpartum psychosis is commonly thought of as occurring along the bipolar spectrum, mood stabilizers are the most commonly used treatment option. No large-scale studies of atypical antipsychotics have been conducted in the puerperium, but case reports suggest that risperidone *(163)* and olanzapine *(177)* are effective treatments. The safety and efficacy of mood stabilizers in lactating mothers still needs to be clarified *(232)*.

Antidepressants should be used very cautiously in treating postpartum psychosis, even when depressive symptoms are present, because of the risk of precipitating rapid cycling *(231)*. ECT, especially when bilaterally administrated, has also been shown to be highly effective in the treatment of postpartum psychosis *(220,233,234)*, particularly in cases refractory to standard treatment *(235)*. Estrogen has also been suggested as a treatment for postpartum psychosis because symptoms have been shown to improve with reversal of estrogen deficiency *(47)*. However, the role of estrogen in postpartum psychosis has been even less studied than estrogen's contribution to PPD. Prophylaxic use of mood stabilizers has been shown to be beneficial in lowering risk of postpartum psychosis relapse *(236)*. Many women with BPAD may decide to remain on their mood stabilizers during pregnancy because the rate of relapse during pregnancy and the puerperium is alarmingly high *(237)*.

3.6. Specific Recommendations for Treatment

3.6.1. BABY BLUES

As discussed, the baby blues are self-limited and are unlikely to require psychotropic intervention, with the exception of the occasional sleep aid for women who are having difficulty sleeping even when the baby is asleep. Zolpidem (Ambien 5–10 mg) or a benzodiazepine with a medium half-life such a lorazepam (Ativan 0.5–2 mg) for several nights may help to break a cycle of insomnia that is independent from the infant's waking. Emotional and physical support for the mother as she integrates caring for the newborn with her previous responsibilities is crucial. Because the baby blues can be a harbinger of PPD, all patients should be instructed to contact their primary care provider if the symptoms of the blues cause significant distress, limit their ability to function as mothers, or extend past the first postpartum week.

3.6.2. POSTPARTUM DEPRESSION

Individual psychotherapy should be considered as a treatment option for all women with PPD, and this treatment alone may suffice in women with mild to moderate symptom severity. First-line treatment for more severe and/or prolonged PPD includes administration of an SSRI and possible supplementation with a benzodiazepine when extreme anxiety or insomnia is a presenting feature. Although several studies suggest that exogenous estrogen may alleviate symptoms of PPD, it is not yet considered to be first-line therapy because these early findings await confirmation in additional controlled clinical trials. Refractory or severe cases of PPD may be referred for ECT. Nonpharmacological options that may be of some help include nursing or doula visits, bright light therapy, family or group therapy, and general self-care. Certainly, rallying the woman's family and social network to provide emotional and practical support can be vital for recovery.

3.6.3. POSTPARTUM PSYCHOSIS

Because of the unacceptably high risk of harm to either mother or child, postpartum psychosis is a psychiatric emergency that almost always requires in-patient hospitalization. Because of the scarcity of studies focusing on psychosis occurring specifically in the postpartum period and the similarities between postpartum psychosis and bipolar disorder, the current acute treatment for postpartum psychosis typically involves mood stabilizer, antipsychotic, and anxiolytic medications. Immediate formal evaluation by a psychiatrist is always recommended whenever postpartum psychosis is part of the differential diagnosis.

4. CONCLUSION

Childbirth represents an enormous developmental transition for women, which, in the best of circumstances, is accompanied by mild mood changes and psychosocial/interpersonal adjustment. The patient's psychological status during pregnancy and the early puerperium should be discussed openly during prenatal visits so that full disclosure of past psychiatric history and other potential risk factors for PPD or psychosis can be obtained. Screening for PPD can be enhanced by the incorporation of formal mood assessments during obstetrical appointments. These rating scales can be completed by the patient while waiting for the physician or midwife and provide a clear indication of the practitioner's interest in the patient's psychological well-being. An active and up-to-date list of mental health care providers who will take new patients with various means of payment will save the office staff time and ensure that the patient is evaluated in a timely fashion.

The pathogenesis of PPD is not well elucidated, and treatment studies focusing specifically on depression during the puerperium are scant at best. Thus, at the present time treatment of PPD and other mood disorders during the postnatal period are based on treatments for nonpuerperal depression and psychosis. Luckily, most of the antidepressants and anxiolytics used as first-line treatments appear to be relatively safe for the nursing infant. A challenge for the future will be to develop safe methods for critically evaluating the efficacy of medications and/or hormones in postpartum depressed women who may or may not be nursing. In addition, future studies of the pathogenesis of postpartum mood disorders must begin to focus on the hormone/neurotransmitter interface as well as factors, such as genetics, that mediate individual vulnerability to mood disorders during this special time in a woman's life.

ACKNOWLEDGMENTS

Writing of this chapter was supported in part by the following grants: NIH MH18030 and MH064845 (Epperson); T32-MH19961 (Ballew); Dana Foundation (Epperson).

REFERENCES

1. Epperson, C. N. (1999) Postpartum major depression: detection and treatment. Am. Fam. Physician 59, 2247–2254, 2259–2260.
2. O'Hara, M. W., Neunaber, D. J., and Zekoski, E. M. (1984) Prospective study of postpartum depression: prevalence, course, and predictive factors. J. Abnorm. Psychol. 93, 158–171.
3. Cox, J. L., Holden, J. M., and Sagovsky, R. (1987) Detection of postnatal depression. Development of the 10-item Edinburgh Postnatal Depression Scale. Br. J. Psychiatry 150, 782–786.
4. Peindl, K. S., Wisner, K. L., and Hanusa, B. H. (2004) Identifying depression in the first postpartum year: guidelines for office-based screening and referral. J. Affect. Disord. 80, 37–44.
5. Glasser, S., Barell, V., Boyko, V., et al. (2000) Postpartum depression in an Israeli cohort: demographic, psychosocial and medical risk factors. J. Psychosom. Obstet. Gynecol. 21, 99–108.
6. Wickberg, B. and Hwang, C. P. (1996) The Edinburgh Postnatal Depression Scale: validation on a Swedish community sample. Acta Psychiatr. Scand. 94, 181–184.
7. Beck, C. T. and Gable, R. K. (2000) Postpartum depression screening scale: development and psychometric testing. Nurs. Res. 49, 272–282.
8. Beck, C. T. and Gable, R. K. (2001) Comparative analysis of the performance of the Postpartum Depression Screening Scale with two other depression instruments. Nurs. Res. 50, 242–250.

 9. Spitzer, R. L., Williams, J. B., Kroenke, K., et al. (1994) Utility of a new procedure
    for diagnosing mental disorders in primary care. The PRIME-MD 1000 study.
    JAMA 272, 1749–1756.
10. Spitzer, R. L., Williams, J. B., Kroenke, K., et al. (2000) Validity and utility of the
    PRIME-MD patient health questionnaire in assessment of 3000 obstetric-gyneco-
    logic patients: the PRIME-MD Patient Health Questionnaire Obstetrics–Gynecol-
    ogy Study. Am. J. Obstet. Gynecol. 183, 759–769.
11. Gerstein, H. C. (1990) How common is postpartum thyroiditis? A methodologic
    overview of the literature. Arch. Intern. Med. 150, 1397–400.
12. Kokandi, A. A., Parkes, A. B., Premawardhana, L. D., et al. (2003) Association of
    postpartum thyroid dysfunction with antepartum hormonal and immunological
    changes. J. Clin. Endocrinol. Metab. 88, 1126–1132.
13. Lazarus, J. H. Thyroid dysfunction: reproduction and postpartum thyroiditis.
    (2002) Semin. Reprod. Med. 20, 381–388.
14. Muller, A. F., Drexhage, H. A., and Berghout, A. (2001) Postpartum thyroiditis
    and autoimmune thyroiditis in women of childbearing age: recent insights and
    consequences for antenatal and postnatal care. Endocr. Rev. 22, 605–630.
15. Oretti, R.G., Harris, B., Lazarus, J. H., et al. (2003) Is there an association between
    life events, postnatal depression and thyroid dysfunction in thyroid antibody posi-
    tive women? Int. J. Soc. Psychiatry 49, 70–76.
16. Harris, B., Oretti, R., Lazarus, J., et al. (2002) Randomised trial of thyroxine to
    prevent postnatal depression in thyroid-antibody-positive women. Br. J. Psychia-
    try 180, 327–330.
17. Kuijpens, J. L., Vader, H. L., Drexhage, H. A., et al. (2001) Thyroid peroxidase
    antibodies during gestation are a marker for subsequent depression postpartum.
    Eur. J. Endocrinol. 145, 579–584.
18. Hendrick, V., Altshuler, L., and Whybrow, P. (1998) Psychoneuroendocrinology
    of mood disorders. The hypothalamic-pituitary-thyroid axis. Psychiatr. Clin. North
    Am. 21, 277–292.
19. O'Hara, M..W., Zekoski ,E.M., Philipps, L. H., and Wright, E. J. (1990) Controlled
    prospective study of postpartum mood disorders: comparison of childbearing and
    nonchildbearing women. J. Abnorm. Psychol. 99, 3–15.
20. Stein, G. (1982) The maternity blues. In: Brockington, I. F. and Kumar, R.,eds.
    Motherhood and Mental Illness. New York: Grune and Stratton, pp. 119–154.
21. Handley, S. L., Dunn, T. L., Waldron, G., et al. (1980) Tryptophan, cortisol and
    puerperal mood. Br. J. Psychiatry 136, 498–508.
22. Hannah, P., Adams, D., Lee, A., et al. (1992) Links between early post-partum
    mood and post-natal depression. Br. J. Psychiatry 160, 777–780.
23. Cox, J. L., Connor, Y. M., Henderson, I., et al. (1983) Prospective study of the psychi-
    atric disorders of childbirth by self report questionnaire. J. Affect. Disord. 5, 1–7.
24. Diagnostic and Statistical Manual of Mental Disorders, 4th ed. (DSM-IV). (1994)
    Washington, DC: American Psychiatric Association.
25. Wisner, K. L., Peindl, K., and Hanusa, B. H. (1994) Symptomatology of affective
    and psychotic illnesses related to childbearing. J. Affect. Disord. 30, 77–87.
26. Brockington, I. F., Cernik, K. F., Schofield, E. M., et al. (1981) Puerperal psycho-
    sis. Phenomena and diagnosis. Arch. Gen. Psychiatry 38, 829–833.
27. Wisner, K L., Peindl, K. S., Gigliotti, T., et al. (1999) Obsessions and compulsions
    in women with postpartum depression. J. Clin. Psychiatry 60, 176–180.
28. Stanton, J., Simpson, A., and Wouldes, T. (2000) A qualitative study of filicide by
    mentally ill mothers. Child Abuse Neglect 24, 1451–1460.

29. Chandra, P. S., Venkatasubramanian, G., and Thomas, T. (2002) Infanticidal ideas and infanticidal behavior in Indian women with severe postpartum psychiatric disorders. J. Nerv. Ment. Dis. 190, 457–461.

30. Jennings, K. D., Ross, S., Popper, S., et al. (1999) Thoughts of harming infants in depressed and nondepressed mothers. J. Affect. Disord. 54(1–2), 21–28.

31. O'Hara, M. W., Schlechte, J. A., Lewis, D. A., et al. (1991) Prospective study of postpartum blues. Biologic and psychosocial factors. Arch. Gen. Psychiatry 48, 801–806.

32. Sugawara, M., Toda, M. A., Shima, S., et al. (1997) Premenstrual mood changes and maternal mental health in pregnancy and the postpartum period. J. Clin. Psychol. 53, 225–232.

33. Campbell, J. C., Poland, M. L., Waller, J. B., et al. (1992) Correlates of battering during pregnancy. Res. Nurs. Health 15, 219–226.

34. Cox, J. L. (1982) Medical management, culture, and mental illness. Br. J. Hosp. Med. 27, 533–537.

35. O'Hara, M. W. (1986) Social support, life events, and depression during pregnancy and the puerperium. Arch. Gen. Psychiatry 43, 569–573.

36. O'Hara, M. W., Rehm, L. P., and Campbell S. B. (1983) Postpartum depression. A role for social network and life stress variables. J. Nerv. Ment. Dis. 171, 336–341.

37. Paykel, E. S., Emms, E. M., Fletcher, J., et al. (1980) Life events and social support in puerperal depression. Br. J. Psychiatry 136, 339–346.

38. Kendell, R. E. (1985) Emotional and physical factors in the genesis of puerperal mental disorders. J. Psychosom. Res. 29, 3–11.

39. Turton, P., Hughes, P., Evans, C. D. H., et al. (2001). Incidence, correlates and predictors of post-traumatic stress disorder in the pregnancy after stillbirth. Br. J. Psychiatry 178, 556–560.

40. O'Hara, M. W., Rehm, L. P., and Campbell, S. B. (1982) Predicting depressive symptomatology: cognitive-behavioral models and postpartum depression. J. Abnorm. Psychol. 91, 457–461.

41. Playfair, H. R. and Gowers, J. I. (1981) Depression following childbirth — a search for predictive signs. J. Roy. Coll. Gen. Pract. 31, 201–208.

42. Alder, E. M. and Cox, J. L. (1983) Breast feeding and post-natal depression. J. Psychosom. Res. 27, 139–144.

43. Parry, B. L., Sorenson, D. L., Meliska, C. J., et al. (2003) Hormonal basis of mood and postpartum disorders. Curr. Women's Health Rep. 3, 230–235.x

44. Bloch, M., Schmidt, P. J., Danaceau, M., et al. (2000) Effects of gonadal steroids in women with a history of postpartum depression. Am. J. Psychiatry 157, 924–930.

45. Wieck, A., Kumar, R., Hirst, A. D., et al. (1991) Increased sensitivity of dopamine receptors and recurrence of affective psychosis after childbirth. Br. Med. J. 303(6803), 613–616.

46. Ahokas, A. and Aito, M. (1990) Role of estradiol in puerperal psychosis. Psychopharmacology 147, 108–110.

47. Ahokas, A., Aito, M., and Rimon, R. (2000) Positive treatment effect of estradiol in postpartum psychosis: a pilot study. J. Clin. Psychiatry 61, 166–169.

48. Ahokas, A., Kaukoranta, J., Wahlbeck, K., et al. (2001) Estrogen deficiency in severe postpartum depression: successful treatment with sublingual physiologic 17beta-estradiol: a preliminary study. J. Clin. Psychiatry 62, 332–336.

49. Ross L. E., Sellers E. M., Gilber Evans S. E., et al. (2004) Mood changes during pregnancy and the postpartum period: development of a biopsychosocial model. Acta Psychiatr. Scand. 109, 457–466.

50. Lawrie T. A., Hofmeyr G. J., De Jager, M., et al. (1998) A double-blind randomised placebo controlled trial of postnatal norethisterone enanthate: the effect on postnatal depression and serum hormones. Br. J. Obstet. Gynaecol. 105, 1082–1090.

51. Butler, J. and Leonard, B. E. (1986) Post-partum depression and the effect of nomifensine treatment. Int. Clin. Psychopharmacol. 1, 244–252.

52. Ballinger, C. B., Kay, D. S., Naylor, G. J., et al. (1982) Some biochemical findings during pregnancy and after delivery in relation to mood change. Psychol. Med. 12, 549–556.

53. Heidrich, A., Schleyer, M., Spingler, H., et al. (1994) Postpartum blues: relationship between not-protein bound steroid hormones in plasma and postpartum mood changes. J. Affect. Disord. 30, 93–98.

54. Harris, B., Johns, S., Fung, H., et al. (1989) The hormonal environment of postnatal depression. Br. J. Psychiatry 154, 660–667.

55. Harris, B., Lovett, L., Newcombe, R. G., et al. (1994) Maternity blues and major endocrine changes: Cardiff puerperal mood and hormone study II. Br. Med. J. 308, 949–953.

56. Nott, P.N., Franklin, M., Armitage, C, et al. (1976) Hormonal changes and mood in the puerperium. Br. J. Psychiatry 128, 379–383.

57. Singh, B., Gilhotra, M., Smith, R, et al. (1986) Post-partum psychoses and the dexamethasone suppression test. J. Affect. Disord. 11, 173–177.

58. Harris, B., Lovett, L., Smith, J., et al. (1996) Cardiff puerperal mood and hormone study. III. Postnatal depression at 5 to 6 weeks postpartum, and its hormonal correlates across the peripartum period. Br. J. Psychiatry 168, 739–744.

59. Magiakou, M. A., Mastorakos, G., Rabin, D., et al. (1996) Hypothalamic corticotropin-releasing hormone suppression during the postpartum period: implications for the increase in psychiatric manifestations at this time. J. Clin. Endocrinol. Metab. 81, 1912–1917.

60. Stewart, D. E., Addison, A. M., Robinson, G. E., et al. (1988) Thyroid function in psychosis following childbirth. Am. J. Psychiatry 145, 1579–1581.

61. Bokhari, R., Bhatara, V. S., Bandettini, F., et al (1998) Postpartum psychosis and postpartum thyroiditis. Psychoneuroendocrinology 23, 643–650.

62. Smith, J. E. (1990) Pregnancy complicated by thyroid disease. J. Nurse-Midwifery 35, 143–149.

63. Glover, V., Liddle, P., Taylor, A., et al. (1994) Mild hypomania (the highs) can be a feature of the first postpartum week. Association with later depression. Br. J. Psychiatry 164, 517–521.

64. Harris, B. Oretti, R., Lazarus, J., et al. (2002) Randomised trial of thyroxine to prevent postnatal depression in thyroid-antibody-positive women. Br. J. Psychiatry 180, 327–330.

65. Epperson, C. N., Haga, K., Mason, G. F., et al. (2002) Cortical gamma-aminobutyric acid levels across the menstrual cycle in healthy women and those with premenstrual dysphoric disorder: a proton magnetic resonance spectroscopy study. Arch. Gen. Psychiatry 59, 851–858.

66. Epperson, C. N., Jatlow, P. I., Czarkowski, K., et al. (2003) Maternal fluoxetine treatment in the postpartum period: effects on platelet serotonin and plasma drug levels in breast-feeding mother-infant pairs. Pediatrics 112, e425.

67. Demarest, K. T., Riegle, G. D., and Moore, K. E. (1984) Adenohypophysial dopamine content during physiological changes in prolactin secretion. Endocrinology 115, 2091–2097.

68. Van Hartesveldt, C. and Joyce, J. N. (1986) Effects of estrogen on the basal ganglia. Neurosci. Biobehav. Rev. 10, 1–14.
69. Wieck, A. (1989) Endocrine aspects of postnatal mental disorders. Baillieres Clin. Obstet. Gynaecol. 3, 857–877.
70. Ettigi, P., Lal, S., Martin, J. B, et al. (1975) Effect of sex, oral contraceptives, and glucose loading on apomorphine-induced growth hormone secretion. J. Clin. Endocrinol. Metab. 40, 1094–1098.
71. Cookson, J. C. (1985) The neuroendocrinology of mania. J. Affect. Disord. 233–241.
72. O'Hara, M. W., Schlechte, J. A., Lewis D. A., et al. (1991) Controlled prospective study of postpartum mood disorders: psychological, environmental, and hormonal variables. J. Abnorm. Psychol. 100, 63–73.
73. Pedersen, C. A., Stern, R. A., Pate, J., et al. (1993) Thyroid and adrenal measures during late pregnancy and the puerperium in women who have been major depressed or who become dysphoric postpartum. J. Affect. Disord.. 29(2–3), 201–211.
74. Ryan, A. S., Pratt, W. F., Wysong, J. L., et al. (1991) A comparison of breast-feeding data from the National Surveys of Family Growth and the Ross Laboratories Mothers Surveys. Am. J. Public Health 81, 1049–1052.
75. Anonymous. (1997) Breast-feeding and the use of human milk. American Academy of Pediatrics work group on breast-feeding. Pediatrics 100, 1035–1039.
76. Wright, A. L., Holberg, C. J., Martinez, F. D., et al. (1989) Breast feeding and lower respiratory tract illness in the first year of life. Group Health Medical Associates. Br. Med. J. 299, 946–949.
77. Pisacane, A., Graziano, L., Mazzarella, G., et al. (1992) Breast-feeding and urinary tract infection. J. Pediatr. 120, 87–89.
78. Aniansson, G., Alm, B., Andersson, B., et al. (1994) A prospective cohort study on breast-feeding and otitis media in Swedish infants. Pediatr. Infect. Dis. J. 13, 183–188.
79. Takala, A. K. (1989) Epidemiologic characteristics and risk factors for invasive Haemophilus influenzae type b disease in a population with high vaccine efficacy. Pediatr. Infect. Dis. J. 8, 343–346.
80. Halken, S., Host, A., Hansen, L. G., et al. (1992) Effect of an allergy prevention programme on incidence of atopic symptoms in infancy. A prospective study of 159 "high-risk" infants. Allergy 47, 545–553.
81. Ford, R. P., Taylor, B. J., Mitchell, E. A., et al. (1993) Breast-feeding and the risk of sudden infant death syndrome. Int. J. Epidemiol.. 22, 885–890.
82. Mayer, E., Hamman, R., Gay, E., et al. (1988) Reduced risk of IDDM among breastfed children. Diabetes 37, 1625–1632.
83. Fergusson, D. M., Beautrais, A. L., and Silva, P. A. (1982) Breast-feeding and cognitive development in the first seven years of life. Soc. Sci. Med. 16, 1705–1708.
84. Lucas, A., Morley, R., Cole, T., et al. (1992) Breast milk and subsequent intelligence quotient in children born preterm. Lancet 339, 261–264.
85. Vestergaard, M., Obel, C., Henriksen, T., et al. (1999) Duration of breast-feeding and developmental milestones during the latter half of infancy. Acta Paediatr. 88, 1327–1332.
86. Winans, E. A. (2001) Antipsychotics and breast-feeding. J. Hum. Lactation 17, 344–347.
87. Craig, M. and Abel, K. (2001) Drugs in pregnancy. Prescribing for psychiatric disorders in pregnancy and lactation. Best Pract. Res. Clin. Obstet. Gynaecol. 15, 1013–1030.

88. Buist, A. (2001) Treating mental illness in lactating women. Medscape Womens Health 6, 3.
89. Spencer, J. P., Gonzalez, L. S., 3rd., and Barnhart, D. J. (2001) Medications in the breast-feeding mother. Am. Fam. Physician 64, 119–126.
90. Burt, V. K., Suri, R., Altshuler, L. L., et al. (2001) The use of psychotropic medications during breast-feeding. Am. J. Psychiatry 158, 1001–1009.
91. Dodd, S., Maguire, K. P., Burrows, G. D., et al. (2000) Nefazodone in the breast milk of nursing mothers: a report of two patients. J. Clin. Psychopharmacol. 20, 717–718.
92. Tenyi, T., Csabi, G., and Trixler, M. (2000) Antipsychotics and breast-feeding: a review of the literature. Paediatr. Drugs 2, 23–28.
93. Ito, S. (2000) Drug therapy for breast-feeding women. N. Engl. J. Med. 343, 118–126.
94. Briggs, G., Freeman, R. K., and Yaffe, S. J., eds. (2002) Drugs in Pregnancy and Lactation: A Reference Guide to Fetal and Neonatal Risk, 6th ed. Baltimore: Williams and Wilkins.
95. Stowe, Z. N., Owens, M. J., Landry, J. C, et al. (1997) Sertraline and desmethyl-sertraline in human breast milk and nursing infants [see comment]. Am. J. Psychiatry 154, 1255–1260.
96. Stowe, Z. N., Cohen, L. S., Hostetter, A., et al. (2000) Paroxetine in human breast milk and nursing infants. Am. J. Psychiatry 157, 185–189.
97. Hendrick, V., Stowe, Z. N., Altshuler, L. L., et al. (2001) Fluoxetine and norfluoxetine concentrations in nursing infants and breast milk. Biol. Psychiatry 50, 775–782.
97a. Dodd, S., Stocky, A., Buist, A., Burrows, G. D., and Norman, T. R. (2001) Sertraline analysis in the plasma of breast-fed infants. Australian & New Zealand J. Psych. 35(4), 545–546.
98. Weissman, A. M., Barcey, T. L., Hartz, A. J., et al. (2004) Pooled analysis of antidepressant levels in lactating mothers, breast milk and nursing infants. Am. J. Psychiatry 161, 1066–1078.
99. Hendrick, V., Fukuchi, A., Altshuler, L., et al. (2001) Use of sertraline, paroxetine and fluvoxamine by nursing women. Br. J. Psychiatry 179, 163–166.
100. Dodd, S., Buist, A., and Norman, T. R. (2000) Antidepressants and breast-feeding: a review of the literature. Paediatr. Drugs 2, 183–192.
101. Frey, O. R., Scheidt, P., and von Brenndorff, A. I. (1999) Adverse effects in a newborn infant breast-fed by a mother treated with doxepin. Ann. Pharmacother. 33, 690–693.
102. Ilett, K. F., Hackett, L. P., Dusci, L. J., et al. (1998) Distribution and excretion of venlafaxine and O-desmethylvenlafaxine in human milk. Br. J. Clin. Pharmacol. 45, 459–462.
103. Yoshida, K., Smith, B., and Kumar, R. C. (1997) Fluvoxamine in breast-milk and infant development. Br. J. Clin. Pharmacol.. 44, 210–211.
104. Epperson, C. N., Anderson, G. M., and McDougle, C. J. (1997) Sertraline and breast-feeding. N. Engl. J. Med. 336, 1189–1190.
105. Wisner, K. L. and Perel, J. M. (1996) Nortriptyline treatment of breast-feeding women. Am. J. Psychiatry 153, 295.
106. Breyer-Pfaff, U., Nill, K., Entenmann K. N., et al. (1995) Secretion of amitriptyline and metabolites into breast milk. Am. J. Psychiatry 152, 812–813.
107. Wisner, K. L., Perel, J. M., and Foglia, J. P. (1995) Serum clomipramine and metabolite levels in four nursing mother-infant pairs. J. Clin. Psychiatry 56, 17–20.

108. Buist, A., Norman, T. R., and Dennerstein, L. (1993) Mianserin in breast milk. Br. J. Clin. Pharmacol. 36, 133–134.
109. Wisner, K. L. and Perel J. M. (1991) Serum nortriptyline levels in nursing mothers and their infants. Am. J. Psychiatry 148, 1234–1236.
110. Isenberg, K. E. (1990) Excretion of fluoxetine in human breast milk. J. Clin. Psychiatry 51, 169.
111. Stancer, H. C. and Reed, K. L. (1986) Desipramine and 2-hydroxydesipramine in human breast milk and the nursing infant's serum. Am. J. Psychiatry 143, 1597–600.
112. Kemp, J., Ilett, K. F., Booth J., et al. (1985) Excretion of doxepin and N-desmethyldoxepin in human milk. Br. J. Clin. Pharmacol. 20, 497–499.
113. Brixen-Rasmussen, L., Halgrener, J., and Jorgensen, A. (1982) Amitriptyline and nortriptyline excretion in human breast milk. Psychopharmacology 76, 94–95.
114. Bader, T. F. and Newman, K. (1980) Amitriptyline in human breast milk and the nursing infant's serum. Am. J. Psychiatry 137, 855–856.
115. Erickson, S. H., Smith, G. H., and Heidrich, F. (1979) Tricyclics and breast feeding. Am. J. Psychiatry 136, 1483–1484.
116. Chambers, C. D., Anderson, P. O., Thomas, R. G., et al. (1999) Weight gain in infants breastfed by mothers who take fluoxetine. Pediatrics 104(5), e61.
117. Brent, N. B. and Wisner K. L. (1998) Fluoxetine and carbamazepine concentrations in a nursing mother/infant pair. Clin. Pediatr. 37, 41–44.
118. Oo, C. Y., Kuhn, R. J., Desai, N., Wright, C. E, et al. (1995) Pharmacokinetics in lactating women: prediction of alprazolam transfer into milk. Br. J. Clin. Pharmacol. 40, 231–236.
119. Lebedevs, T. H., Wojnar-Horton R. E., Yapp, P., et al. (1992) Excretion of temazepam in breast milk. Br. J. Clin. Pharmacol. 33, 204–206.
120. Soderman, P. and Matheson, I. (1988) Clonazepam in breast milk. Eur. J. Pediatr. 147, 212–213.
121. Wretlind, M. (1987) Excretion of oxazepam in breast milk. Eur. J. Clin. Pharmacol. 33, 209–210.
122. Summerfield, R. J. and Nielsen, M. S. (1985) Excretion of lorazepam into breast milk. Br. J. Anaesth. 57, 1042–1043.
123. Wesson, D. R., Camber, S., Harkey, M., et al. (1985) Diazepam and desmethyldiazepam in breast milk. J. Psychoactive Drugs 17, 55–56.
124. Fisher, J. B., Edgren, B. E., Mammel, M. C., et al. (1985) Neonatal apnea associated with maternal clonazepam therapy: a case report. Obstet. Gynecol. 66(3 Suppl.), 34S–35S.
125. Humpel, M., Stoppelli, I., Milia, S., et al. (1982) Pharmacokinetics and biotransformation of the new benzodiazepine, lormetazepam, in man. III. Repeated administration and transfer to neonates via breast milk. Eur. J. Clin. Pharmacol. 21, 421–425.
126. Kok, T. H., Taitz, L. S., Bennett, M. J., et al. (1982) Drowsiness due to clemastine transmitted in breast milk. Lancet 1, 914–915.
127. Brandt, R. (1976) Passage of diazepam and desmethyldiazepam into breast milk. Arzneimittel-Forschung 26, 454–457.
128. Erkkola, R. and Kanto, J. (1972) Diazepam and breast-feeding. Lancet 1(7762), 1235–1236.
129. Liporace, J., Kao, A., and D'Abreu, A. (2004) Concerns regarding lamotrigine and breast-feeding. Epilepsy Behav. 5, 102–105.
130. Frey, B., Braegger, C. P., and Ghelfi, D. (2002) Neonatal cholestatic hepatitis from carbamazepine exposure during pregnancy and breast feeding. Ann. Pharmacother. 36, 644–647.

131. Ohman, I., Vitols, S., and Tomson, T. (2000) Lamotrigine in pregnancy: pharmaco-kinetics during delivery, in the neonate, and during lactation. Epilepsia 41, 709–713.
132. Piontek, C. M., Baab, S., Peindl, K. S., et al. (2000) Serum valproate levels in 6 breast-feeding mother-infant pairs. J. Clin. Psychiatry 61, 170–172.
133. Wisner, K. L. and Perel, J. M. (1998) Serum levels of valproate and carbamazepine in breast-feeding mother-infant pairs. J. Clin. Psychopharmacol. 18, 167–169.
134. Rambeck, B., Kurlemann, G., Stodieck, S. R., et al. (1997) Concentrations of lamotrigine in a mother on lamotrigine treatment and her newborn child. Eur. J. Clin. Pharmacol. 51, 481–484.
135. Tomson, T., Ohman, I., and Vitols, S. (1997) Lamotrigine in pregnancy and lac-tation: a case report. Epilepsia 38, 1039–1041.
136. Stahl, M. M., Neiderud, J., and Vinge, E. (1997) Thrombocytopenic purpura and anemia in a breast-fed infant whose mother was treated with valproic acid. J. Pediatr. 130, 1001–1003.
137. Frey, B., Schubiger, G., and Musy, J. P. (1990) Transient cholestatic hepatitis in a neonate associated with carbamazepine exposure during pregnancy and breast-feeding. Eur. J. Pediatr. 150, 136–138.
138. Schou, M. (1990) Lithium treatment during pregnancy, delivery, and lactation: an update. J. Clin. Psychiatry 51, 410–413.
139. Tsuru, N., Maeda, T., and Tsuruoka, M. (1988) Three cases of delivery under sodium valproate — placental transfer, milk transfer and probable teratogenicity of sodium valproate. Jpn. J. Psychiatry Neurol. 42, 89–96.
140. Bardy, A. H., Hiilesmaa, V. K., and Teramo, K. A. (1987) Serum phenytoin during pregnancy, labor and puerperium. Acta Neurol. Scand. 75, 374–375.
141. Pittard, W. B., 3rd. and O'Neal, W., Jr. (1986) Amitriptyline excretion in human milk. J. Clin. Psychopharmacol. 6, 383–384.
142. von Unruh, G. E., Froescher, W., Hoffmann, F., et al. (1984) Valproic acid in breast milk: how much is really there? Ther. Drug Monit. 6, 272–276.
143. Froescher, W., Eichelbaum, M., Niesen, M., et al. (1984) Carbamazepine levels in breast milk. Ther. Drug Monit. 6, 266–271.
144. Kuhnz, W., Jager-Roman, E., Rating, D., et al. (1983) Carbamazepine and carbamazepine-10,11- epoxide during pregnancy and postnatal period in epileptic mother and their nursed infants: pharmacokinetics and clinical effects. Pediatr. Pharmacol. 3(3–4), 199–208.
145. Philbert, A. and Dam, M. (1982) The epileptic mother and her child. Epilepsia 23, 85–99.
146. Nau, H,. Rating, D., Koch, S., et al. (1981) Valproic acid and its metabolites: placental transfer, neonatal pharmacokinetics, transfer via mother's milk and clini-cal status in neonates of epileptic mothers. J. Pharmacol. Exp. Ther.. 219, 768–777.
147. Niebyl, J. R., Blake, D. A., Freeman, J. M., et al. (1979) Carbamazepine levels in pregnancy and lactation. Obstet. Gynecol. 53, 139–140.
148. Sovner, R. and Orsulak, P. J. (1979) Excretion of imipramine and desipramine in human breast milk. Am. J. Psychiatry 136(4A), 451–452.
159. Alexander, F. W. (1979) Sodium valproate and pregnancy. Arch. Dis. Child. 54, 240.
150. Dickinson, R. G., Harland, R. C., Lynn, R. K., et al. (1979) Transmission of valproic acid (Depakene) across the placenta: half-life of the drug in mother and baby. J. Pediatr. 94, 832–835.
151. Pynnonen, S., Kanto, J., Sillanpaa, M., et al. (1977) Carbamazepine: placental transport, tissue concentrations in foetus and newborn, and level in milk. Acta Pharmacol. Toxicol. 41, 244–253.

152. Skausig, O. B. and Schou, M. (1977) [Breast feeding during lithium therapy. [Danish] Ugeskr. Laeg. 139, 400–401.
153. Sykes, P. A., Quarrie, J., and Alexander, F. W. (1976) Lithium carbonate and breast-feeding. Br. Med. J. 2, 1299.
154. Pynnonen, S. and Sillanpaa, M. (1975) Letter: carbamazepine and mother's milk. Lancet 2(7934), 563.
155. Schou, M. and Amdisen, A. (1973) Lithium and pregnancy. 3. Lithium ingestion by children breast-fed by women on lithium treatment. Br. Med. J. 2, 138.
156. Tunnessen, W. W., Jr. and Hertz, C. G. (1972) Toxic effects of lithium in newborn infants: a commentary. J. Pediatr. 81, 804–807.
157. Fries, H. (1970) Lithium in pregnancy. Lancet 1, 1233.
158. Weinstein, M. R. and Goldfield, M. (1969) Lithium carbonate treatment during pregnancy; report of a case. Dis. Nerv. Syst. 30, 828–832.
159. Ilett, K. F., Hackett, L. P., Kristensen, J. H., et al. (2004) Transfer of risperidone and 9-hydroxyrisperidone into human milk. Ann. Pharmacother. 38, 273–276.
160. Ambresin, G., Berney, P., Schulz, P., et al. (2004) Olanzapine excretion into breast milk: a case report. J. Clin. Psychopharmacol. 24, 93–95.
161. Gardiner, S. J., Kristensen, J. H., Begg, E. J., et al. (2003) Transfer of olanzapine into breast milk, calculation of infant drug dose, and effect on breast-fed infants. Am. J. Psychiatry 160(8), 1428–1431.
162. Tenyi, T., Csabi, G., and Trixler, M. (2000) Antipsychotics and breast-feeding: a review of the literature. Paediatr. Drugs 2, 23–28.
163. Hill, R. C., McIvor, R. J., Wojnar-Horton, R. E., et al. (2000) Risperidone distribution and excretion into human milk: case report and estimated infant exposure during breast-feeding. J. Clin. Psychopharmacol. 20, 285–286.
164. Barnas, C., Bergant, A., Hummer, M., et al. (1994) Clozapine concentrations in maternal and fetal plasma, amniotic fluid, and breast milk. Am. J. Psychiatry 151, 945.
165. Olesen, O. V., Bartels, U., and Poulsen, J. H. (1990) Perphenazine in breast milk and serum. Am. J. Psychiatry 147, 1378–1379.
166. Whalley, L. J., Blain, P. G., and Prime, J. K. (1981) Haloperidol secreted in breast milk. Br. Med. J. Clin. Res. Ed. 282, 1746–1747.
167. Stewart, R. B., Karas, B., and Springer, P. K. (1980) Haloperidol excretion in human milk. Am. J. Psychiatry 137, 849–850.
168. Wiles, D. H., Orr, M. W., and Kolakowska, T. (1978) Chlorpromazine levels in plasma and milk of nursing mothers. Br. J. Clin. Pharmacol. 5, 272–273.
169. Birnbaum, C. S., Cohen, L. S., Bailey, J. W., et al. (1999) Serum concentrations of antidepressants and benzodiazepines in nursing infants: a case series. Pediatrics 104(1), e11.
170. Dusci, L. J., Good, S. M., Hall, R. W., et al. (1990) Excretion of diazepam and its metabolites in human milk during withdrawal from combination high dose diazepam and oxazepam. Br. J. Clin. Pharmacol. 29, 123–126.
171. Patrick, M. J., Tilstone, W. J., and Reavey, P. (1972) Diazepam and breast-feeding. Lancet 1, 542–544.
172. Pons, G., Francoual, C., Guillet P., et al. (1989) Zolpidem excretion in breast milk. Eur. J. Clin. Pharmacol. 37, 245–248.
173. Darwish, M., Martin, P. T., Cevallos, W. H., et al. (1999) Rapid disappearance of zaleplon from breast milk after oral administration to lactating women. J. Clin. Pharmacol. 39, 670–674.
174. Chaudron, L. H. and Jefferson, J. W. (2000) Mood stabilizers during breast-feeding: a review. J. Clin. Psychiatry 61, 79–90.

175. Iqbal, M. M., Gundlapalli, S. P., Ryan, W. G., et al. (2001) Effects of antimanic mood-stabilizing drugs on fetuses, neonates, and nursing infants. South. Med. J. 94, 304–322.

176. Yoshida, K., Smith, B., Craggs, M., et al. (1998) Neuroleptic drugs in breast-milk: a study of pharmacokinetics and of possible adverse effects in breast-fed infants. Psychol. Med. 28, 81–91.

177. Goldstein, D. J., Corbin, L. A., and Fung, M. C. (2000) Olanzapine-exposed pregnancies and lactation: early experience. J. Clin. Psychopharmacol. 20, 399–403.

178. Stowe, Z. N., Hostetter, A. L., Owens, M. J., et al. (2003) The pharmacokinetics of sertraline excretion into human breast milk: determinants of infant serum concentrations. J. Clin. Psychiatry 64, 73–80.

179. Epperson, N., Czarkowski, K. A., Ward-O'Brien, D., et al. (2001) Maternal sertraline treatment and serotonin transport in breast-feeding mother-infant pairs. Am. J. Psychiatry 158, 1631–1637.

180. Wisner, K. L., Perel, J. M., and Blumer, J. (1998) Serum sertraline and N-desmethylsertraline levels in breast-feeding mother-infant pairs. Am. J. Psychiatry 155, 690–692.

181. Kristensen, J. H., Ilett, K. F, Dusci, L. J., et al. (1998) Distribution and excretion of sertraline and N-desmethylsertraline in human milk. Br. J. Clin. Pharmacol. 45, 453–457.

182. Mammen, O. K., Perel, J. M., Rudolph, G., et al. (1997) Sertraline and norsertraline levels in three breastfed infants. J. Clin. Psychiatry 58, 100–103.

183. Altshuler, L. L., Burt, V. K., McMullen, M., et al. (1995) breast-feeding and sertraline: a 24-hour analysis. J. Clin. Psychiatry 56, 243–245.

184. Suri, R., Stowe, Z. N., Hendrick, V., et al. (2002) Estimates of nursing infant daily dose of fluoxetine through breast milk. Biol. Psychiatry 52, 446–451.

185. Kristensen, J. H, Ilett, K. F., Hackett, L. P., et al. (1999) Distribution and excretion of fluoxetine and norfluoxetine in human milk. Br. J. Clin. Pharmacol. 48, 521–527.

186. Yoshida, K., Smith, B., Craggs, M., et al. (1998) Fluoxetine in breast-milk and developmental outcome of breast-fed infants. Br. J. Psychiatry 172, 175–178.

187. Taddio, A., Ito, S., and Koren, G. (1996) Excretion of fluoxetine and its metabolite, norfluoxetine, in human breast milk. J. Clin. Pharmacol. 36, 42–47.

188. Lester, B. M., Cucca, J., Andreozzi, L., et al. (1993) Possible association between fluoxetine hydrochloride and colic in an infant. J. Am. Acad. Child Adolesc. Psychiatry 32, 1253–1255.

189. Burch, K. J. and Wells, B. G. (1992) Fluoxetine/norfluoxetine concentrations in human milk. Pediatrics 89(4 Pt. 1), 676–677.

190. Merlob, P., Mor, N., and Litwin, A. (1992) Transient hepatic dysfunction in an infant of an epileptic mother treated with carbamazepine during pregnancy and breast-feeding. Ann. Pharmacother. 26, 1563–1565.

191. Hendrick, V., Stowe, Z. N., Altshuler, L. L., et al. (2000) Paroxetine use during breast-feeding. J. Clin. Psychopharmacol. 20, 587–589.

192. Begg, E. J., Duffull, S. B., Saunders, D. A., et al. (1999) Paroxetine in human milk. Br. J. Clin. Pharmacol. 48, 142–147.

193. Ohman, R., Hagg, S., Carleborg, L., et al. (1999) Excretion of paroxetine into breast milk. J. Clin. Psychiatry 60, 519–523.

194. Misri, S., Kim, J., Riggs, K.W., et al. (2000) Paroxetine levels in postpartum depressed women, breast milk, and infant serum. J. Clin. Psychiatry 61, 828–832.

195. Spigset, O., Carleborg, L., Norstrom, A., et al. (1996) Paroxetine level in breast milk. J. Clin. Psychiatry 57, 39.

196. Lee, A., Woo, J., and Ito, S. (2004) Frequency of infant adverse events that are associated with citalopram use during breast-feeding. Am. J. Obstet. Gynecol. 190, 218–221.
197. Heikkinen, T., Ekblad, U., Kero, P., et al. (2002) Citalopram in pregnancy and lactation. Clin. Pharmacol Ther. 72, 184–191.
198. Schmidt, K., Olesen, O. V., and Jensen, P. N. (2000) Citalopram and breast-feeding: serum concentration and side effects in the infant. Biol. Psychiatry 47, 164–165.
199. Rampono, J., Kristensen, J. H., Hackett, L. P., et al. (2000) Citalopram and demethylcitalopram in human milk; distribution, excretion and effects in breast fed infants. Br. J. Clin. Pharmacol. 50, 263–268.
200. Jensen, P. N., Olesen, O. V,. Bertelsen, A., et al. (1997) Citalopram and desmethylcitalopram concentrations in breast milk and in serum of mother and infant. Ther. Drug Monit. 19, 236–239.
201. Spigset, O., Carieborg, L., Ohman, R., et al. (1997) Excretion of citalopram in breast milk. Br. J. Clin. Pharmacol. 44, 295–298.
202. Kristensen, J. H., Hackett, L. P., Kohan, R., et al. (2002) The amount of fluvoxamine in milk is unlikely to be a cause of adverse effects in breastfed infants. J. Hum. Lactation 18, 139–143.
203. Piontek, C. M., Wisner, K. L., Perel, J. M., et al. (2001) Serum fluvoxamine levels in breastfed infants. J. Clin. Psychiatry 62, 111–113.
204. Yoshida, K., Smith, B., Craggs, M., et al. (1997) Investigation of pharmacokinetics and of possible adverse effects in infants exposed to tricyclic antidepressants in breast-milk. J. Affect. Disord. 43, 225–237.
205. Wright, S., Dawling, S., and Ashford, J. J. (1991) Excretion of fluvoxamine in breast milk. Br. J. Clin. Pharmacol. 31, 209.
206. Briggs, G. G., Samson, J. H., Ambrose, P. J., et al. (1993) Excretion of bupropion in breast milk. Ann. Pharmacother. 27, 431–433.
206a. Baab, S. W., Peindl, K. S., Piontek, C. M., and Wisner, K. L. (2002) Serum bupropion levels in 2 breastfeeding mother-infant pairs. J. Clin. Psych. 63, 910–911.
206b. Chaudron, L. H. and Schoenecker, C. J. (2004) Bupropion and breastfeeding: A case of a possible infant seizure. J. Clin. Psych. 65, 881–882.
206c. Hendrick, V., Altshuler, L., Wertheimer, A., and Dunn, W. A. (2001) Venlafaxine and breast-feeding. Am. J. Psychiatry 158(12), 2089–2090.
207. Ilett, K. F., Kristensen, J. H., Hackett, L. P., et al. (2002) Distribution of venlafaxine and its O-desmethyl metabolite in human milk and their effects in breastfed infants. Br. J. Clin. Pharmacol. 53, 17–22.
208. Hart, S., Field, T., Jones, N., et al. (1999) Intrusive and withdrawn behaviours of mothers interacting with their infants and boyfriends. J. Child Psychol. Psychiatry Allied Disciplines 40, 239–245.
209. Hammen, C., Burge, D., and Adrian, C. (1991) Timing of mother and child depression in a longitudinal study of children at risk. J. Consult. Clin. Psychol. 59, 341–345.
210. Caplan, H. L., Cogill, S. R., Alexandra, H., et al. (1989) Maternal depression and the emotional development of the child. Br. J. Psychiatry 154, 818–822.
211. Breznitz, Z. and Sherman, T. (1987) Speech patterning of natural discourse of well and depressed mothers and their young children. Child Dev. 58, 395–400.
212. Jones, N. A., Field T., and Davalos, M. (2000) Right frontal EEG asymmetry and lack of empathy in preschool children of depressed mothers. Child Psychiatry Hum. Dev. 30, 189–204.

213. Field, T., Lang, C., Yando, R., et al. (1995) Adolescents' intimacy with parents and friends. Adolescence 30, 133–140.
214. Warner, R., Appleby, L., Whitton, A., et al. (1996) Demographic and obstetric risk factors for postnatal psychiatric morbidity. Br. J. Psychiatry 168, 607–611.
215. O'Hara, M. W., Stuart, S, Gorman, L. L., et al. (2000) Efficacy of interpersonal psychotherapy for postpartum depression. Arch. Gen. Psychiatry 57, 1039–1045.
216. Epperson, C. N., Wisner, K. L., and Yamamoto, B. (1999) Gonadal steroids in the treatment of mood disorders. Psychosom. Med. 61, 676–697.
217. Gregoire, A. J., Kumar, R., Everitt, B., et al. (1996) Transdermal oestrogen fo treatment of severe postnatal depression. Lancet 347, 930–933.
218. Stowe, Z. N., Casarella J., Landry J., et al. (1995) Sertraline in the treatment of women with postpartum major depression. Depression 3, 49–55.
219. Granger, A. C. and Underwood, M. R. (2001) Review of the role of progesterone in the management of postnatal mood disorders. J. Psychosom. Obstet. Gynecol. 22, 49–55.
220. Rabheru, K. (2001) The use of electroconvulsive therapy in special patient populations. Can. J. Psychiatry 46, 710–719.
221. Gruen, D. S. (1993) A group psychotherapy approach to postpartum depression. Int. J. Group Psychother. 43, 191–203.
222. Armstrong, K. L, Van Haeringen, A. R., Dadds, M. R., et al. (1998) Sleep deprivation or postnatal depression in later infancy: separating the chicken from the egg. J. Paediatr. Child Health 34, 260–262.
223. Corral, M., Kuan, A., and Kostaras, D. (2000) Bright light therapy's effect on postpartum depression. Am. J. Psychiatry 157, 303–304.
224. Field, T., Grizzle, N., Scafidi F., et al. (1996) Massage and relaxation therapies' effects on depressed adolescent mothers. Adolescence 31, 903–911.
225. Stamp, G. E.., Williams, A. S., Crowther, C. A. (1995) Evaluation of antenatal and postnatal support to overcome postnatal depression: a randomized, controlled trial. Birth 22, 138–143.
226. Zlotnick, C., Johnson, S. L., Miller, I. W., et al. (2001) Postpartum depression in women receiving public assistance: pilot study of an interpersonal-therapy-oriented group intervention. Am. J. Psychiatry 158, 638–640.
227. Murray, L., Cooper, P., and Hipwell, A. (2003) Mental health of parents caring for infants. Arch. Women's Mental Health 6 (Suppl. 2), S71–77.
228. Wisner, K. L., Perel, J. M., Peindl, K. S., et al. (2004) Timing of depression recurrence in the first year after birth. J. Affect. Disord. 78, 249–252.
229. Wisner, K. L., Perel, J. M., Peindl, K. S., et al. (2001) Prevention of recurrent postpartum depression: a randomized clinical trial. J. Clin. Psychiatry 62, 82–86.
230. Hibbeln, J. R. (2002) Seafood consumption, the DHA content of mothers' milk and prevalence rates of postpartum depression: a cross-national, ecological analysis. J. Affect. Disord. 69(1-3), 15–29.
231. Chaudron, L. H. and Pies, R. W. (2003) The relationship between postpartum psychosis and bipolar disorder: a review. J. Clin. Psychiatry 64, 1284–1292.
232. Burgess, P., Pirkis, J., Morton, J., et al. (2000) Lessons from a comprehensive clinical audit of users of psychiatric services who committed suicide. Psychiatr. Serv. 51, 1555–1560.
233. Nurnberg, H. G. (1989) An overview of somatic treatment of psychosis during pregnancy and postpartum. Gen. Hosp. Psychiatry 11, 328–338.
234. Hamilton, M. (1984) Depression and endogenicity. Acta Psychiatr. Belg. 84, 240–248.

235. Reed, P., Sermin, N., Appleby, L., et al. (1999) A comparison of clinical response to electroconvulsive therapy in puerperal and non-puerperal psychoses. J. Affect. Disord. 54, 255–260.

236. Cohen, L. S., Sichel, D. A., Robertson, L. M., et al. (1995) Postpartum prophylaxis for women with bipolar disorder. Am. J. Psychiatry 152, 1641–1645.

237. Viguera, A. C., Nonacs, R., Cohen, L. S., et al. (2000) Risk of recurrence of bipolar disorder in pregnant and nonpregnant women after discontinuing lithium maintenance. Am. J. Psychiatry 157, 179–184.

4

Treatment of Anxiety Disorders in Pregnancy and the Postpartum

Jonathan S. Abramowitz, Karin Larsen, and Katherine M. Moore

Summary

This chapter begins with a review of the prevalence, assessment, and clinical presentation of anxiety in the perinatal period. Next, we discuss two forms of treatment for anxiety that have been found effective in clinical research: cognitive-behavioral therapy and certain classes of medication. The effectiveness of these treatments with each of the anxiety disorders is discussed, as is the issue of how medication might affect the unborn and breast-feeding infant. Finally, we present a case study of a representative patient with postpartum obsessive-compulsive disorder who was evaluated and treated in our anxiety disorders program.

Key Words: Anxiety; postpartum; pregnancy; cognitive-behavioral therapy; pharmacotherapy.

1. INTRODUCTION

Whereas the perinatal period is an exciting and joyful time for many women as they anticipate the birth of a baby and then bond with the infant, some experience the onset or intensification of severe emotional distress. Much has been written on the prevalence and treatment of depression in the perinatal period, but less is known about the nature and treatment of anxiety disorders during this time. Although early research suggested that women might experience freedom from psychiatric disorders during pregnancy *(1,2)*, more recent evidence suggests that the opposite may in fact be true, especially where anxiety disorders are concerned *(3,4)*. In this chapter, we review the prevalence, assessment,

From: *Current Clinical Practice: Psychiatric Disorders in Pregnancy and the Postpartum: Principles and Treatment*
Edited by: V. Hendrick © Humana Press, Totowa, NJ

and clinical presentation of anxiety in the perinatal period before turning to a discussion of two effective forms of treatment: cognitive-behavioral therapy (CBT) and medication. The chapter concludes with a case study of a patient with postpartum obsessive-compulsive disorder (OCD) who was evaluated and treated in our anxiety disorders program.

2. PREVALENCE OF PERINATAL ANXIETY DISORDERS

The prevalence of perinatal anxiety disorders ranges widely from study to study (8.7–30%) *(5–7)*. One explanation for this diversity is that the screening and diagnostic instruments used in these studies varied in sensitivity. A second reason for the variability in findings is that the studies assessed women at different time points. Recently, Wenzel and colleagues *(8)* conducted a comprehensive investigation of the prevalence of postpartum anxiety disorders. They administered a standardized clinical interview to a community sample of 147 women approx 8 wk after giving birth and found that the most common forms of clinical and subsyndromal postpartum anxiety problems were generalized anxiety disorder (GAD) (19.7%) and social anxiety (15.0%). About half of the women meeting criteria for an anxiety (or depressive) disorder reported a postpartum onset of these symptoms. Moreover, the overall rates of postpartum anxiety disorders were higher than that of postpartum depression (PPD). Interestingly, lower socioeconomic status and poor relationship (e.g., marital) quality were predictive of increased anxiety symptoms. Changing hormone levels occurring in the perinatal period may also influence the prevalence of anxiety disorders during the perinatal period, but the link between hormone levels and psychiatric status requires further investigation *(9)*. Other possible risk factors include personal or family history of an anxiety disorder or a partner who is experiencing a psychiatric disorder *(10)*.

In general, anxiety disorders and depression are highly co-morbid conditions, and this co-morbidity may be common in the perinatal period as well *(5,7,10)*. Based on these findings, Matthey and colleagues *(10)* have suggested that anxiety and depression represent a false distinction and should be subsumed into one diagnostic classification termed "perinatal mood disorder." No matter how one feels about such diagnostic issues, the clinical implications of these findings are clear: pregnant and postpartum women who are diagnosed with an anxiety disorder should also be evaluated for a mood disorder and vice versa.

3. IDENTIFICATION AND ASSESSMENT

Approximately 30% of women will experience an anxiety disorder over the course of their lives, and prenatal visits provide an ideal opportunity for health care providers to assess and treat these disorders *(11)*. Furthermore, during the prenatal and postpartum periods, women may look to their obstetrician as their primary care provider. Therefore, obstetrical visits may be the best opportunity for a provider to assess a woman's psychological well-being. Unfortunately, however, studies suggest that pregnant women do not discuss their emotional difficulties with their health care providers, even when significant levels of anxiety and depression are present *(6,12)*. Recognition of psychiatric morbidity in obstetric clinics may occur in as few as 26% of cases, suggesting that most women requiring psychological services are overlooked and untreated *(12)*.

Despite the failure to actually raise such concerns, research suggests most women are willing to discuss their psychiatric symptomatology with their obstetrician, and that many would agree to see a mental health provider if such a referral was made *(5)*. Nevertheless, problems such as lack of provider time, the assumption that women will spontaneously report any psychological difficulties, and lack of knowledge regarding treatment and/or referral for psychiatric disorders likely hinder the identification of psychological morbidity in perinatal women. The degree to which pregravid anxiety disorder predicts the occurrence of postpartum anxiety is also unknown. In summary, clinicians need to be proactive in asking women about any emotional difficulties and referring them as needed to mental health care providers.

4. PRESENTATION OF ANXIETY DISORDERS IN PREGNANCY AND THE POSTPARTUM

Although the fourth edition of the *Diagnostic and Statistical Manual of Mental Disorders (13)* includes a specifier indicating postpartum onset of a mood disorder, there is no such specifier for the anxiety disorders. As with the mood disorders, diagnosis of an anxiety disorder is made on the basis of the same set of criteria whether it occurs in the perinatal period or some other stage of life. However, it is important to consider the effects of somatic symptoms accompanying pregnancy and the postpartum period (i.e., fatigue, sleep disturbance) when making a diagnosis *(14)*. More is known about perinatal panic disorder, OCD, and posttraumatic stress disorder (PTSD) than the other anxiety disorders.

4.1. Panic Disorder

Panic disorder is diagnosed when women experience unexpected panic attacks characterized by intense fear and the abrupt onset of physical symptoms such as shortness of breath, racing heart, and dizziness.

The diagnostic criteria also include (a) anticipatory worry over the possibility of additional attacks, (b) worry about the consequences of the attack (e.g., "I will die or go crazy"), and (c) change in behavior as a result of the attacks (e.g., avoidance). Agoraphobia may be diagnosed along with panic disorder if there is clinically significant avoidance of situations in which panic attacks are feared (e.g., being home alone, being in crowds).

Because the physiological changes associated with pregnancy may result in occasional tachycardia, sweating, dizziness, and shortness of breath, perinatal women may be at an increased risk for onset or recurrence of panic disorder (1,15). That is, women with panic disorder often misinterpret these normal physiological sensations in catastrophic ways, believing that they are experiencing a significant medical event (e.g., heart attack) or mental health crisis (e.g., "going crazy"). For those with a history of panic attacks, the perinatal period may be a time of increased risk for recurrence, whereas other women may experience a reduction in symptoms during pregnancy and a return of symptoms postpartum (16). One study reported a prevalence rate of 2% for panic disorder during pregnancy (12). Rates of panic disorder in the postpartum period have been reported, ranging from 1.4 to 2.7% (8,10).

4.2. OCD

A number of studies have examined postpartum OCD symptoms. OCD involves (a) unwanted intrusive thoughts, ideas, images, doubts, or impulses that evoke anxiety (obsessions); and (b) urges to neutralize these mental stimuli with some other behavioral or mental act (compulsive rituals). A growing number of studies suggest that the perinatal period is a time of risk for the development or intensification of OCD symptoms (17). Although our own research indicates that more than half of women (and, interestingly, their spouses) experience subclinical obsessional intrusions in the postpartum period (18), the prevalence rate of clinically severe OCD in the postpartum is largely unknown. One recent study reported a postpartum prevalence rate of 2.7% (8).

Often, pregnancy and postpartum-onset obsessions concern the baby's well-being, such as persistent thoughts of the baby dying of sudden infant death syndrome (SIDS) or unwanted impulses to intentionally harm the child (18,19). However, in contrast to women experiencing clinical OCD, those with nonclinical intrusions ("normal obsessions") (20) do not describe their intrusive thoughts as significantly time consuming, distressing, or negatively impacting their functioning (18). Because women with postpartum OCD often experience obsessions that they might harm their baby, they may avoid their infants to reduce their fear of acting on such thoughts. For this reason, their symptoms often impair their ability to care for their infants.

4.2.1. RELATIONSHIP BETWEEN POSTPARTUM OCD AND POSTPARTUM DEPRESSION

There is evidence of a relationship between postpartum depression (PPD) and OCD symptoms, particularly unwanted intrusive thoughts of hurting the newborn (21,22). However, it is not known whether these OCD symptoms represent a cause or an effect of PPD. Given that depression involves unwanted and/or self-destructive thoughts, it is possible that obsessional problems (e.g., unwanted aggressive thoughts) are symptoms of PPD. Alternatively, it is plausible that the presence of unwanted obsessional thoughts is distressing to the point that they give rise to depressive symptoms. Indeed, many individuals with OCD report secondary depressive symptoms (23). Finally, OCD and depression could occur coincidentally, each being the result of a third variable (e.g., biological and psychosocial factors). Our research group is currently conducting a longitudinal study to better clarify this relationship. Results from this investigation will have a bearing on the clinical management of these disorders.

4.2.2. POSTPARTUM OCD VS POSTPARTUM PSYCHOSIS

It is very important to distinguish between the symptoms of OCD in the postpartum and those of postpartum psychosis because either may involve ideation regarding harming the newborn. Fortunately, despite this superficial similarity in thought content, obsessional phenomena are grossly distinct from psychotic symptoms. First, actual hallucinations (e.g., "I saw smoke and fire coming from the baby's nose and ears") and delusions (e.g., "The Devil is out to get the baby"), which characterize postpartum psychosis, are quite rare (24) and not be observed in OCD. Second, postpartum psychosis usually includes other typical psychotic features such as confusion, mood lability, agitation, and other bizarre behaviors as well. Most importantly, the aggressive ideation in psychosis is experienced as consistent with the person's delusional thinking and behavior (ego-syntonic), is not associated with fears or rituals, and is associated with an increased risk of aggressive behavior.

In contrast, postpartum obsessions (even those with violent and horrific content; e.g., the thought to put the baby in the microwave) are not associated with an increased risk of committing harm. This is because obsessional thoughts are experienced as senseless, unwanted, and inconsistent with the person's typical personality or behavior (ego-dystonic). The woman with OCD symptoms recognizes that the intrusive thoughts are contrary to her judgment and reports a fear of engaging in unacceptable behavior (including fears of thinking about it). This is in contrast to delusional thinking, where the person accepts the delusion as true.

Moreover, postpartum OCD patients engage in excessive resistance, avoidance, and ritualizing in attempt to control or suppress their thoughts and ensure that feared consequences do not occur. In short, women with postpartum OCD present with severe anxiety complaints (e.g., worry over whether or not they will harm), as opposed to general psychotic symptoms, such as loss of touch with reality and aggressive, unpredictable behavior.

4.3. PTSD

Individuals who experience intense distress upon being subject to or witnessing a life-threatening event and (a) re-experience the event (e.g., through nightmares or flashbacks), (b) avoid cues eliciting memories of the event, and (c) experience hyperarousal (e.g., irritability, insomnia) are suffering from PTSD. Estimates of PTSD prevalence in pregnant women range widely from 1.7 to 8.1% *(12,25),* based on self-report symptom measures. Researchers interviewing low-income women found that 3.5– 7.7% of pregnant women met the criteria for PTSD *(12,26).* Some evidence suggests that women who experience traumatic labor are at increased risk for developing PTSD *(25,27).* In a prospective study of 289 pregnant women, 8.1% met the criteria for PTSD during pregnancy. When these women were excluded from further analysis, 2.8% of the remaining sample met criteria for PTSD at 6 wk postpartum and 1.5% met these criteria at 6 mo postpartum. This suggests that PTSD can develop as a result of childbirth *(25).*

4.4. GAD

GAD is diagnosed when an individual experiences excessive and uncontrollable worry for more than half the days over a period of 6 mo or longer. These worries may concern a number of life domains, such as work, relationships, health, and finances, and are accompanied by a variety of physical symptoms, such as restlessness, irritability, and muscle tension. Of course, the perinatal period might be further complicated by physical symptoms such as sleep disturbance and muscle aches, as well as by psychosocial stressors such as role changes, neonatal health concerns, and financial issues. Whereas most women manage to cope with these stressors and are able to distract themselves from the concerns mentioned earlier, women suffering from GAD have great difficulty attempting to control their worry and therefore spend significant time and psychological resources devoted to worrying. Very little research has examined GAD in the perinatal period. Wenzel and colleagues *(8)*, in the United States found that 8.2% of postpartum women met diagnostic criteria for GAD. An Australian study found that 1.9–3.1% of postpartum women were experiencing symptoms of generalized anxiety with postpartum onset *(10)*.

4.5. Social Phobia

Individuals with social phobia experience marked distress in social and/or performance situations because they fear being embarrassed or negatively judged by others. When confronted with such situations these individuals either avoid the situation entirely or endure it with intense distress. For individuals with social anxiety the avoidance and/or distress experienced in these situations interferes significantly with their normal occupational or social functioning. Because perinatal women may be avoiding social gatherings for multiple reasons, including health (e.g., secondhand smoke), fatigue, or child care, social phobia should only be diagnosed if the woman reports avoiding social situations due to fear of criticism or embarrassment. The prevalence of social phobia in the perinatal period is largely unknown, but one study reported a prevalence rate of 4.1% in the postpartum period *(8)*.

4.6. Anxiety Problems Associated With Miscarriage

Pregnancy loss may be a risk factor for elevated symptoms of anxiety or the development of an anxiety disorder *(28–30)*. Most studies of women's psychological functioning following miscarriage have focused on depression rather than the anxiety disorders. However, one study compared rates of anxiety disorder in a matched comparison group of community women who had not been pregnant in the past year and a group of women who attended a hospital following a miscarriage *(28)*. Results indicated that women experiencing miscarriage were at a greater risk for a recurrent episode of OCD (relative risk = 8.0), whereas the incidence of panic disorder, phobic disorders, or agoraphobia was not statistically different between groups *(28)*. Studies with larger samples are warranted so that the prevalence of anxiety disorders in this population may be better understood.

5. TREATMENT

5.1. Psychological Treatment

5.1.1. Overview

The psychological treatment of choice for clinical anxiety problems is CBT, and there is no theoretical or practical reason why this choice should not extend to perinatal anxiety problems. CBT is a skills-based approach that is derived from an empirically based conceptual model of anxiety. In contrast to psychodynamic or psychoanalytic psychotherapy, CBT is not concerned with intrapsychic conflicts or uncovering the "root causes" of the patient's problems. In fact, CBT assumes that the causes of anxiety are manifold and cannot be easily determined. As opposed to supportive therapy, which emphasizes giving advice, CBT is a goal-oriented treatment involving the learning of theoretically derived strategies to reverse processes that maintain pathological anxiety. The therapist assumes the role of a teacher or coach, and the patient, the role of student. CBT incorporates "homework assignments" in which the patient practices the necessary skills between treatment sessions. Here we describe the basic theory underlying the use of CBT before turning to the specific treatment procedures used and reviewing the evidence for their efficacy with anxiety disorders.

5.1.2. THEORETICAL RATIONALE FOR CBT

The basic principle of CBT is that emotional responses are caused not by situations *per se*, but by the person's beliefs and interpretations about such situations; moreover, specific emotions are linked to certain types of beliefs and interpretations *(31)*. To illustrate, consider that you have invited a friend to dinner at 6 PM, but it is now 6:45 and there is no sign of your friend. If you think to yourself that your friend isn't coming because he or she doesn't like you anymore, you will feel sad or depressed. Alternatively, if you tell yourself that the person is out of line and inconsiderate because people just should not be late, you will feel anger. If your immediate thought is that the friend has been in a terrible accident, you will feel worried and perhaps call the local police. On the other hand, if you tell yourself that the friend will probably show up shortly with a good story as to why he or she is late, this will not produce any strong negative emotional or behavioral consequences. The implication here is that the same situation, depending on how it is interpreted, can produce different emotions (and behavioral reactions), meaning that beliefs, not situations, cause emotions. Thus, the success of CBT hinges on the understanding that anxiety arises from the belief about the situation rather than from the situation itself. This understanding is critical because, although we cannot control the external world, we can learn to control our thoughts and beliefs about the situations around us—and this is an important assumption in CBT.

As illustrated previously, anxiety is evoked when a person interprets a situation as involving a high probability of threat or harm. Some situations, such as being chased by an assailant, realistically warrant threat-related interpretations. However, individuals with pathological anxiety (i.e., anxiety disorders) habitually misinterpret as threatening situations and stimuli that are not objectively dangerous. For example, those with social phobia misperceive social situations—such as forgetting someone's name in conversation—as highly threatening (e.g., "Other people will think I am stupid."). According to CBT, each anxiety disorder is characterized by a particular erroneous belief or set of beliefs. Table 1 shows the kinds of beliefs that are presumed to underlie the major anxiety disorders.

But if anxiety patients misperceive ostensibly safe situations as threatening, why don't they (like most people) recognize this, correct their beliefs, and stop their pathological fears and anxieties? According to CBT, learned habits termed "safety-seeking behaviors" interfere with the natural correction of mistaken beliefs for people with anxiety disorders. For instance, as shown in Table 1, panic attacks involve the catastrophic misinterpretation of the benign body sensations (e.g., sympathetic arousal) as indicating a serious physical problem such as a heart attack. A common safety behavior for panic patients is to take a benzodiazepine (e.g., Klonopin), which reduces the level of sympathetic arousal. Although this is an understandable response, which indeed works in the short term to reduce the person's distress, the immediate escape from sympathetic arousal has an unfortunate long-term side effect. It prevents the person from learning that these internal sensations are not at all dangerous and that they dissipate over time. Thus, the person comes to believe (erroneously) that he or she narrowly escaped catastrophe (i.e., if I had not taken the Klonopin, I would have had a heart attack, gone crazy, etc.), rather than learn that these sensations are not dangerous. Thus, safety behaviors complete a self-perpetuating vicious cycle that maintains pathological (irrational) anxiety.

5.1.3. TREATMENT PROCEDURES IN CBT

Understanding the cognitive and behavioral factors that underlie anxiety disorders is critical to formulating an effective treatment strategy. It follows from this model that treatment must (a) help patients recognize and modify their anxiety-producing catastrophic beliefs and (b) eliminate barriers to the self-correction of these faulty beliefs. Here, we describe specific CBT procedures recommended for individuals with pregnancy or postpartum anxiety disorders.

5.1.3.1. Proper Medical Evaluation. Before treatment can commence, a thorough review of the patient's medical records and complete medical evaluation is required. The possibility of any co-existing or confounding

Table 1
Characteristic Beliefs and Safety Behaviors Present in Each Anxiety Disorder

Disorder	Feared situation/stimuli	Characteristic erroneous belief(s)	Characteristic safety behavior(s)
Social phobia	Social situations (e.g., public speaking, the opposite sex, authority figures)	"They won't like me." "They'll think I am stupid." "I'll be embarrassed and never get over it."	Avoidance, rehearsal
Panic disorder/ agoraphobia	Normal internal sensations associated with anxiety (e.g., racing heart)	"I'm dying." "I'm going crazy."	Avoidance, sitting down, take pulse, benzodiazepine use
OCD	Intrusive unwanted thoughts, images, and urges (obsessions [e.g., violent urges, thoughts about germs])	"Thoughts are equivalent to actions." "I am responsible for preventing harm."	Compulsive rituals (checking, washing), avoidance, concealment of thoughts
PTSD	Memories of traumatic experiences (e.g., a rape, assault, natural disaster)	"It will probably happen to me again."	Avoidance, keep nearby a "safe person"
Specific phobia	Animals, elevators, thunderstorms, enclosed spaces, etc.	"I'll be bitten." "There will be an accident." "I'll run out of air."	Avoidance
GAD	Health, work situations, disagreement with significant other, etc.	"I'll become ill." "I'll be fired and never find another job." "We'll break up and I'll be alone forever."	Reassurance-seeking

OCD, obsessive-compulsive disorder; PTSD, posttraumatic stress disorder; GAD, generalized anxiety disorder.

organic basis for anxiety-related symptoms must be ruled out. Additionally, because severe depression may interfere with response to CBT, co-morbid mood disorders should be assessed and, if present, pharmacological management considered.

5.1.3.2. Formulation of an Idiosyncratic Model. The initial step in CBT involves the development of a conceptual model of the patient's particular anxiety symptoms that will guide the use of specific therapeutic strategies. This "blueprint," typically developed in collaboration with the patient, diagrams how the patient's beliefs evoke fear and are maintained by maladaptive safety-seeking behaviors. An example of such a model and a treatment plan for one patient seen in our clinic is provided later.

5.1.3.3. Education. Education about the physiology of anxiety is an important component of CBT. For individuals with panic attacks, time is spent reviewing how anxiety is a normal and adaptive reaction to perceived threat that includes behavioral, mental, and physiological responses. For patients with PTSD, education focuses on the normalcy of intrusive memories of traumatic experiences. For those with OCD, education focuses on the universality of unwanted intrusive thoughts (e.g., images of the newborn baby dead in his crib).[*] Patients are also given an introduction to the cognitive-behavioral model of anxiety, including how beliefs influence anxiety and how maladaptive "coping" strategies (i.e., safety-seeking behaviors) maintain erroneous beliefs.

5.1.3.4. Modifying Erroneous Beliefs. The main goal of CBT is to modify patients' erroneous beliefs about danger that lead to pathological anxiety. Most patients make catastrophic overestimates of the probability of harm (e.g., "The baby will probably be born with a birth defect.") and/or overestimates of the severity of harm (e.g., "What if the baby has meningitis!?") A number of procedures may be employed in CBT to help modify patients' exaggerated catastrophic beliefs and assumptions. One method, termed "cognitive restructuring," involves helping the anxious individual identify evidence for and against her catastrophic beliefs. For example, one patient with postpartum-onset panic disorder feared that her unexpected feelings of dizziness meant that she was losing control and "becoming schizophrenic." She noted that when she sat down, the dizziness (and her fear) subsided. The therapist helped this patient to

---

[*]Copies of educational materials provided to patients in our clinic are available by contacting the first author (abramowitz.jonathan@mayo.edu).

understand what this meant by asking, "Would a psychiatrist prescribe frequent sitting for someone with schizophrenia? If sitting would not stop schizophrenia, what role might it play in your symptoms? If the problem was an erroneous belief about what the dizziness really means, would sitting help you?" This patient realized that sitting down merely allowed her to slow her breathing, thereby alleviating her hyperventilation-induced lightheadedness.

5.1.3.5. Exposure and Response Prevention. Crucial to the successful modification of catastrophic beliefs is direct confrontation with situations or stimuli that evoke irrational fear, but that are objectively low risk. In exposure exercises, patients test their predictions as to whether or not, for example, the physical sensations they experience are part of a severe illness or merely symptoms of anxious arousal that dissipate after a brief period of time. For such panic patients, exposure involves confrontation with interoceptive cues. Individuals with postpartum-onset OCD might be helped to test catastrophic beliefs about the meaning of intrusive thoughts. For example, if the patient believes thinking about harming the baby will lead to actually committing harm, an exposure exercise might involve practicing bathing the child while purposely thinking about drowning him or her. Importantly, in order to modify beliefs, the situations or stimuli (e.g., thoughts) that are confronted during exposure must match closely with the patient's actual fears.

During exposure, it is also important for patients to engage in response prevention, which means refraining from performing any safety behaviors that might obstruct the modification of catastrophic beliefs. Thus, the patient with panic described earlier would be instructed to refrain from going to the emergency room, taking a benzodiazepine, or measuring her heart rate. The woman with obsessions would be instructed to stop having her husband nearby "just in case she lost control" and acted on her violent thoughts. Implementing response prevention ensures that the only explanation for the nonoccurrence of feared consequences of exposure is that such consequences are unlikely.

5.1.4. COURSE OF CBT

CBT is a brief, time-limited treatment. In the case of anxiety disorders, therapy typically includes 12–16 weekly treatment sessions. As mentioned previously, therapy sessions are spent learning and implementing skills for modifying beliefs (e.g., exposure, cognitive restructuring). In between sessions, the patient practices these skills. CBT is generally delivered by a trained licensed mental health professional, such as a behaviorally oriented clinical psychologist; although there has been a recent emphasis on training paraprofessionals and those involved in primary care to administer CBT.

5.1.5. EFFECTIVENESS OF CBT

Although the effectiveness of CBT for anxiety disorders is well established *(32)*, few researchers have investigated its efficacy with perinatal women. Nevertheless, researchers from the fields of psychiatry and clinical psychology suggest that CBT be the first line of therapy for pregnant and postpartum women with anxiety disorders *(33–36)*. One of the few studies examining the effects of CBT for anxiety disorders in the perinatal period only included women diagnosed with PPD and a co-morbid anxiety disorder *(37)*. Women were randomly assigned to receive either paroxetine only or the combination of paroxetine and CBT. Following 12 wk of treatment, both groups showed substantial and statistically significant improvement on measures of anxious and depressive symptoms, with 75– 84% of women experiencing a 50% reduction in anxiety symptoms as measured by the Hamilton Rating Scale for Anxiety. No group differences in response to treatment were found, and follow-up data were not reported. These findings suggest that CBT may not provide additional benefit for women who are also receiving pharmacotherapy. However, because no women received a CBT monotherapy intervention, it is unclear whether CBT may have proven more efficacious alone than when combined with medication. In the remainder of this section, we review the literature supporting the use of CBT for the anxiety disorders and direct the reader to resources describing treatment approaches. To our knowledge, there are no contraindications for CBT in perinatal populations, although it has been suggested that psychopharmacological therapy be considered for more severely ill patients *(38)*.

The efficacy of CBT in reducing panic attacks and disorder is one of the most consistent findings across the mental health literature *(32)*. Evidence suggests that as few as 12 sessions of CBT is significantly more effective than wait-list controls as well as credible placebo treatments such as progressive muscle relaxation. Furthermore, some research suggests that combining pharmacotherapy with CBT does not enhance the outcome of CBT and may, in fact, attenuate treatment response *(39–41)*. Importantly, despite its intuitive appeal, progressive muscle relaxation therapy does not provide gains above those found with CBT incorporating the cognitive restructuring and exposure procedures described earlier *(42,43)*.

Research also strongly supports the efficacy of CBT for OCD *(38,44)*. Effective components of this intervention include exposure to obsession-evoking material and abstinence from compulsive rituals or other neutralizing strategies (safety behaviors) performed to reduce anxiety. Exposure-based therapy for OCD is more effective than relaxation *(45)*, anxiety management *(46)*, and the antidepressant clomipramine *(47)*. Because patients with postpartum OCD symptoms often evidence unwanted violent or aggressive obsessional thoughts that are appraised as dangerous and threatening (e.g., "I will act on my bad thoughts"), exposure necessarily involves repeated and prolonged direct confrontation with such thoughts *(48)*. That is, the patient repeatedly evokes the thought (or listens to it verbalized on an audio tape) until the associated distress subsides (i.e., habituates). The cognitive component of CBT for OCD focuses on teaching patients about the normalcy of such thoughts and helping them challenge erroneous appraisals of these intrusions. For example, cognitive therapy for a woman who repeats prayers to ensure that her infant will not die of SIDS might address the statistical probability that thinking this thought will cause this event to occur.

Social anxiety also responds well to treatments that include cognitive restructuring and exposure, and these interventions are more efficacious than no treatment or nonspecific therapies *(39)*. Some evidence suggests that group therapy for social anxiety, a format that provides access to other patients for role-play and models for learning intervention strategies, is effective; however, whether it is more effective than individual treatment is unclear *(49)*. At present, no studies of interventions developed specifically for women experiencing social anxiety in the perinatal period have been conducted. However, during this period women may experience increased attention from others, for example, when their pregnancy is quite evident or when they are with their infant. For a woman with social phobia, this increased notice may be negatively interpreted. Thus, cognitive therapy might include challenging the woman's perception that others evaluate her condition in a negative manner or are overly concerned with her appearance or behavior in general.

Women diagnosed with PTSD often benefit from interventions including stress inoculation training as well as traditional CBT. Stress inoculation includes cognitive techniques ("thought-stopping," challenging negative self-cognitions) as well as relaxation techniques, modeling, and role-playing. Some research supports the efficacy of stress inoculation training in reducing PTSD symptoms *(50)*. Exposure for PTSD involves gradual confrontation with traumatic memories for the purposes of reducing cognitive avoidance of these memories and of environmental stimuli (e.g., pictures, places) that evoke such memories *(51)*. Because no research has addressed the treatment of PTSD in perinatal women, the efficacy of these interventions within this population remains unknown.

The effective components of CBT for GAD are less clear than for the other anxiety disorders. Cognitive therapy that focuses on teaching strategies to identify worries, identify potential solutions, and test these solutions appears to offer more improvement than nondirective therapies or psychodynamic therapies. Arousal-reduction techniques, including relaxation techniques, may not offer substantial long-term benefit *(39)*.

5.1.6. PROS AND CONS OF CBT

The treatment for anxiety disorders during the perinatal period must accomplish two goals: maintain the emotional stability of the mother and minimize the risks to the fetus or newborn. It is important for the clinician to weigh the pros and cons of various treatment approaches and to discuss these with the patient. The most important advantage of a CBT approach is the demonstrated effectiveness of this form of treatment over a relatively brief period of time, as discussed earlier. Moreover, CBT has durable effects. Research indicates that patients often maintain their improvement up to several years after the end of formal therapy. This is likely because CBT involves learning and perfecting the use of skills. In essence, the patient learns to become his or her own therapist and develops the ability to manage similar fears that might arise after the completion of treatment.

Of course, CBT also has its disadvantages. One consideration is that whereas medication treatment requires little effort, CBT demands a firm commitment from the patient. The patient must attend regular treatment sessions and complete "homework assignments" between visits. A second disadvantage of this approach is that, in most cases, the patient must confront the very situations that evoke his or her anxiety—situations he or she has been taking great pains to avoid. Importantly, the anxiety that is evoked during exposure is temporary, and the therapist works collaboratively with the patient to minimize his or her distress (e.g., by using a graded approach). However, CBT involves "investing anxiety now in a calmer future." A final disadvantage of CBT is that it might be difficult to find. At present, knowledgeable treatment providers who are trained to deliver this kind of therapy are somewhat few and far between. Excellent resources for clinicians seeking to refer patients for CBT include the Anxiety Disorders Association of America, the Obsessive Compulsive Foundation, and the Association for Behavioral and Cognitive Therapies (formerly Association for the Advancement of Behavior Therapy). These organizations have websites with helpful links for locating therapists.

5.2. Pharmacotherapy

The literature on the pharmacological treatment of anxiety disorders occurring in pregnancy and the postpartum is very limited; what is available focuses on treatments of panic disorder and OCD. A larger body of literature has developed on the treatment of depression during pregnancy and in the puerperium. It is from this work that most of the available information regarding the use of antidepressant medication of the selective serotonin reuptake inhibitor (SSRI) type in the perinatal period is gleaned. Because this class of medications is easy to administer and carries a low risk of toxicity in overdose, the SSRIs are recommended as first-line pharmacological treatments for PPD *(52)*, as well as for postpartum panic disorder and OCD *(53)*.

Nevertheless, the decision to use psychotropic medications during pregnancy should be approached on an individual basis, with discussion between the patient, her partner (if appropriate) and her health care provider. Given the beneficial effects of CBT for anxiety described above, psychological treatment should be recommended as the first-line approach. If pharmacotherapy is considered, the relative risks and benefits associated with it must be weighed and discussed openly and carefully with the patient. Treatment should be reserved for those cases in which the risks to the mother and fetus from the disorder are felt to exceed the risk of medication usage. General guidelines for treatment include using the lowest effective dose of medication and avoiding exposure during the first trimester of pregnancy (again, strongly considering nonpharmacological interventions), if possible.

A growing controversy is the possibility of perinatal syndromes related to SSRI use during the third trimester of pregnancy. In Summer 2004, based on the recommendation of the Pediatric Advisory Subcommittee of the US Food and Drug Administration (FDA), the FDA opted to instruct the makers of the SSRI and selective norepinephrine reuptake inhibitor (SNRI) antidepressants to place warnings on the package inserts describing the possible occurrence of neurobehavioral symptoms in neonates exposed to these medications late in the third trimester and through labor and delivery. Troublesome symptoms have included feeding difficulties, agitation, irritability, sleep disturbance, respiratory distress, cyanosis, apnea, seizures, hypertonia, hyperflexia, and tremor. It is not clear at this time whether these symptoms represent a type of withdrawal reaction or serotonin overstimulation. The subcommittee also recommended changes to the dosage and administration section of the drug label advising physicians to consider taper and discontinuation of these agents prior to labor and delivery. This has significant implications for women being treated for mood and anxiety disorders, as the postpartum period has been identified as a time of increased vulnerability to the recurrence of these problems. If an agent is tapered around the time of labor and delivery, strong consideration should be given to reinstituting it immediately after delivery.

Here we consider some issues in the pharmacological treatment of panic disorder and OCD during pregnancy and the postpartum.

5.2.1. PANIC DISORDER

If conception is planned, the preferred approach to pharmacotherapy for panic disorder is to taper the medication slowly as soon as possible (54). The use of concomitant CBT may assist patients in discontinuing their medications or increasing the interval of wellness prior to relapse (55). If the taper is unsuccessful, resumption of the medication regimen may be indicated. The use of SSRIs or tricyclic antidepressants (TCAs) would be preferable over that of benzodiazepines because first-trimester benzodiazepine exposure has been associated with an increased risk of oral clefts relative to that in the general population (56). For patients on anxiolytic medications who present with unplanned pregnancies, abrupt discontinuation is generally not recommended.

As discussed previously, the course of panic disorder during pregnancy is variable. A retrospective evaluation by Cohen et al. (57) suggested that some women experience an amelioration of anxiety symptoms when pregnant. The clinical course of 49 women with pregravid panic disorder was evaluated over three trimesters of pregnancy. Within this sample, 17 women had attempted discontinuation of their panic medication prior to pregnancy, and 9 of those experienced a return of symptoms on discontinuation. Of the nine failures, six tried again to discontinue after their pregnancy was confirmed. At that point, three of these six women remained off medication treatment during the remainder of pregnancy. This indicates that although some women are able to discontinue medication during pregnancy, others are not.

5.2.2. OCD

The SSRIs are the mainstay of pharmacological treatment for OCD. Although TCAs, particularly clomipramine, are additional options, drawbacks of these agents include their potential to aggravate orthostatic hypotension and their association with neonatal seizures (58). However, clomipramine use in pregnant women with severe OCD is not absolutely contraindicated. Misri and Mills (59) reported a small, open-label trial of the novel antipsychotic agent quetiapine as augmentation of SSRIs or

SNRIs in treatment-resistant postpartum OCD patients. Of the 17 patients who received quetiapine augmentation, 14 completed the 12-wk trial and only 3 withdrew early as a result of side effects (sedation was the most commonly described side effect). Of the completer sample, 11 showed a clinically meaningful response (mean improvement of 59.6% on the Yale-Brown Obsessive Compulsive Scale) with a mean dose of 112.5 mg/d.

5.2.3. PHARMACOTHERAPY AND BREAST-FEEDING

A major consideration regarding the use of pharmacological agents in the puerperium includes whether the woman will be breast-feeding. A more detailed discussion of the use of specific medications in this case is undertaken later.

For nonlactating women, standard treatment approaches may be utilized *(60)*. For women with a past history of anxiety disorder, medication may have been stopped prior to conception or during pregnancy, and it is important to for these women to be reassessed at their obstetrical follow-up visits for any emerging signs and symptoms of anxiety in the postpartum period. Regimens that were previously beneficial should be restarted if symptoms are present in the nonlactating patient.

There are recognized benefits to breast-feeding, and the American Academy of Pediatrics recommends breast-feeding as an exclusive source of nutrition for infants up through the first year of life. However, breast-feeding also complicates the decision as to whether to use psychotropic medication. All psychotropic agents are secreted into the breast milk. Data regarding plasma drug concentrations in breast-fed infants are limited, as is any information regarding potential long-term adverse neurobehavioral effects on the baby from medication exposure. These unknowns have to be weighed against the potential negative effects that untreated anxiety may have on both the mother's and infant's health. Each case should be considered individually. There are no controlled studies on the safety of psychotropic medications in nursing mothers. Treatment guidelines regarding the use of psychotropic medication in breast-feeding women are based on case reports and small case series. In a comprehensive review of psychotropic medication use during breast-feeding, Burt et al. *(61)* recommend that the baseline clinical status of the infant be reviewed and that the child's pediatrician be educated about the potential side effects of medication exposure and interactions with other medications typically used in the infant population. Whereas obtaining infant drug levels is not recommended (the association between these values and clinical status is unclear), ongoing clinical monitoring of the infant is advised.

Although specific data regarding the treatment of postpartum anxiety disorders in lactating women are very sparse, SSRIs can be considered the first-line agents on the basis of their safety and efficacy in nongravid populations *(60)*. Weissman et al. *(62)* conducted a pooled analysis of antidepressant levels in nursing mothers, breast milk, and nursing infants. They reported that breast-feeding infants exposed to nortriptyline, paroxetine, or sertraline appeared unlikely to develop detectable or elevated plasma levels. On the other hand, infants exposed to fluoxetine or citalopram appeared to be at higher risk of developing elevated levels. Fluoxetine produced the highest proportion (22%) of elevated infant levels. This may be particularly true if there has been prenatal exposure. Citalopram produced elevated levels in 17% of infants. However, more data are clearly needed before firm conclusions can be reached. For instance, plasma levels may provide limited information in terms of what the specific biochemical effects of an antidepressant are on an infant's developing brain. Accordingly, Weissman et al. *(62)* do not recommend clinical monitoring of maternal plasma or breast milk anti-depressant levels as a means of estimating infant plasma levels.

Benzodiazepines are frequently prescribed for anxiety symptoms in the general population. It has been suggested that occasional low doses of short-acting benzodiazepines (i.e., oxazepam or temazepam) are likely safe in breast-feeding *(63)*. Given reports of adverse effects with diaz-epam and withdrawal related to alprazolam use, these agents are not recommended as first-line benzodiazepine choices *(61)*.

6. CONCLUSION

Recognition of anxiety disorders during pregnancy and the postpar-tum period is extremely important because symptoms may affect not only the mother, but also the infant and the mother–infant relationship. Clinicians should therefore assume an active role in assessing for symp-toms in their pregnant and postpartum patients. There are effective treat-ments for anxiety disorders, and this fact should be communicated to patients. CBT is an attractive option because of its substantial benefits, limited duration, the lack of any drug exposure to a fetus or infant, and its durability of effect.

Nevertheless, CBT is not always easy to find and also requires sub-stantial time and energy from the patient. Pharmacotherapy, primarily in the form of SSRIs, has been shown to be useful in the treatment of anxiety disorders in the general population as well as in pregnant and postpartum women. The widespread availability and ease of administra-tion make SSRIs an appealing option. Pharmacological intervention certainly may be indicated in cases of more severe anxiety and should be considered for patients who are not interested in CBT and/or who may not be able to access a quality provider.

However, much remains unknown regarding the effects of SSRIs on the fetus and breast-feeding baby. Accordingly, each case should be approached on an individualized basis, assessing the severity of symptoms, obtaining past history and response to any previous treatments (if any), understanding the patient's preferences, and educating the patient about the potential benefits and potential risks of each treatment.

7. CASE REPORT

Jen, a 27-yr-old elementary school teacher, had given birth to her son Alex less than 3 mo previously. Although she had no previous psychiatric history, she informed her child's pediatrician that she now was feeling depressed most of the day and sometimes felt afraid of interacting with Alex. The pediatrician briefly described the pros and cons of medication and psychological treatment for anxiety and depression before referring Jen to our anxiety disorders clinic for evaluation. At her initial assessment, Jen described recurrent unwanted thoughts of harming Alex, including the idea that she could suffocate him, put him in the microwave, or stab him with a knife. These intrusive thoughts were unacceptable to Jen, who considered herself a "gentle person" and reported no history or intent of violent behavior. Jen was spending inordinate amounts of time praying for these thoughts to go away and was avoiding being alone with her infant. These rituals and her avoidance of being alone with Alex for fear of "losing control" were interfering with her family functioning as well as her relationship with her newborn.

Jen was breast-feeding and told our evaluation team that she would prefer to begin CBT rather than use medication. During the first therapy session, Jen's therapist assessed Jen's intrusive thoughts, inquiring about (a) the content of the thoughts and stimuli that triggered them, (b) her interpretations of the unwanted thoughts, and (c) her responses to them. Jen reported that she believed the thoughts meant that she was "evil at heart" and that their presence was a sign that she might act on them at any moment. She believed she had to take precautions, such as having others nearby to stop her if she lost control. When the thoughts came to mind, Jen repeated certain prayers in sets of three, which she believed kept her from acting out her violent thoughts. She had also been concealing the content and frequency of her obsessions from others (including her husband) for fear that they would think she was an "evil monster." Because Jen's mood symptoms began only after she had been experiencing obsessions, her depression was conceptualized as secondary to the OCD symptoms. The hypothesis was made that successful treatment of her obsessions would lead to reduced mood symptoms.

Psychoeducation began after the assessment and case formulation was complete. The therapist normalized the experience of intrusive "bad" thoughts by teaching Jen that practically everyone, from time to time, experiences ideas, images, or impulses that are upsetting or inconsistent with their personality. The therapist even gave examples of his own unwanted thoughts. Jen had never considered that others had similar experiences and was somewhat relieved to find this out. The therapist discussed how Jen's concealment of her thoughts, although understandable given Jen's beliefs about the thoughts, prevented her from finding out how common such experiences are. Jen was helped to see that her mistaken *appraisals* of these thoughts as dangerous, immoral, and needing to be controlled were the real problem. Normal intrusions can escalate into obsessions if they are misappraised as dangerous. By trying to suppress and control these thoughts, Jen was making herself even more scared and preoccupied, which accounts for their persistence and development of a "life of their own."

Jen was also taught that she was very unlikely to act on her unwanted thoughts if she didn't *wish* to act on them. A discussion of the relationship between thoughts and actions was followed by an experiment in which Jen was asked to hold a paperweight from the therapist's desk. The therapist turned his back and then asked Jen to vividly imagine throwing this object at the therapist. Of course, Jen did not throw the paperweight, even after visualizing this action for several minutes in different ways. The results of this experiment (i.e., thoughts themselves don't lead to actions) were discussed in terms of the probability that Jen would act on thoughts to harm Alex (which was deemed to be acceptably low).

Although Jen found herself feeling less distressed over her intrusive thoughts, the intrusions still evoked moderate levels of anxiety, and Jen was still fearful of having the thoughts while she was with Alex. Moreover, she continued to use prayer rituals to reduce her fears of disastrous consequences. Thus, the therapist introduced the techniques of *exposure* and *response prevention* as a way of weakening Jen's pattern of becoming anxious when such thoughts arose and of using rituals to reduce her anxiety. After providing a rationale for purposely confronting her unwanted thoughts without engaging in any prayer rituals, Jen and the therapist constructed a hierarchy consisting of situations for Jen to practice both in-session and at home (Table 2). Jen agreed to practice the situations without saying the prayers. She realized that she needed to

Table 2
Jen's Exposure Therapy Hierarchy

Situation	Anxiety level (%)
1. Think about stabbing Alex	40
2. Think about stabbing Alex while holding a knife with Alex nearby	50
3. Think about putting Alex in the microwave	55
4. Hold Alex in the kitchen while thinking about putting him in the microwave	65
5. Think about suffocating Alex	65
6. Watch Alex sleeping, hold a pillow, and think about suffocating him	75

prove to herself that these thoughts were not indicative of danger and that her prayers were not actually keeping her from acting.

During the first exposure session, Jen and the therapist collaboratively created a tape-recorded scenario of Jen's intrusive thought about stabbing Alex. The scenario was as follows:

You've just started cutting the vegetables and you see little Alex lying on the floor on his blanket. He's cooing and very content. Then you have the idea that you could easily stab him to death with the knife you are using. He is so small and defenseless. He wouldn't be able to stop you. Then you feel yourself trying to push those thoughts away — but you can't. They keep coming back to mind. You feel the urge growing stronger and stronger. You want to say the prayers, but you know you are not supposed to because of the therapy instructions. So, you refrain from praying. But then you feel yourself going over to Alex and you begin stabbing him over and over. There is blood everywhere. What are you doing . . . this is your own son! Alex is crying, but then he goes limp as he dies on the blanket. You can't believe what you've just done. What will your husband say? If only you had said those prayers. Now, Alex is dead.

Jen practiced listening to the scenario on a loop-tape in the session. The therapist kept track of Jen's anxiety level on a scale from 0 (*none*) to 100 (*extreme*). As the exposure began, Jen's anxiety reached 75%, but after 15 min of listening to the loop-tape, it decreased to 40%. After another 10 min the tape evoked mild anxiety (25%). Next, Alex (who had been in the waiting room with his father) was brought into the office and Jen retrieved a large knife that she had brought from home. Alex was placed on the floor next to Jen, and Jen practiced holding the knife while listening to the tape. At first, Jen felt uncomfortable, but after about 15 min her distress subsided even while she held the knife. She reported also refraining from any prayer rituals. Then, after obtaining Jen's permission, the therapist left Jen and Alex alone in the office. Again, Jen's distress level temporarily increased, but soon decreased (after about 10 min) as she realized that she was unlikely to act on the upsetting thoughts. Jen felt very good about completing the exercise and was instructed to practice the same tasks once each day between sessions.

Over the course of the next month, Jen practiced similar exposure exercises and practiced refraining from rituals and avoidance strategies. This was extremely helpful. After only 2 mo of treatment (eight therapy sessions), Jen no longer avoided being alone with Alex, and her prayer rituals were reduced substantially. Although Jen still experienced occasional unwanted intrusive violent thoughts, these thoughts no longer produced anxiety. Jen reported "knowing in her gut" that she didn't have to worry about these experiences. Her depressive symptoms had also abated, and she reported being much happier about being a new mother. For the next 3 mo, the therapist saw Jen on a monthly basis for follow-up sessions. Jen continued to remain improved through this time, and treatment was therefore terminated.

REFERENCES

1. Cowley, D. S. and Roy-Byrne, P. P. (1989) Panic disorder during pregnancy. J. Psychosom. Obstet. Gynaecol. 10, 193–210.
2. Elliot, S. A., Rugg, A. J., Watson, J. P., and Brough, D. I. (1983) Mood changes during pregnancy and after the birth of a child. Br. J. Psychiatry 22, 295–308.
3. Altshuler, L. L., Hendrick, V., and Cohen, L. S. (1998) Course of mood and anxiety disorders during pregnancy and the postpartum period. J. Clin. Psychiatry 59 (Suppl. 2), 29–33.
4. Shear, K. M. and Mammen, O. (1995) Anxiety disorders in pregnant and postpartum omen. Psychopharmacol. Bull. 31, 693–703.
5. Birndorf, C. A., Madden, A., Portera, L., et al. (2001) Psychiatric symptoms, functional impairment, and receptivity toward mental health treatment among obstetrical patients. Int. J. Psychiatry Med. 31, 355–365.
6. Kelly, R. H., Zatzick, D. F., and Anders, T. F. (2001) The detection and treatment of psychiatric disorders and substance use among pregnant women cared for in obstetrics. Am. J. Psychiatry 158, 213–219.
7. Stuart, S., Couser, G., Schilder, K., et al. (1998) Postpartum anxiety and depression: Onset and comorbidity in a community sample. J. Nerv. Ment. Dis. 186, 420–424.
8. Wenzel, A., Haugen, E. N., Jackson, L. C., and Brendle, J. R. (2005) Anxiety symptoms and disorders at eight weeks postpartum. J. Anxiety Disord. 19, 295–311.
9. Rapkin, A. J., Mikacich, J. A., Moatakef-Imani, B., and Rasgon, N. (2002) The clinical nature and formal diagnosis of premenstrual, postpartum, and perimenopausal affective disorders. Curr. Psychiatry Rep. 4, 419–428.

10. Matthey, S., Barnett, B., Howie, P., and Kavanagh, D. J. (2003) Diagnosing post-partum depression in mothers and fathers: Whatever happened to anxiety? J. Affect. Disord. 74, 139–147.
11. Kessler, R. C., McGonagle, K. A., Zhao, S., et al. (1994) Lifetime and 12-month prevalence of DSM-III-R psychiatric disorders in the United States: results from the National Comorbidity Survey. Arch. Gen. Psychiatry 51, 8–19.
12. Smith, M. V., Rosehheck, R. A., Cavaleri, M. A., et al. (2004) Screening for and detection of depression, panic disorder, and PTSD in public-sector obstetrics clinics. Psychiatr. Serv. 55, 407–414.
13. American Psychiatric Association. (1994) Diagnostic and Statistical Manual of Mental Disorders, 4th ed., rev. Washington, DC: American Psychiatric Association.
14. Salamero, M., Marcos, T., Gutierrez, F., and Rebull, E. (1994) Factorial study of the BDI in pregnant women. Psychol. Med. 24, 1031–1035.
15. Wisner, K. L., Peindl, K. S., and Hanusa, B. H. (1996) Effects of childbearing on the natural history of panic disorder with comorbid mood disorder. J. Affect. Disord. 41, 173–180.
16. Levine, R. E., Oandasan, A. P., Primeau, L. A., and Berenson, A. B. (2003) Anxiety disorders during pregnancy and postpartum. Am. J. Perinatol. 20, 239–248.
17. Abramowitz, J. S., Schwartz, S. A., Moore, K. M., and Luenzmann, K. R. (2003) Obsessive-compulsive symptoms in pregnancy and the puerperium: a review of the literature. J. Anxiety Disord. 17, 461–478.
18. Abramowitz, J. S., Schwartz, S. A., and Moore, K. M. (2003) Obsessional thoughts in postpartum females and their partners: content, severity and relationship with depression. J. Clin. Psychol. Med. Settings 10, 157–164.
19. Sichel, D. A., Cohen, L. S., Dimmock, J. A., et al. (1993) Postpartum obsessive compulsive disorder: a case series. J. Clin. Psychiatry 54, 156–159.
20. Rachman, S. J. and de Silva, P. (1978) Abnormal and normal obsessions. Behav. Res. Ther. 16, 233–238.
21. Jennings, K. D., Ross, S., Pepper, S., et al. (1999) Thoughts of harming infants in depressed and nondepressed mothers. J. Affect. Disord. 54, 21–28.
22. Wisner, K. L., Peindl, K. S., Gigliotti, T., et al. (1999) Obsessions and compulsions in women with postpartum depression. J. Clin. Psychiatry 60, 176–180.
23. Ricciardi, J. N. and McNally, R., J. (1995) Depressed mood is related to obsessions but not compulsions in obsessive-compulsive disorder. J. Anxiety Disord. 9, 249–256.
24. Suri, R. and Burt, V. (1997) The assessment and treatment of postpartum psychiatric disorders. J. Pract. Psychiatry Behav. Health 3, 67–77.
25. Ayers, S. and Pickering, A. D. (2001) Do women get posttraumatic stress disorder as a result of childbirth? A prospective study of incidence. Birth 28, 111–118.
26. Cook, C. A. L., Flick, L. H., Homan, S. M., et al. (2004) Posttraumatic stress disorder in pregnancy: prevalence, risk factors and treatment. Obstet. Gynecol. 103, 710–717.
27. Ballard, C. G., Stanley, A. K., and Brockington, I. F. (1995) Post-traumatic stress disorder (PTSD) after childbirth. Br. J. Psychiatry 166, 525–528.
28. Geller, P. A., Klier, C. M., and Neugebauer, R. (2001) Anxiety disorders following miscarriage. J. Clin. Psychiatry 62, 432–438.
29. Frost, M., and Condon, J. T. (1996) The psychological sequelae of miscarriage: a critical review of the literature. Aust. NZ J. Psychiatry 30, 54–62.
30. Geller, P. A., Kerns, D., and Klier, C. M. (2004) Anxiety following miscarriage and the subsequent pregnancy: a review of the literature and future directions. J. Psychosom. Res. 56, 35–45.

31. Beck, A. T. (1976) Cognitive Therapy of the Emotional Disorders. New York: International Universities Press.

32. Barlow, D. H. (2002) Anxiety and Its Disorders. New York: Guilford.

33. Shear, K. and Mammen, O. (1995) Anxiety disorders in pregnant and postpartum women. Psychopharmacol. Bull. 31, 693–703.

34. Brown, C. S. (2001) Depression and anxiety disorders. Obstet. Gynecol. Clin. North Am. 28, 241–268.

35. Weisberg, R. B. and Paquette, J. A. (2002) Screening and treatment of anxiety disorders in pregnant and lactating women. Women's Health Issues 12, 32–36.

36. McGrath, C., Buist, A., and Norman, T. R. (1999) Treatment of anxiety during pregnancy: effects of psychotropic drug treatment on the developing fetus. Drug Safety 20, 171–186.

37. Misri, S., Reebye, P., Corral, M., et al. (2004) The use of paroxetine and cognitive-behavioral therapy in postpartum depression and anxiety: a randomized controlled trial. J. Clin. Psychiatry 65, 1236–1241.

38. Burt, V. K. and Hendrick, V. C. (2005) Clinical Manual of Women's Mental Health. Washington, DC: American Psychiatric Publishing Inc.

39. Barlow, D. H., Raffa, S. D., and Cohen, E. M. (2002) Psychosocial treatments for panic disorders, phobias, and generalized anxiety disorder. In: Nathan, P. E. and Gorman, J. M., eds. A Guide to Treatments That Work, 2nd ed., New York: Oxford University Press, pp. 301–335.

40. Foa, E. B., Franklin, M. E., and Moser, J. (2002) Context in the clinic: how well do cognitive-behavioral therapies and medications work in combination? Biol. Psychiatry 52, 987–997.

41. Westra, H. and Stewart, S. (1998) Cognitive behavioural therapy and pharmaco-therapy: Complementary or contradictory approaches to the treatment of anxiety? Clin. Psychol. Rev. 18, 307–340.

42. Craske, M. G., Brown, T. A., and Barlow, D. H. (1991) Behavioral treatment of panic disorder: a two-year follow-up. Behav. Ther. 22, 289–304.

43. Beck, J. G., Stanley, M. A., Baldwin, L. E., et al. (1994) Comparison of cognitive therapy and relaxation training for panic disorder. J. Consult. Clin. Psychol. 62, 818–826.

44. Abramowitz, J. S. (1996) Variants of exposure and response prevention in the treatment of obsessive compulsive disorder: a meta-analysis. Behav. Ther. 27, 583–600.

45. Fals-Stewart, W., Marks, A. P., and Schafer, J. (1993) A comparison of behavioral group therapy and individual behavior therapy in treating obsessive-compulsive disorder. J. Nerv. Ment. Dis. 181, 189–193.

46. Lindsay, M., Crino, R., and Andrews, G. (1997) Controlled trial of exposure and response prevention in obsessive-compulsive disorder. Br. J. Psychiatry 171, 135–139.

47. Foa, E. B., Liebowitz, M. R., Kozak, M. J., et al. (2005) Treatment of obsessive-compulsive disorder by exposure and ritual prevention, clomipramine, and their combination: a randomized, placebo controlled trial. Am. J. Psychiatry. 162, 151–161.

48. Freeston, M. H. and Ladouceur, R. (1999) Exposure and response prevention for obsessive thoughts. Cogn. Behav. Pract. 6, 362–383.

49. Turk, C. L., Heimberg, R. G., and Hope, D. A. (2001) Social anxiety disorder. In: Barlow D. E., ed., Clinical Handbook of Psychological Disorders: A Step-by-Step Treatment Manual, 3rd ed. New York: Guilford Press, pp.114–153.

50. Resick, P. A. and Calhoun, K. S. (2001) Posttraumatic stress disorder. In: Barlow, D. E., ed. Clinical Handbook of Psychological Disorders: A Step-by-Step Treatment Manual, 3rd ed. New York: Guilford Press, pp. 60–113.
51. Foa, E., Keane, T., and Friedman, M., eds. (1999) Effective Treatments for PTSD. New York: Guilford.
52. Wisner, K. L., Parry, B. L., and Pointek, C. M. (2002) Postpartum depression. N. Engl. J. Med. 347, 194–199.
53. Boerner, R. and Moeller, H. (1999) The importance of new antidepressants in the treatment of anxiety and depressive disorders. Pharmacopsychiatry 32, 119–126.
54. Cohen, L. S. and Rosenbaum, J. F. (1998) Psychotropic drug use during pregnancy: weighing the risks. J. Clin. Psychiatry 59(Suppl. 2), 18–28.
55. Robinson, L., Walker, J., and Anderson, D. (1992) Cognitive-behavioral treatment of panic disorder during pregnancy and lactation. Can. J. Psychiatry 37, 623–626.
56. Altshuler, L., Cohen, L., Szuba, M., et al. (1996) Pharmacologic management of psychiatric illness in pregnancy: dilemmas and guidelines. Am. J. Psychiatry 153, 592–606.
57. Cohen, L., Sichel, D., Dimmock, J., et al. (1994) Postpartum course in women with preesisting panic disorder. J. Clin. Psychiatry 55, 289–292.
58. Cowe, L., Lloyd, D., and Dawling, S. (1982) Neonatal convulsions caused by withdrawal from maternal clomipramine. Br. Med. J. 284, 1837–1838.
59. Misri, S. and Mills, L. (2004) Obsessive-compulsive disorder in the postpartum: open label trial of quetiapine augmentation. J. Clin. Psychopharmacol. 24, 624–627.
60. Shear, K. M. and Mammen, O. (1995) Anxiety disorders in pregnant and postpartum women. Psychopharmacol. Bull. 31, 693–704.
61. Burt, V., Suri, R., Altshuler, L., et al. (2001) The use of psychotropic medications during breast-feeding. Am. J. Psychiatry 158, 1001–1009.
62. Weissman, A. M., Levy, B., Hartz, A., et al. (2004) Pooled analysis of antidepressant levels in lactating mothers, breast milk, and nursing infants. Am. J. Psychiatry 161, 1066–1078.
63. American Academy of Pediatrics Committee on Drugs. (1989) Transfer of drugs and other chemicals into human milk. Pediatrics 84, 924–936.

5

Bipolar Disorder

*Special Issues in Pregnancy
and the Postpartum*

Lori L. Altshuler and Carol Kiriakos

Summary

This chapter reviews knowledge regarding the management of bipolar illness during pregnancy and in the postpartum (lactation) period. The natural
course of bipolar illness during pregnancy and postpartum is discussed. Additionally, the chapter reviews information on the effects of medication exposure
in utero and during lactation on the fetus and infant. General guidelines about
treating bipolar disorder are given.

Key Words: Bipolar; pregnancy; postpartum; mood stabilizer; anticonvulsant.

1. INTRODUCTION

Bipolar disorder affects 0.5–1.5% of individuals in the United States,
and women and men are affected equally. The age of onset for bipolar
disorder is typically in the early 20s. Thus, the onset of bipolar illness
coincides with the active reproductive life of many women.

Pregnancy is generally considered to be a time of emotional well-being.
However, very little is known about the impact of pregnancy on the natural
course of bipolar disorder. For patients with major depressive disorder
(MDD), prevalence estimates of depression in pregnancy are the same as in
the nongravid state *(1)*, and many women who stop their antidepressants
in pregnancy relapse during pregnancy back into depression *(2,3)*. Thus
pregnancy *per se* does not appear to be protective against MDD episodes.
Whether pregnancy is protective against mood episodes for women with
bipolar disorder is not well established *(4–8)*. In one study *(9)*, the number
of hospital admissions for bipolar illness during pregnancy was only

From: *Current Clinical Practice: Psychiatric Disorders in
Pregnancy and the Postpartum: Principles and Treatment*
Edited by: V. Hendrick © Humana Press, Totowa, NJ

three-fourths the number during nonpregnancy-related periods, suggesting some protective effect of pregnancy on mood episodes. However, during the first month postpartum, admissions were eight times as common as during nonpregnancy-related periods, and from months 2–12 postpartum, admissions were twice as common. This is consistent with other studies that have shown the postpartum period to be a time of extreme vulnerability to relapse for women with bipolar disorder *(5,10–13)*. Certainly for many women, pregnancy *per se* is not protective against a manic or depressive episode *(7)*. Discontinuation of stable maintenance mood stabilizers increases the risk of relapse in nonpregnant and pregnant women with bipolar I and II disorder *(8)*. The risk of relapse is high in nongravid patients with bipolar disorder who discontinue such medication abruptly (i.e., in less than 2 wk) *(8,14,15)*.

Several recent excellent reviews have been published on the treatment of bipolar disorder in pregnancy and following delivery *(16–20)*. In this chapter we review the impact on the fetus of medications used to treat bipolar disorder in pregnancy. We additionally review information on the risk of breast-feeding associated with medication use in the postpartum for patients for bipolar illness.

2. NATURAL COURSE OF BIPOLAR DISORDER IN PREGNANCY

Although there are no systematic data on the effects of untreated manic, depressive, or mixed states on fetal development in patients with bipolar disorder, systematic studies have shown that other forms of psychopathology during pregnancy are associated with adverse effects on offspring. Maternal depression during pregnancy has been associated with preterm delivery and low birthweight *(21,22)* and anxiety in pregnancy has been associated with an increased risk of both preterm delivery *(23)* and behavioral problems in early childhood *(24,25)*. Rodent and primate research has shown a link between maternal antenatal stress and persistent impaired behavioral adjustment and emotional reactivity in offspring that is accompanied by changes in hypothalamic–pituitary–adrenal axis functioning *(24,26)*. Thus, it is possible that episodes of mania or bipolar depression during pregnancy could have long-term deleterious effects on the infant. The risks of the impact on the fetus of a woman who experiences mania or depression during pregnancy must be weighed against the risk of the impact of medication exposure to the fetus in a woman who stays on medication in an attempt to maintain euthymia—stable mental health—during pregnancy. The risks of medication exposure on the developing fetus are discussed here.

3. IMPACT OF PSYCHOTROPIC
MEDICATIONS ON OFFSPRING

All psychotropic medications diffuse readily across the placenta during pregnancy. Thus, the fetus is exposed to medication and its potential complications. Risks of medication exposure can include organ malformation (teratogenicity), obstetrical complications, perinatal syndromes (neonatal toxicity), and long-term postnatal behavioral sequelae (behavioral teratogenicity) *(3)*. Teratogenicity is defined as an organ malformation/congenital deformity that occurs with a significantly greater risk over the baseline risk of malformations. In the United States, the baseline risk of malformations (i.e., the risk in the population at large) is 2–3% *(27)*. Obstetrical complications include preterm delivery, low birth rate, and delivery complications such as low Apgar scores. Perinatal syndromes (neonatal toxicity) include behavioral symptoms noticed shortly after birth such as jitteriness. Postnatal behavioral sequelae (behavioral teratogenicity) include long-term neurobehavioral effects in children who are exposed to medication *in utero*. The data for the risks of teratogenicity, prenatal toxicity, and behavioral teratogenicity are discussed here. Each of these risks is possible and must be balanced against the risk of untreated bipolar illness in pregnancy *(3,16,17)*. In the following, we review each medication used to treat bipolar illness and its known impact on neonatal development.

3.1. Lithium

3.1.1. TERATOGENICITY

The Register of Lithium Babies noted a 400-fold higher rate of cardiovascular malformations, most notably Ebstein's anomaly, in offspring exposed *in utero*, compared with the general population *(17)*. This congenital anomaly, characterized by downward displacement of the tricuspid valve into the right ventricle and variable levels of right ventricular hypoplasia, occurs at a rate of 1:20,000 in the general population *(28)*. The risk among offspring of lithium users of Ebstein's anomaly was 1:1000 (0.1%) to 2:1000 (0.05%), or 20–40 times higher than the rate in the general population *(16,19,21,22,29)*. Thus, the relative risk for Ebstein's anomaly with prenatal lithium exposure is significantly higher than in the general population; however, the absolute risk—that is, the likelihood that a baby exposed to lithium *in utero* will be born with Ebstein's anomaly—remains small (1–2 in 1000 births).

3.1.2. NEONATAL TOXICITY

Toxicities experienced by offspring exposed to lithium during labor include "floppy baby" syndrome, characterized by cyanosis and hypotonicity *(16)*. Neonatal hypothyroidism and nephrogenic diabetes insipidus have also been described *(16)*. Close monitoring of lithium levels in the mother during labor is now routine.

3.1.3. NEUROBEHAVIORAL TERATOGENICITY

In a follow-up study of 60 children who were exposed to lithium *in utero* and born without malformations, children did not differ behaviorally from their nonexposed siblings *(30)*.

3.2. Anticonvulsants

Sodium valproate and carbamazepine are used in the acute treatment of bipolar disorder. More recently, lamotrigine has become commonly used to treat bipolar disorder.

3.2.1. VALPROATE

3.2.1.1. Teratogenicity. Sodium valproate is considered a human teratogen. Use of this compound during the first trimester is associated with neural tube defect rates of 5–9% *(23,31,32)*, and risk is dose-related *(33,34)*. Fetal exposure to carbamazepine and valproate, even late in the pregnancy, is associated with craniofacial abnormalities and cognitive dysfunction *(29,35–37)*, as well as minor malformations that resolve with time, such as rotated ears, depressed nasal bridge, short nose, elongated upper lip, and fingernail hypoplasia *(34,35,38–40)*.

3.2.1.2. Neonatal Toxicity. Heart rate decelerations *(34)* and withdrawal symptoms of irritability, jitteriness, feeding difficulties, and abnormal tone *(41)* have been reported in neonates in association with valproate use near the time of delivery. Other complications among neonates include liver toxicity *(42)* and hypoglycemia *(43)*. Reductions in neonatal fibrinogen levels have also been reported *(44)*.

3.2.1.3. Neurobehavioral Teratogenicity. Mental retardation has been reported after *in utero* exposure to valproate. However, the data to support this are not definitive *(45)*.

3.2.2. CARBAMAZEPINE

3.2.2.1. Teratogenicity. Use of carbamazepine in the first trimester has been associated with teratogenic effects. The rate for neural tube defects has ranged between 0.5 and 1% *(37,40)*. Other findings include craniofacial defects (11%) and fingernail hypoplasia (26%) *(46)*. The teratogenic potential of carbamazepine has been reported to be increased when it is given with other agents and in particular with valproate *(46)*.

3.2.2.2. Neonatal Toxicity. Carbamazepine has been associated with transient hepatic toxicity (cholestatic hepatitis *[47]* and direct hyperbilirubinemia *[48]*) in case reports of neonates exposed to the drug during pregnancy. In both cases, hepatic dysfunction resolved.

3.2.2.3. Neurobehavioral Teratogenicity. The impact of carbamazepine on neonatal development remains to be elucidated. In one study, children who had a history of prenatal exposure to carbamazepine showed no neurodevelopmental problems compared with controls *(49)*. In another study, developmental delays were found in 20% of live-born offspring *(40)*.

3.2.3. LAMOTRIGINE

3.2.3.1. Teratogenicity. Lamotrigine is now approved by the US Food and Drug Administration (FDA) for maintenance treatment for bipolar disorder *(50,51)*. To date, 1274 prospectively followed pregnancies involving exposure to lamotrigine were registered with GlaxoSmith-Kline *(52)* (personal communication, GlaxoSmith-Kline, 2005). An estimated 2.9% of these infants were born with major malformations, a rate similar to the general population rate for major malformations. There was no pattern in the type of defects seen. (Defects included anencephaly and ventral septal defects.)

3.2.3.2. Neonatal Toxicity. Lamotrigine is metabolized exclusively by means of glucuronidation, a metabolic process that is very immature in the fetus and neonate. Although to our knowledge there are no known cases of neonatal toxicity, hepatotoxicity is a theoretical concern as measurement of the clearance of lamotrigine in neonates after the first 72 h of life decreased by 25% relative to umbilical cord blood concentrations *(52)*.

3.2.3.3. Neurobehavioral Teratogenicity. A single follow-up of 23 infants whose mothers used lamotrigine in pregnancy for control of epilepsy demonstrated no alterations in development at 12 mo of age *(53)*.

3.3. Antipsychotic Agents

3.3.1. TYPICAL ANTIPSYCHOTICS

3.3.1.1. Teratogenicity. The effects of using antipsychotic medications on women with bipolar disorder and on infant outcome have not been well studied. Data regarding fetal outcome using antispychotics have been best studied in the condition of hyperemesis gravidarum using such antipsychotics as chlorpromazine *(54,55)*. In a survey of more than

50,000 mother–child pairs that identified 142 first-trimester exposures to chlorpromazine, there was no elevation in the rate of physical malformations in those children exposed to chlorpromazine *(55)*. To our knowledge, no systematic studies regarding the use of typical antipsychotics in women with bipolar disorder have been reported. One study involving schizophrenic women on typical antipsychotic medication in pregnancy suggested that psychiatric illness (psychosis) may influence pregnancy outcomes more than antipsychotic medication. Sobel compared psychotic women with and without histories of chlorpromazine exposure during pregnancy *(56)*. The rates of fetal malformation or death in the offspring of the exposed and nonexposed women with psychosis were similar but were approximately two times the rate in the general population. The author suggested that a spectrum of factors other than prenatal exposure to antipsychotics *per se* might account for the higher rates of malformation in the offspring of psychotic patients.

3.3.1.2. Neonatal Toxicity. Neonatal symptoms, including irritability, abnormal hand posturing, and extremity tremors, have been reported in neonates with haloperidol exposure. These symptoms last up to 6 mo *(57)*. Extrapyramidal symptoms, including hypertonicity, tremors, motor restlessness, spasticity, and difficulty with feeding, have been found in infants exposed to chlorpromazine *(58)*. Such symptoms have been reported to last up to 10 mo, but most resolve within days.

3.3.1.3. Behavioral Teratogenicity. No behavioral teratogenicity has been reported with either phenothiazines or butyrophenones *(55)*. Children with and without histories of antipsychotic exposure showed no differences in behavioral functioning or IQ when followed up to 5 yr of age *(59)*.

3.3.2. ATYPICAL ANTIPSYCHOTIC AGENTS

Many atypical antipsychotics, including olanzapine, quetiapine, risperidone, aripiprazole, and ziprasidone, are currently FDA approved for the treatment of mania. Olanzapine and aripiprazole are additionally approved for the maintenance treatment of bipolar disorder. Although clozapine is not FDA approved, it has been used to treat mania as well. Because experience with all of these medications in pregnant women is limited, they will be reviewed together here.

3.3.2.1. Teratogenicity. A single preliminary study has shown no increased risk of teratogenicity in 23 cases during which olanzapine was used in antenatally *(60)*. Another case report also showed no adverse outcome regarding teratogenicity, although the pregnancy was complicated by the development of hypertension and pre-eclampsia in the mother *(61)*. Very few case reports have been written regarding *in utero* use of clozapine. These limited case reports to date have not shown a clear teratogenic effect *(62–64)*. Several studies have suggested an increased risk for hyperglycemia in pregnant women related to using atypical antipsychotic therapy during gestation *(65)*. One study in schizophrenic women suggested that atypical antipsychotics are associated with a higher risk of neural tube defects in the infants of 21 women with schizophrenia *(66)*. However, in another study *(67)*, women who had been exposed to atypical antipsychotics were matched to a comparison group of pregnant women who had not been exposed to these agents. The study evaluated 151 pregnancy outcomes that involved 60 exposures to olanzapine, 49 exposures to risperidone, 36 exposures to quetiapine, and 6 exposures to clozapine. Rates of malformation were 0.9%. Thus, in this controlled study there were no significant differences in the rates of teratogenicity in the exposed vs the comparison group. However, there was a higher rate of low birthweight (10% of children exposed in the medicated group vs 2% in the comparison group).

3.3.2.2. Neonatal Toxicity and Behavioral Teratogenicity. To our knowledge no data exist that suggest neonatal toxicity or behavioral teratogenicity in association with the use of atypical antipsychotic medications during pregnancy. However, clearly more data are needed.

3.4. Benzodiazepines and Other Sedative Hypnotic Agents

Benzodiazepines are used commonly as adjunctive medications for mood stabilization or for anxiety, agitation, and sleep problems. Knowledge regarding the use of this class of medication during pregnancy and its impact on outcome is reviewed below.

3.4.1. TERATOGENICITY

Oral clefts develop in the first trimester, with closure being complete by the 10th week of gestation *(68,69)*. The risk for the anomaly cleft palate in the general population appears to be 6 in 10,000 (0.06%) *(31)*. The extent to which benzodiazepines heighten risk for oral cleft or other anomalies in humans remains controversial. In more than 14 different studies in which the relationship between first-trimester exposure to benzodiazepines and risk for congenital anomalies was assessed, no more than 4 studies used the same design to answer any particular question, and often a number of different benzodiazepines were reported on together *(31,70–83)*. These differences contribute to the confusion and controversy regarding the safety of benzodiazepine use during pregnancy.

One meta-analysis found a positive association between first-trimester *in utero* exposure to benzodiazepines and a specific anomaly, oral cleft *(3)*. A more recent meta-analysis found an association between oral cleft and benzodiazepine use among case–control studies (odds ratio = 1.79, 95% confidence interval =1.13–2.82) but not in cohort studies *(84)*. The difference in findings among studies is probably a result of the greater sensitivity of case–control studies in analyzing rare events. Results from case–control studies of the relationship between benzodiazepine exposure and cleft lip or palate have suggested a risk rate of about 11:10,000 births, a significant increase over the base risk rate of 6:10,000 births in the general population, but still an absolute risk that is rare *(3,84)*.

Another case–control study of 13,703 cases reported no increased risk for any malformations associated with the overall use of benzodiazepines in the first trimester of pregnancy *(85)*. However, when the benzodiazepines were examined individually, a significant association was found between lorazepam and anal atresia *(85)*. Other studies of individual benzodiazepines have reported that clonazepam was not linked with birth defects, although it has been associated with neonatal hypotonia when used in combination with imipramine near term *(26)*. (This suggests that coadministration of benzodiazepines with other psychotropic medications may require close neonatal observation.) The reproductive safety of diazepam is controversial. Early reports described an increased risk of oral clefts after first-trimester exposure to diazepam *(71)*, but later studies have not supported this association *(31,86)*.

3.4.2. NEONATAL TOXICITY

Acute side effects from benzodiazepines occur in association with therapy near term. Case reports have described impaired temperature regulation, apnea, lower Apgar scores at both 1 and 5 min, muscular hypotonia, and failure to feed *(87–93)*. Infants born to mothers who chronically used benzodiazepines may evidence withdrawal symptoms, including tremor, irritability, diarrhea, vomiting, vigorous sucking, and hypertonicity In one small study of a series of infants whose mothers (*N* = 39) had taken clonazepam (0.5–3.5 mg/d) for treatment of panic disorder during pregnancy, neonatal toxicity was not found *(26)*.

3.4.3. BEHAVIORAL TERATOGENICITY

Systematically derived data on the long-term neurobehavioral effects of benzodiazepine exposure are sparse. Motor and developmental delays have been reported, although these reports have been criticized for having significant ascertainment biases *(94)*. Other investigators have found no association between benzodiazepine exposure and developmental delay *(82)*.

3.5. Antidepressants

This class of drugs and their impact on the developing fetus and obstetrical outcome is reviewed in Chapter 2 and, thus, are not reviewed here.

4. ELECTROCONVULSIVE THERAPY

Electroconvulsive therapy (ECT), which is highly effective for bipolar manic, depressive, and mixed states, has not been associated with deleterious effects on pregnant women or neonates *(95,96)*, although more data are needed.

4.1. Teratogenicity

Although there have been occasional reports of congenital malformations in offspring exposed to ECT *in utero (33),* neither the number nor the pattern of these findings implicates ECT as a causal factor.

4.2. Neonatal Toxicity

No instances of neonatal toxicity have been reported in the literature.

4.3. Neurobehavioral Teratogenicity

A few case reports have described developmental delays or mental retardation in offspring exposed to ECT *in utero (33).* However, neither the number nor the pattern of these reports suggests a causal relationship between ECT and the developmental delays. No systematic, long-term follow-up studies of neurobehavioral parameters have been conducted in offspring whose mothers received ECT during pregnancy.

5. TREATMENT GUIDELINES

To minimize risk to mother and child, the best type of conception is a planned conception. Some patients and their clinicians may feel comfortable attempting to taper off of medications prior to attempts to get pregnant and to see if the woman is at a phase of her illness that may be quiescent. Because of the severity of prior episodes, other women may feel that this will not be safe for them and will prefer to be put on the safest medication possible while attempting to get pregnant. Tapering off or transitioning to medications can be done in a thoughtful and conservative way if clinicians and patients are given the time. Often, however, patients will find that they are pregnant while on a medication and feel the need to abruptly discontinue their treatment. It is clear that an abrupt discontinuation of antimanic agents, at least of lithium, rather than a slow taper, is associated with an increased risk for relapse *(14,15).*

Clearly, the biggest concern is first-trimester exposure because this is the period associated with the highest risk for teratogenicity. Although second- and third-trimester exposure are not associated with teratogenic risks, they are potentially associated with other problems, including minor malformations and behavioral effects. Most of these risks are theoretical because, to our knowledge, there are no controlled data concerning the frequency of such effects in women treated with antimanic medications.

Compared with other antimanic agents, such as the anticonvulsants, lithium appears to be the least teratogenic and, therefore, has the greater relative safety in terms of teratogenicity when compared with divalproex sodium or carbamazepine. Additionally, data regarding lamotrigine suggest low risk for teratogenic effects. However, if a woman has had a poor antimanic response to lithium or lamotrigine in the past, switching to lithium—even though it may be safer from a teratogenic point of view—may actually put the woman at risk for relapse.

If a woman is to remain on carbamazepine or divalproex sodium in the first trimester of pregnancy, her infant will have an increased risk for neural tube defects. Therefore, using the lowest dose that may control her mood might decrease the risk for spina bifida. Lower maternal folic acid levels have been associated with neural tube defects (97). A higher dosage of folic acid (3–4 mg/d) should be prescribed for women on anticonvulsants in pregnancy, and close coordination of care between the psychiatrist and the obstetrician/gynecologist is recommended.

ECT is another option for patients who developed either a mania or depression in pregnancy, but for most patients this is not a first choice. There has been no indication that ECT is associated with any teratogenic effects (96). Therefore, ECT should presently be viewed as a safe and effective treatment for episodes of either mania or depression during pregnancy, especially for severe or life-threatening mood and psychotic episodes. When used in pregnant patients, ECT may pose fewer risks than untreated mood episodes or pharmacotherapy with a teratogenic agent.

Overall, little is known about the direct or indirect effects of nonpharmacological interventions on mania, and no controlled clinical trials have evaluated these strategies during pregnancy. Thus, a purely psychotherapeutic approach for treating mania in pregnancy is not recommended. Cognitive therapies aimed at preventing a manic episode have focused on increasing adherence to treatment with medication (98), improvement of social and occupational functioning, minimizing sleep deprivation (because sleep deprivation can precipitate mania) (3,16), improving other circadian rhythm patterns (99), and preventing relapse.

Cognitive-behavioral strategies may be extremely effective at treating the depressed phase of the illness. In a recent uncontrolled study using a modified version of interpersonal psychotherapy for 13 women with depression and pregnancy, all subjects responded with remission of their depressive symptoms *(100)*. Thus, for bipolar depression in pregnancy, especially if the depression is mild, psychotherapeutic strategies may be an alternative to medication intervention *(100)*.

6. BIPOLAR DISORDER AND THE POSTPARTUM PERIOD

More systematic research exists on the course of bipolar disorder during the postpartum period than during pregnancy. This period is recognized as a time of significantly heightened risk for bipolar relapse, conferring the greatest risk for exacerbation of this illness than at any other time in a woman's life *(101,102)*. Recurrence rates of bipolar disorder within the first 3–6 postpartum months have ranged from 20 to 80% among women with bipolar illness *(7,12,103–108)*. In the four most recent studies, these rates have ranged from 67 to 82% *(7,8,108,109)*. The rate of postpartum depression (PPD) in women with bipolar disorder has been estimated at 33–50% (compared with 12–16% in postpartum women without a diagnosis of a mood disorder) and is even higher when mood-stabilizing medications are discontinued during pregnancy or not administered within 48 h of delivery *(15,110)*. Bipolar women who discontinue lithium in the postpartum period have a threefold higher relapse risk than nonpregnant and nonpostpartum women with the illness *(6,8)*. Although data are limited, the rate of postpartum relapse appears to drop to 10% when mood-stabilizing prophylaxis is initiated during pregnancy or soon after delivery *(111)*.

The pathophysiology of bipolar exacerbation during the postpartum period is not understood. Proposed contributors to the destabilization of mood include disturbances in the hypothalamic–pituitary–thyroid axis and major withdrawal of steroid hormones after birth *(112–115)*. The changes in reproductive hormone status are considered important in regulating mood, and rapid and steep decline in estrogen after delivery may trigger mood changes in vulnerable women regardless of their diagnosis *(110,116)*. The efficacy of hormone replacement therapy for bipolar disorder during the postpartum period has not been adequately assessed *(112,113)*.

Women with bipolar disorder have a high risk of symptom emergence that can occur within a few days to weeks after childbirth *(4–6,16)*. Additionally, postpartum women are approximately seven times more likely to be hospitalized for a first bipolar episode and two times more likely to be hospitalized for a recurrent bipolar episode when compared with nonpostpartum and nonpregnant women *(6,16)*. In the largest study to date, the risk of psychiatric admission in the first 30 d after childbirth was 21.4% for women with a history of bipolar disorder, manic, or cyclical type and 13.3% for women with a history of bipolar disorder, depressed type *(117)*.

Worsening mood symptoms during pregnancy may be predictive of the development of PPD in many women with bipolar disorder, whereas lack of change or improvement in mood symptoms may be somewhat protective against PPD *(110)*. PPD symptoms are similar to those in MDD. However, psychotic symptoms or suicidal ideation may also be present, and the suicidality can extend to thoughts of killing the newborn infant.

Sleep loss may be a contributor to the development of hypomanic and manic episodes in the postpartum period *(115,118,119)*. For women who have primary responsibility for the care and feeding of their newborns, sleep disruption might be as frequent as every 2 h. This is a significant component of the psychosocial stress from the adaptation required to meet the requirements of parenthood *(16)*. Whenever possible, women with bipolar disorder should be helped to minimize sleep deprivation during the postpartum period *(112–114)*.

7. RELATIONSHIP BETWEEN POSTPARTUM PSYCHOSIS AND BIPOLAR AFFECTIVE DISORDER

Many researchers believe that postpartum psychosis is either a variant or a manifestation of a manic/mixed episode and in many women demarcates the onset of bipolar disorder *(110,120,121)*. Postpartum psychosis is a rare condition affecting 0.1–0.2% of all women experiencing childbirth *(110,122)*. Women with bipolar disorder have a significantly higher risk than women without a psychiatric disorder of developing postpartum psychosis *(5,12,17,18,104–108,123)*. Recent studies have found that for women with bipolar disorder, the risk of developing postpartum psychosis is increased to 20–50%, particularly when mood-stabilizing medications (i.e., lithium) are discontinued during pregnancy and not reinstated within 48 h of delivery *(5,110,116,122)*. Furthermore, additional research has demonstrated that many women with postpartum psychosis will later develop bipolar disorder *(7,12,17,104–108,111,124–128)*.

One study found that one-third of 486 women admitted psychiatrically with postpartum psychosis in the first 3 mo following delivery had a prior diagnosis of bipolar illness *(5)*. Several studies suggest that recurrent bipolar disorder usually follows an episode of postpartum psychosis *(5,110,120)*. In addition, primiparity, family history of bipolar disorder, and psychosocial stressors increase the risk of the disorder *(110)*.

Studies have consistently found that more than two-thirds of women who develop postpartum psychosis do so within the first 2 wk following childbirth *(107,117,129,130)*. Symptoms of postpartum psychosis typically occur rapidly, within 48–72 h of delivery, and share features with manic or mixed episodes—elated mood alternating rapidly with depressed mood, irritability, restlessness or motor excitement, sleep and appetite disturbance, disorganized behavior, and psychotic symptoms (i.e., auditory hallucinations) *(5,110)*. The delusions often revolve around the infant or children and must be carefully assessed because women with postpartum psychosis may have thoughts of harming their infants and sometimes act on these thoughts *(117,131–133)*. Risks of infanticide have been estimated as high as 4% *(110,134)*. Many authors have reported a "delirious" or "perplexed" state with waxing and waning confusional presentation *(17,117,129,131,132)*.

Studies that support a link between bipolar illness and postpartum psychosis found that the risk of having an affective episode among first-degree relatives of women with postpartum psychosis is similar to the risk among first-degree relatives of patients with bipolar disorder *(117,130,135,136)*. A single large study that used direct interview of relatives suggested that familial factors play a role in the vulnerability to postpartum triggering itself. Episodes of postpartum psychosis occurred in 74% ($n = 20$) of the 27 parous women with bipolar disorder who had a family history of postpartum psychosis in a first-degree relative but in only 30% ($n = 38$) of the 125 women with bipolar disorder with no such family history *(137)*. This study also reported that there is significant evidence ($p < 0.003$) that variation at the serotonin transporter gene exerts a substantial and important influence on susceptibility to bipolar affective postpartum psychosis *(137,138)*.

8. PSYCHOTROPIC MEDICATIONS IN THE MANAGEMENT OF POSTPARTUM BIPOLAR DISORDER

The high rate of postpartum recurrence of bipolar disorder underscores the importance of prophylactic intervention at or before delivery *(17,111,124–128,139,140)*. This risk appears to be reduced by mood-stabilizing treatments. However, virtually all medications are secreted in breast milk during lactation, posing further treatment dilemmas in the female patient who wants to breast-feed *(18)*.

Consideration of medication use while breast-feeding must take into account the mother's history of medication response, side effects, and infant-related factors *(117,141)*. Breast-feeding almost guarantees sleep deprivation, a condition that may induce psychiatric instability in bipolar patients *(18)*. The benefits of breast-feeding to the infant and the mother with bipolar disorder must be balanced with the mother's need to manage bipolar illness during the high-risk postpartum period *(112)*.

The American Academy of Pediatrics (AAP) Committee on Drugs has published guidelines on the use of medications by nursing mothers *(112,117,142,143)*. It is important to note that recommendations for breast-feeding while being treated with psychotropic medications have generally been made based on limited data. Most of the data come from epileptic women *(144)*. The frequency of severe complications related to neonatal exposure to psychotropic medications appears to be low, but the effects of even small amounts of psychoactive medications on an infant's developing brain are not well known *(110)*. Therefore, it is recommended that, in order to minimize risk of exposure, the mother take the medication just after she has breast-fed the infant or just before the infant is due to have a lengthy sleep period *(18)*.

8.1. Lithium

Although research data demonstrate that introducing lithium prophylaxis within 48 h postdelivery has been effective in reducing the risk of postpartum relapse, earlier reintroduction of a mood stabilizer 2–4 wk prior to expected delivery date may be a more prudent option that allows time to optimize the medication dosage prior to the woman entering a period of high relapse risk *(17)*. Postpartum prophylaxis appears to reduce the rate of relapse from near 50% to less than 10% *(16,111,125)*. In an open-label study of 21 women given lithium prophylaxis in the third trimester of pregnancy or immediately after delivery, only 2 women experienced a recurrence of their bipolar illness *(125)*.

Among women who elect to discontinue lithium during the postpartum, the estimated relapse risk is three times higher than for nonpregnant, nonpostpartum women *(145)*. When lithium is given several weeks prior to delivery or immediately postpartum, the risk of postpartum recurrences of bipolar disorder is reduced on average two- to fivefold, compared with untreated women *(17,111,124–128,139,146)*.

8.1.1. LACTATION SAFETY

The AAP has changed lithium's categorization from contraindicated to "should be given to nursing mothers with caution" *(117,142)*. A case-specific approach to breast-feeding women who require treatment with lithium has been recommended *(115,117,139)*.

8.1.2. SIDE EFFECTS

There is a concern of rapid dehydration in neonates if they develop febrile illness that could cause the levels of lithium in the infant to increase *(16)*. Symptoms of lithium toxicity in the infant include lethargy, hypotonia, hypothermia, cyanosis, and T-wave changes on electrocardiogram *(18,144,147)*. The long-term effects on infants with sustained lithium levels are unknown at this time.

A prevalence of clinical hypothyroidism during lithium treatment of 14% in women vs 5.5% in men has been reported *(148)*. Lithium-treated women may also be at higher risk of lithium-induced thyroiditis *(18)*.

8.1.3. MONITORING GUIDELINES

It is important to monitor lithium serum concentration and administer a complete blood panel in the breast-fed infant *(16)*. Some advise avoiding lithium until the infant is at least 5 mo of age because of decreased renal clearance, although careful monitoring of infant clinical status and serum lithium concentrations is recommended regardless of when this medication is started *(141,144)*. Nursing infants of mothers taking lithium should be monitored for hypotonia, lethargy, and cyanosis *(13,66)*. Hydration status should also be monitored, as dehydration can increase the risk of lithium-related adverse events *(145)*. There appear to be no drug–drug interactions with oral contraceptive pills, which is useful information for bipolar women who are trying to avoid becoming pregnant *(18,149)*.

8.2. Anticonvulsant Mood Stabilizers

8.2.1. VALPROATE

8.2.1.1. Lactation Safety. Valproate has been classified as "usually compatible" with breast-feeding by the AAP *(117,142)*. This is also supported by the Academy of Neurology—which states that breast-feeding is acceptable for mothers who are maintained on antiepileptic agents *(16,150)*.

8.2.1.2. Side Effects. No adverse effects to infants have been reported when mothers are treated with valproate solely during breast-feeding *(16,151)*. In a case series of six breast-feeding bipolar disorder mother–infant pairs, no adverse clinical effects were observed in the infants *(18)*.

There is at least one case report of thrombocytopenia purpura and anemia in a 3-mo-old infant whose mother used valproate during pregnancy and lactation. However, the symptoms resolved after the discontinuation of breast-feeding *(152)*.

Some experts recommend avoiding valproate because of increased risk of hepatotoxicity with use in children younger than 2 yr *(150,151)*. There is at least one case report of hepatic dysfunction in a nursing child exposed to valproate through breast milk *(151)*.

8.2.1.3. Monitoring Guidelines. It is recommended that pediatric clinical status, liver enzymes, and platelets in the breast-fed infant be monitored *(141,144)*. No drug–drug interactions have been reported with concurrent oral contraceptive pill use *(18,153)*.

8.2.2. CARBAMAZEPINE

To our knowledge, no data are available on the use of carbamazepine in treating or preventing postpartum bipolar illness.

8.2.2.1. Lactation Safety. Carbamazepine has been classified as "usually compatible" with breast-feeding by the AAP *(117,142)*.

8.2.2.2. Side Effects. There are at least two reports of an increased risk of hepatotoxicity in nursing infants *(18)*. Other case studies have reported drowsiness and poor feeding *(147)*. In rare instances, there have also been findings of seizure-like activity, irritability, and high-pitched cry in infants whose mothers take this medication while nursing *(18,154)*. There have been at least three reports of poor feeding and two reports of hyperexcitability *(144,155,156)*. By contrast, one study from 1979 reported no adverse events in 94 infants exposed to carbamazepine during lactation *(157)*.

Generally, many of the women in the case series reported above were on anticonvulsant polytherapy, which makes interpretation and generalization of the data difficult to extrapolate to the management of bipolar illness.

8.2.2.3. Monitoring Guidelines. When using carbamazepine during breast-feeding, careful monitoring of the infant clinically and via laboratory monitoring (liver enzymes, complete blood count, platelets) to rule out possible hepatotoxicity or hematological toxicity *(157)* is recommended. Nursing should be discontinued if any adverse reactions are observed *(144)*. This medication induces hepatic cytochrome P450 and thus decreases levels of oral contraceptive pills *(18,157)*.

8.2.3. LAMOTRIGINE

To our knowledge, no studies or case reports are available on the use of lamotrigine for the treatment or prevention of bipolar illness.

8.2.3.1. Lactation Safety. This medication is designated as a drug "for which the effect on nursing infants is unknown but may be of concern" by the AAP *(142,144)*.

8.2.3.2. Side Effects. The adverse effects of this medication are unknown. However, there are at least four case reports in nursing epileptic patients, which have reported no adverse effects on infants *(18,52,158)*. There is potential theoretical concern regarding reports of life-threatening rash, such as Stevens-Johnson syndrome or toxic epidermal necrolysis, in epileptic children treated with this medication *(147)*.

8.2.3.3. Monitoring Guidelines. Because it is unknown at this time whether the same risk factors exist for exposed nursing infants, the manufacturer does not recommend breast-feeding while taking lamotrigine *(123)*. Although no adverse effects have been noted thus far, it is still advised to monitor for the outbreak of any new rash *(4,159)*. One report found that oral contraceptive pills reduced lamotrigine plasma levels by 41–64% (mean 49%). Therefore, caution is advised in women who are concurrently taking oral contraceptives *(160)*.

8.3. Antipsychotics

8.3.1. Lactation Safety

8.3.1.1. First-Generation Antipsychotic Agents (i.e., Haloperidol, Chlorpromazine). There are at least 10 reports in which 28 infants were exposed to this class of drugs. In the majority of these cases, there was no evidence of adverse effects *(16,161)*.

8.3.1.2. Atypical Antipsychotics. Available evidence regarding the safety of atypical antipsychotics in lactation is minimal *(65)*. Presently, this class of drugs does not demonstrate any class advantages over typical antipsychotics *(65,162)* when used in lactating women. The manufacturers recommend that women receiving olanzapine, clozapine, risperidone, quetiapine, ziprasidone and aripiprazole should not breast-feed until more information is known *(18,142,144,144,163–165)*.

8.3.2. Side Effects

Data are reported here on any observation to our knowledge that exists in the literature on the impact of an antipsychotic on a breast-fed infant.

8.3.2.1. Haloperidol. Haloperidol has been associated with lower developmental scores in nursing infants in one study *(112)*. However, this particular study was of children of schizophrenic mothers with no controls who might have had lower developmental scores owing to the course of their psychotic illness even without haloperidol exposure. In another study that examined the effects of five breast-feeding infants exposed to haloperidol, there was no evidence of any acute or delayed adverse effects *(166)*. In the same study, three other breast-fed infants exposed to both haloperidol and chlorpromazine showed a decline in their developmental scores at 12–18 mo.

8.3.2.2. Olanzapine. Two retrospectively reported cases of infants exposed during lactation suggest no harm to one infant and no relationship of olanzapine to another infant's problems *(60)*. Of 20 reports of breast-fed infants exposed to olanzapine, 4 noted adverse events, including (a) jaundice, sedation, cardiomegaly, and a heart murmur; (b) shaking, poor sucking, and lethargy; (c) protruding tongue; and (d) rash, diarrhea, and sleeping disorder. However, no definitive conclusions were made regarding the role of olanzapine in contributing to these events *(144)*. In another study, no adverse events were reported in two retrospectively ascertained cases of lactation exposure *(60)*.

8.3.2.3. Clozapine. This medication has been associated with sedation, decreased suckling, restlessness or irritability, seizures, and cardiovascular instability in nursing infants *(154)*. Unlike in older patients, the theoretical risks of leukopenia and agranulocytosis have not been demonstrated in neonates exposed to clozapine via breast milk *(144)*.

8.4. Antidepressants

Some investigators recommend treatment with antidepressants in conjunction with a mood stabilizer after delivery to reduce the risk of developing PPD in women with recurrent depressive disorder *(5,7,110)*. Postpartum prophylaxis with an antidepressant agent immediately after delivery has been noted to reduce depression rates dramatically in women with recurrent depression, with a 6.2% rate in women receiving the medication vs 62% in women not on prophylaxis treatment. It is not known whether this finding also applies to women with bipolar disorder *(7,110)*. The use of antidepressants in lactation is reviewed in Chapter 3, thus it is not reviewed here.

Antidepressants may precipitate mania or rapid cycling in women who suffer from PPD or postpartum psychosis with prominent depressive features *(112,117,167)*. If an antidepressant is used in managing postpartum psychosis, it should, of course, be used only in conjunction with a mood stabilizer *(168,169)*.

Further details on the use of antidepressants in nursing are reviewed in Chapter 3.

8.5. Benzodiazepines

The AAP categorizes benzodiazepines as "drugs for which the effect on nursing infants is unknown, but may be of concern" *(162)*. There are no controlled studies in breast-feeding women; however, the risk of untoward effects to the breast-fed infant is possible *(162)*. No described complications have been observed with lorazepam and clonazepam *(6)*. However, alprazolam, clonazepam, diazepam, and lorazepam fall under the "moderately safe" lactation risk category: there has been at least one case report associated with diazepam causing sedation in neonates *(170)*. Other studies show that diazepam during lactation is not recommended because of potential for sedation, lethargy, and weight loss in nursing infants *(162,171)*.

No adverse effects have been reported with use of lorazepam during lactation *(162,171)*.

Short-acting benzodiazepines (alprazolam, lorazepam) may be safer for use during lactation as long as their use is short term, intermittent, low dose, or occurs after the first week postpartum *(162)*.

The available literature suggests that in order to minimize the risks of benzodiazepine therapy among nursing infants, it is advised that lactating women use drugs that have established safety profiles at the lowest effective dose for the shortest possible duration *(171)*.

As for the use of newer benzodiazepine-like agents (zolpidem and zaleplon), there are no studies on the use of zolpidem, but one study examined five lactating women who were administered a therapeutic dose of zaleplon (10 mg): very small quantities were transferred through breast milk to the nursing infant, which are unlikely to be clinically important *(172)*.

9. ECT

There are no rigorously controlled studies on the use of ECT in the treatment of postpartum psychosis. However, it is recommended as an alternative, especially in refractory or rapidly progressing cases of bipolar illness or postpartum psychosis *(117,173)*. Women with postpartum psychosis require aggressive treatment and careful supervision in an inpatient setting owing to the associated high risk of suicide and infanticide *(110)*. Immediate treatment with a mood stabilizer and antipsychotic agent or ECT is required for management of postpartum psychosis *(5)*.

10. PSYCHOTHERAPY

There are no published controlled studies on the role of psychotherapy in the management of bipolar disorder in women during the postpartum period.

11. TREATMENT GUIDELINES

In treatment planning, it also helps to conceptualize pregnancy and the postpartum period as two distinct risk periods because the use of medications may have a specific set of treatment implications, depending on whether the patient is pregnant, postpartum, or nursing *(17)*. Additionally, the treatment approach should be guided by severity of symptoms and the degree of impairment *(110)*.

Pregnant women and their families and acquaintances expect the postpartum period to be a cheerful time, characterized by the happy arrival of the newborn. Unfortunately, for women with bipolar disorder this is not always the case. Because the risk of a psychotic episode or the recurrence of a depressive or manic episode in the postpartum period is undisputedly high for women with bipolar illness, prophylaxis with mood stabilizers should be discussed with all such patients and recommended for maximum protection against relapse. Decisions regarding restarting medications in the third trimester or soon after delivery can be made during pregnancy in women who discontinued medication before or during pregnancy and remained stable off medication *(117)*.

No consensus exists regarding the most suitable time to reintroduce prophylaxis *(117,119)*. The most prudent plan is to use medication(s) to which the individual woman has previously responded well and to prepare a plan for rapid augmentation if breakthrough episodes of hypomania or depression or mixed eipsodes occur during the immediate postpartum period *(115)*. It is well known that women with bipolar disorder who discontinue lithium prior to pregnancy and have remained well during the pregnancy are at significantly increased risk of relapse, which may take the form of manic psychosis or a major depressive episode, within the first month postpartum *(174)*. Although some authors suggest reinstituting mood stabilizers in the second or third trimester of pregnancy when the teratogenic risk is lower, many patients may prefer to defer prophylaxis until immediately after delivery *(117)*. Particularly vulnerable women may require treatment throughout their pregnancies.

Women who are breast-feeding and are on medications must be made aware that all psychotropics, including antidepressants as well as mood stabilizers and benzodiazepines, are secreted in the breast milk at varying concentrations *(116)*. Although consideration of the mood stabilizer may be based on the patient's clinical status and past response, regardless of breast-feeding status, it is important to consider the effect to exposed infants if lactation is a concern *(144)*. Both valproate and carbamazepine are considered "compatible with breast-feeding" by the AAP, although in general the recommendations made by the AAP and other sources are based on very limited information, and there are reports of adverse events, particularly in infants exposed to carbamazepine *(142)*. During lactation, lithium should be used with caution. The newer anticonvulsants and atypical antipsychotics have not been studied sufficiently for any definitive recommendations to be made at present. The most conservative approach is thus to avoid breast-feeding while using these medications until more information is known *(142)*.

The risks and benefits of breast-feeding, of not taking medications, and of nursing while taking medications should be discussed with all new mothers *(144)*. Breast-feeding mothers should be informed about the signs and symptoms of drug toxicity, and formula supplements should be used during any periods of infant illness or dehydration. Polypharmacy should be avoided if possible, and the lowest effective doses should be used *(174)*.

The most important clinical factors that influence treatment planning during pregnancy are illness history and the reproductive risks of medications. This includes prior response to various medications, illness severity, duration of euthymia while taking and not taking medications, time to relapse after medication discontinuation, and time to recovery with the reintroduction of pharmacotherapy.

Issues relating to the course of bipolar illness during the pregnancy and postpartum periods are surrounded by myths and stereotypes, causing concern to both patients and physicians alike. Therefore, adequate clinical knowledge about the course of bipolar disorder during the reproductive period is important to ensure that the right treatment decisions are made and that the patient is informed about periods of increased risk. Informed choices coupled with close psychiatric follow-up and coordinated care with the obstetrician are the elements of an optimal model for the management of psychiatric disorders during pregnancy *(175)*.

REFERENCES

1. Kessler, R. C., McGonagle, K. A., Swartz, M., Blazer, D. G., and Nelson, C. B. (1993) Sex and depression in the National Comorbidity Survey. I: lifetime prevalence, chronicity and recurrence. J. Affect. Disord. 29, 85–96.
2. Cohen, L. S., Altshuler, L. L., Stowe, Z. N., and Faraone, S. V. (2004) Reintroduction of antidepressant therapy across pregnancy in women who previously discontinued treatment. A preliminary retrospective study. Psychother. Psychosom. 73, 255–258.
3. Altshuler, L. L., Cohen, L., Szuba, M. P., Burt, V. K., Gitlin, M., and Mintz, J. (1996) Pharmacologic management of psychiatric illness during pregnancy: dilemmas and guidelines. Am. J. Psychiatry 153, 592–606.
4. Grof, P., Robbins, W., Alda, M., Berghoefer, A., Vojtechovsky, M., Nilsson, A., and Robertson, C. (2000) Protective effect of pregnancy in women with lithium-responsive bipolar disorder. J. Affect. Disord. 61, 31–39.

5. Kendell, R. E., Chalmers, J. C., and Platz, C. (1987) Epidemiology of puerperal psychoses. Br. J. Psychiatry 150, 662–673.
6. Terp, I. M. and Mortensen, P. B. (1998) Post-partum psychoses. Clinical diagnoses and relative risk of admission after parturition. Br. J. Psychiatry 172, 521–526.
7. Freeman, M. P., Smith, K. W., Freeman, S. A., McElroy, S. L., Kmetz, G. E., Wright, R., and Keck, P. E., Jr. (2002) The impact of reproductive events on the course of bipolar disorder in women. J. Clin. Psychiatry 63, 284–287.
8. Viguera, A. C., Nonacs, R., Cohen, L. S., Tondo, L., Murray, A., and Baldessarini, R. J. (2000) Risk of recurrence of bipolar disorder in pregnant and nonpregnant women after discontinuing lithium maintenance. Am. J. Psychiatry 157, 179–184.
9. Kastrup, M., Lier, L., and Rafaelsen, O. J. (1989) Psychiatric illness in relation to pregnancy and childbirth, I: methodologic considerations. Nordisk Psykiatrisk Tidsskrift 45, 531–534.
10. Kendell, R. E., Wainwright, S., Hailey, A., and Shannon, B. (1976) The influence of childbirth on psychiatric morbidity. Psychol. Med. 6, 297–302.
11. Paffenberger, R. S. (1982) Epidemiological aspects of mental illness associated with childbirth. In: Brockington, I. F., Kumar, R., ed. Motherhood and Mental Illness. New York: Grune and Stratton, pp. 19–36.
12. Brockington, I. F., Cernik, K. F., Schofield, E. M., Downing, A. R., Francis, A. F., and Keelan, C. (1981) Puerperal psychosis. Phenomena and diagnosis. Arch. Gen. Psychiatry 38, 829–833.
13. Reich, T. and Winokur, G. (1970) Postpartum psychoses in patients with manic depressive disease. J. Nerv. Ment. Dis. 151, 60-68.
14. Suppes, T., Baldessarini, R. J., Faedda, G. L., and Tohen, M. (1991) Risk of recurrence following discontinuation of lithium treatment in bipolar disorder. Arch. Gen. Psychiatry 48, 1082–1088.
15. Faedda, G. L., Tondo, L., Baldessarini, R. J., Suppes, T., and Tohen, M. (1993) Outcome after rapid vs gradual discontinuation of lithium treatment in bipolar disorders. Arch. Gen. Psychiatry 50, 448–455.
16. Yonkers, K. A., Wisner, K. L., Stowe, Z., Leibenluft, E., Cohen, L., Miller, L., Manber, R., Viguera, A., Suppes, T., and Altshuler, L. (2004) Management of bipolar disorder during pregnancy and the postpartum period. Am. J. Psychiatry 161, 608–620.
17. Viguera, A. C., Cohen, L. S., Baldessarini, R. J., and Nonacs, R. (2002) Managing bipolar disorder during pregnancy: weighing the risks and benefits. Can. J. Psychiatry 47, 426–436.
18. Burt, V. K. and Rasgon, N. (2004) Special considerations in treating bipolar disorder in women. Bipolar. Disord. 6, 2–13.
19. Thomas, P. and Severus W.E. (2003) Managing bipolar disorder during pregnancy and lactation: Is there a safe and effective option? European Psychiatry 18, 3s-8s.
20. Altshuler, L., Richards, M., and Yonkers, K. (2003) Treating bipolar disorder during pregnancy. Current Psychiatry 2, 15–25.
21. Orr, S. T. and Miller, C. A. (1995) Maternal depressive symptoms and the risk of poor pregnancy outcome. Review of the literature and preliminary findings. Epidemiol. Rev. 17, 165–171.
22. Steer, R. A., Scholl, T. O., Hediger, M. L., and Fischer, R. L. (1992) Self-reported depression and negative pregnancy outcomes. J. Clin. Epidemiol. 45, 1093–1099.
23. Hedegaard, M., Henriksen, T. B., Sabroe, S., and Secher, N. J. (1993) Psychological distress in pregnancy and preterm delivery. BMJ 307, 234–239.

24. Glover, V. and O'Connor, T. G. (2002) Effects of antenatal stress and anxiety: Implications for development and psychiatry. Br. J. Psychiatry 180, 389–391.

25. O'Connor, T. G., Heron, J., Golding, J., Beveridge, M., and Glover, V. (2002) Maternal antenatal anxiety and children's behavioural/emotional problems at 4 years. Report from the Avon Longitudinal Study of Parents and Children. Br. J. Psychiatry 180, 502–508.

26. Weinstock, L., Cohen, L. S., Bailey, J. W., Blatman, R., and Rosenbaum, J. F. (2001) Obstetrical and neonatal outcome following clonazepam use during pregnancy: a case series. Psychother. Psychosom. 70, 158–162.

27. Nelson, K. and Holmes, L. B. (1989) Malformations due to presumed spontaneous mutations in newborn infants. N. Engl. J. Med. 320, 19–23.

28. Cohen, L. S., Friedman, J. M., Jefferson, J. W., Johnson, E. M., and Weiner, M. L. (1994) A reevaluation of risk of in utero exposure to lithium. JAMA 271, 146–150.

29. Cohen, L. S. and Rosenbaum, J. F. (1998) Psychotropic drug use during pregnancy: weighing the risks. J. Clin. Psychiatry 59 (Suppl. 2), 18–28.

30. Schou, J. (1976) [Drugs and fetal development]. Ugeskr. Laeger 138: 2174.

31. Heinonen, O. P., Slone, D., and Shapiro, S. (1999) Birth Defects and Drugs in Pregnancy. Littleton, MA: Publishing Sciences Group.

32. Tomson, T. and Battino, D. (2005) Teratogenicity of antiepileptic drugs: state of the art. Curr. Opin. Neurol. 18, 135–140.

33. Impastato, D. J., Gabriel, A. R., and Lardaro, H. H. (1964) Electric and insulin shock therapy during pregnancy. Dis. Nerv. Syst. 25, 542–546.

34. Jager-Roman, E., Deichl, A., Jakob, S., Hartmann, A. M., Koch, S., Rating, D., Steldinger, R., Nau, H., and Helge, H. (1986) Fetal growth, major malformations, and minor anomalies in infants born to women receiving valproic acid. J. Pediatr. 108, 997–1004.

35. Koch, K., Hartman, A., Jager-Roman, E., Rating, D., and Helge, H. (1982) Major malformations of children of epileptic parents-due to epilepsy or its therapy? In: Janz, D., Bossi, L., Dam, M., Helge, H., Richens, A., Schmidt, D., eds. Epilepsy, Pregnancy and the Child. New York: Raven Press, pp. 313–316.

36. Omtzigt, J. G., Los, F. J., Hagenaars, A. M., Stewart, P. A., Sachs, E. S., and Lindhout, D. (1992) Prenatal diagnosis of spina bifida aperta after first-trimester valproate exposure. Prenat. Diagn. 12, 893–897.

37. Rosa, F. W. (1991) Spina bifida in infants of women treated with carbamazepine during pregnancy. N. Engl. J. Med. 324, 674–677.

38. Delgado-Escueta, A. V. and Janz, D. (1992) Consensus guidelines: preconception counseling, management, and care of the pregnant woman with epilepsy. Neurology 42, 149–160.

39. Gaily, E. and Granstrom, M. L. (1992) Minor anomalies in children of mothers with epilepsy. Neurology 42, 128–131.

40. Jones, K. L., Lacro, R. V., Johnson, K. A., and Adams, J. (1989) Pattern of malformations in the children of women treated with carbamazepine during pregnancy. N. Engl. J. Med. 320, 1661–1666.

41. Kennedy, D. and Koren, G. (1998) Valproic acid use in psychiatry: issues in treating women of reproductive age. J. Psychiatry Neurosci. 23, 223–228.

42. Felding, I. and Rane, A. (1984) Congenital liver damage after treatment of mother with valproic acid and phenytoin? Acta Paediatr. Scand. 73, 565-568.

43. Thisted, E. and Ebbesen, F. (1993) Malformations, withdrawal manifestations, and hypoglycaemia after exposure to valproate in utero. Arch. Dis. Child 69, 288–291.

44. Majer, R. V. and Green, P. J. (1987) Neonatal afibrinogenaemia due to sodium valproate. Lancet 2, 740–741.
45. DiLiberti, J. H., Farndon, P. A., Dennis, N. R., and Curry, C. J. (1984) The fetal valproate syndrome. Am. J. Med. Genet. 19, 473–481.
46. Lindhout, D., Meinardi, H., Meijer, J. W., and Nau, H. (1992) Antiepileptic drugs and teratogenesis in two consecutive cohorts: changes in prescription policy paralleled by changes in pattern of malformations. Neurology 42, 94-110.
47. Frey, B., Schubiger, G., and Musy, J. P. (1990) Transient cholestatic hepatitis in a neonate associated with carbamazepine exposure during pregnancy and breastfeeding. Eur. J. Pediatr. 150, 136-138.
48. Merlob, P., Mor, N., and Litwin, A. (1992) Transient hepatic dysfunction in an infant of an epileptic mother treated with carbamazepine during pregnancy and breastfeeding. Ann. Pharmacother. 26, 1563–1565.
49. Scolnik, D., Nulman, I., Rovet, J., Gladstone, D., Czuchta, D., Gardner, H. A., Gladstone, R., Ashby, P., Weksberg, R., Einarson, T., et al. (1994) Neurodevelopment of children exposed in utero to phenytoin and carbamazepine monotherapy. JAMA 271, 767–770.
50. Calabrese, J. R., Suppes, T., Bowden, C. L., Sachs, G. S., Swann, A. C., McElroy, S. L., Kusumakar, V., Ascher, J. A., Earl, N. L., Greene, P. L., and Monaghan, E. T. (2000) A double-blind, placebo-controlled, prophylaxis study of lamotrigine in rapid-cycling bipolar disorder. Lamictal 614 Study Group. J. Clin. Psychiatry 61, 841–850.
51. Calabrese, J. R., Shelton, M. D., Rapport, D. J., Kimmel, S. E., and Elhaj, O. (2002) Long-term treatment of bipolar disorder with lamotrigine. J. Clin. Psychiatry 63 (Suppl. 10), 18–22.
52. Ohman, I., Vitols, S., and Tomson, T. (2000) Lamotrigine in pregnancy: pharmacokinetics during delivery, in the neonate, and during lactation. Epilepsia 41, 709–713.
53. Mackay, F. J., Wilton, L. V., Pearce, G. L., Freemantle, S. N., and Mann, R. D. (1997) Safety of long-term lamotrigine in epilepsy. Epilepsia 38, 881–886.
54. Rumeau-Rouquette, C., Goujard, J., and Huel, G. (1977) Possible teratogenic effect of phenothiazines in human beings. Teratology 15, 57–64.
55. Slone, D., Siskind, V., Heinonen, O. P., Monson, R. R., Kaufman, D. W., and Shapiro, S. (1977) Antenatal exposure to the phenothiazines in relation to congenital malformations, perinatal mortality rate, birth weight, and intelligence quotient score. Am. J. Obstet. Gynecol. 128, 486–488.
56. Sobel, D. E. (1960) Fetal damage due to ECT, insulin coma, chlorpromazine, or reserpine. Arch. Gen. Psychiatry 2, 606–611.
57. Sexson, W. R. and Barak, Y. (1989) Withdrawal emergent syndrome in an infant associated with maternal haloperidol therapy. J. Perinatol. 9, 170–172.
58. Ayd, F. J., Jr. (1968) Is psychiatry in a crisis because of the complications of the psychopharmaceuticals? Dis. Nerv. Syst. 29, Suppl. 5.
59. Edlund, M. J. and Craig, T. J. (1984) Antipsychotic drug use and birth defects: an epidemiologic reassessment. Compr. Psychiatry 25, 32–37.
60. Goldstein, D. J., Corbin, L. A., and Fung, M. C. (2000) Olanzapine-exposed pregnancies and lactation: early experience. J. Clin. Psychopharmacol. 20, 399–403.
61. Littrell, K. H., Johnson, C. G., Peabody, C. D., and Hilligoss, N. (2000) Antipsychotics during pregnancy. Am. J. Psychiatry 157, 1342.
62. Waldman, M. D. and Safferman, A. Z. (1993) Pregnancy and clozapine. Am. J. Psychiatry 150, 168–169.

63. Dickson, R. A. and Hogg, L. (1998) Pregnancy of a patient treated with clozapine. Psychiatr. Serv. 49, 1081–1083.
64. Stone, S. C., Sommi, R. W., Marken, P. A., Anya, I., and Vaughn, J. (1997) Clozapine use in two full-term pregnancies (letter). J. Clin. Psychiatry 58, 364–365.
65. Gentile, S. (2004) Clinical utilization of atypical antipsychotics in pregnancy and lactation. Ann. Pharmacother. 38, 1265–1271.
66. Koren, G., Cohn, T., Chitayat, D., Kapur, B., Remington, G., Reid, D. M., and Zipursky, R. B. (2002) Use of atypical antipsychotics during pregnancy and the risk of neural tube defects in infants. Am. J. Psychiatry 159: 136–137.
67. McKenna, K., Levinson, A. J., Einarson, A., Diav-Citrin, O., Zipursky, R. B., and Koren, G. (2003) Pregnancy outcome in women receiving atypical antipsychotic drugs: A prospective, multicentre, comparative study. Birth Defects Res. 67: 391.
68. Dicke, J. M. (1989) Teratology: principles and practice. Med. Clin. North Am. 73, 567–582.
69. Langman, J. (1975) Medical Embryology: Human Development—Normal and Abnormal, 3rd ed. Baltimore: Williams & Wilkins.
70. Milkovich, L. and van den Berg, B. J. (1974) Effects of prenatal meprobamate and chlordiazepoxide hydrochloride on human embryonic and fetal development. N. Engl. J. Med. 291, 1268–1271.
71. Aarskog, D. (1975) Letter: Association between maternal intake of diazepam and oral clefts. Lancet 2, 921.
72. Crombie, D. L., Pinsent, R. J., Fleming, D. M., Rumeau-Rouquette, C., Goujard, J., and Huel, G. (1975) Letter: fetal effects of tranquilizers in pregnancy. N. Engl. J. Med. 293, 198–199.
73. Hartz, S. C., Heinonen, O. P., Shapiro, S., Siskind, V., and Slone, D. (1975) Antenatal exposure to meprobamate and chlordiazepoxide in relation to malformations, mental development, and childhood mortality. N. Engl. J. Med. 292, 726–728.
74. Safra, M. J. and Oakley, G. P., Jr. (1975) Association between cleft lip with or without cleft palate and prenatal exposure to diazepam. Lancet 2, 478–480.
75. Saxen, I. and Saxen, L. (1975) Letter: association between maternal intake of diazepam and oral clefts. Lancet 2, 498.
76. Czeizel, A. (1976) Letter: diazepam, phenytoin, and aetiology of cleft lip and/or cleft palate. Lancet 1, 810.
77. Czeizel, A. and Racz, J. (1990) Evaluation of drug intake during pregnancy in the Hungarian Case-Control Surveillance of Congenital Anomalies. Teratology 42, 505–512.
78. Czeizel, A. and Lendvay, A. (1987) In-utero exposure to benzodiazepines (letter). Lancet 1, 628.
79. Rosenberg, L., Mitchell, A. A., Parsells, J. L., Pashayan, H., Louik, C., and Shapiro, S. (1983) Lack of relation of oral clefts to diazepam use during pregnancy. N. Engl. J. Med. 309, 1282–1285.
80. Shiono, P. H. and Mills, J. L. (1984) Oral clefts and diazepam use during pregnancy. N. Engl. J. Med. 311, 919–920.
81. Laegreid, L., Olegard, R., Conradi, N., Hagberg, G., Wahlstrom, J., and Abrahamsson, L. (1990) Congenital malformations and maternal consumption of benzodiazepines: a case-control study. Dev. Med. Child Neurol. 32, 432–441.
82. Bergman, U., Rosa, F. W., Baum, C., Wiholm, B. E., and Faich, G. A. (1992) Effects of exposure to benzodiazepine during fetal life. Lancet 340, 694–696.
83. St Clair, S. M. and Schirmer, R. G. (1992) First-trimester exposure to alprazolam. Obstet. Gynecol. 80, 843–846.

84. Dolovich, L. R., Addis, A., Vaillancourt, J. M., Power, J. D., Koren, G., and Einarson, T. R. (1998) Benzodiazepine use in pregnancy and major malformations or oral cleft: meta-analysis of cohort and case-control studies. BMJ 317, 839–843.
85. Bonnot, O., Vollset, S. E., Godet, P. F., d'Amato, T., Dalery, J., and Robert, E. (2003) [In utero exposure to benzodiazepine. Is there a risk for anal atresia with lorazepam?]. Encephale 29, 553–559.
86. McElhatton, P. R. (1994) The effects of benzodiazepine use during pregnancy and lactation. Reprod. Toxicol. 8, 461–475.
87. Fisher, J. B., Edgren, B. E., Mammel, M. C., and Coleman, J. M. (1985) Neonatal apnea associated with maternal clonazepam therapy: a case report. Obstet. Gynecol. 66, 34S–35S.
88. Gillberg, C. (1977) "Floppy infant syndrome" and maternal diazepam. Lancet 2, 244.
89. Mazzi, E. (1977) Possible neonatal diazepam withdrawal: a case report. Am. J. Obstet. Gynecol. 129, 586–587.
90. Rementeria, J. L. and Bhatt, K. (1977) Withdrawal symptoms in neonates from intrauterine exposure to diazepam. J. Pediatr. 90, 123–126.
91. Rowlatt, R. J. (1978) Effect of maternal diazepam on the newborn. Br. Med J. 1, 985.
92. Speight, A. N. (1977) Floppy-infant syndrome and maternal diazepam and/or nitrazepam. Lancet 2, 878.
93. Whitelaw, A. G., Cummings, A. J., and McFadyen, I. R. (1981) Effect of maternal lorazepam on the neonate. Br. Med. J. (Clin. Res. Ed.) 282, 1106–1108.
94. Laegreid, L., Hagberg, G., and Lundberg, A. (1992) Neurodevelopment in late infancy after prenatal exposure to benzodiazepines—a prospective study. Neuropediatrics 23, 60–67.
95. Ferrill, M. J., Kehoe, W. A., and Jacisin, J. J. (1992) ECT during pregnancy: physiologic and pharmacologic considerations. Convuls. Ther. 8, 186–200.
96. Miller, L. J. (1994) Use of electroconvulsive therapy during pregnancy. Hosp. Commun. Psychiatry 45, 444–450.
97. Dansky, L. V., Rosenblatt, D. S., and Andermann, E. (1992) Mechanisms of teratogenesis: folic acid and antiepileptic therapy 1. Neurology 42, 32–42.
98. Cochran, S. D. (1984) Preventing medical noncompliance in the outpatient treatment of bipolar affective disorders. J. Consult. Clin. Psychol. 52, 873–878.
99. Ehlers, C. L., Frank, E., and Kupfer, D. J. (1988) Social zeitgebers and biological rhythms. A unified approach to understanding the etiology of depression. Arch. Gen. Psychiatry 45, 948–952.
100. Spinelli, M. G. (1997) Interpersonal psychotherapy for depressed antepartum women: a pilot study. Am. J. Psychiatry 154, 1028–1030.
101. Kraepelin, E. (1921) Manic-depressive insanity and paranoia. (Translation of: Psychiatrie: Ein Kurzes Lehrbuch für Studierende und Ärtze, 8th ed.) Edinburgh: Livingstone.
102. Kendell, R. E., Wainwright, S., Hailey, A., and Shannon, B. (1976) The influence of childbirth on psychiatric morbidity. Psychol. Med. 6, 297–302.
103. Baldessarini, R. J., Tondo, L., and Viguera, A. C. (1999) Discontinuing lithium maintenance treatment in bipolar disorders: risks and implications. Bipolar Disord. 1, 17–24.
104. Braftos, O. H. J. (1966) Puerperal mental disorders in manic depressive females. Acta Psychiatr. Scand. 42, 285–294.
105. Reich, T. and Winokur, G. (1970) Postpartum psychoses in patients with manic depressive disease. J. Nerv. Ment. Dis. 151, 60–68.

106. Davidson, J. and Robertson, E. (1985) A follow-up study of post partum illness, 1946-1978. Acta Psychiatr. Scand. 71, 451–457.
107. Klompenhouwer, J. L. and van Hulst, A. M. (1991) Classification of postpartum psychosis: a study of 250 mother and baby admissions in The Netherlands. Acta Psychiatr. Scand. 84, 255–261.
108. Rhode, A. and Marneros, A. (2000) Bipolar disorders during pregnancy, postpartum, and in menopause. In: Marners, A. and Angst, J., ed. Bipolar Disorders: 100 Years After Manic-Depressive Insanity. London: Kluwer Academic Publishers, pp. 127–137.
109. Blehar, M., DePaulo, J., and Gershon, E. (1988) Women with bipolar disorder: findings from the NIMH genetics intiative sample. Psychopharmacol. Bull. 34, 239–243.
110. Kruger, S. and Braunig, P. (2002) Clinical issues in bipolar disorder during pregnancy and the posparturm period. Clin. Approaches Bipolar Disord. 1, 65–71.
111. Cohen, L. S., Sichel, D. A., Robertson, L. M., Heckscher, E., and Rosenbaum, J. F. (1995) Postpartum prophylaxis for women with bipolar disorder. Am. J. Psychiatry 152, 1641–1645.
112. Curtis, V. (2005) Women are not the same as men: specific clinical issues for female patients with bipolar disorder. Bipolar Disord. 7 (Suppl 1), 16–24.
113. Leibenluft, E. (2000) Women and bipolar disorder: an update. Bull. Menninger Clin. 64, 5–17.
114. Parry, B. L. (1989) Reproductive factors affecting the course of affective illness in women. Psychiatr Clin. North Am. 12, 207–220.
115. Wisner, K. L., Hanusa, B. H., Peindl, K. S., and Perel, J. M. (2004) Prevention of postpartum episodes in women with bipolar disorder. Biol. Psychiatry 56, 592–596.
116. Altshuler, L. L., Hendrick, V., and Cohen, L. S. (1998) Course of mood and anxiety disorders during pregnancy and the postpartum period. J. Clin. Psychiatry 59 (Suppl. 2), 29–33.
117. Chaudron, L. H. and Pies, R. W. (2003) The relationship between postpartum psychosis and bipolar disorder: a review. J. Clin. Psychiatry 64, 1284–1292.
118. Sharma, V. and Mazmanian, D. (2003) Sleep loss and postpartum psychosis. Bipolar Disord. 5, 98–105.
119. Strouse, T. B., Szuba, M. P., and Baxter, L. R., Jr. (1992) Response to sleep deprivation in three women with postpartum psychosis. J. Clin. Psychiatry 53, 204–206.
120. Dean, C., Williams, R. J., and Brockington, I. F. (1989) Is puerperal psychosis the same as bipolar manic-depressive disorder? A family study. Psychol. Med. 19, 637–647.
121. McNeil, T. F. (1987) A prospective study of postpartum psychoses in a high-risk group. 2. Relationships to demographic and psychiatric history characteristics. Acta Psychiatr. Scand. 75, 35-43.
122. Suri, R. and Burt, V. K. (1997) The assessment and treatment of postpartum psychiatric disorders. J. Pract. Psychiatry Behav. Health 3, 67-77.
123. Pariser, S. F. (1993) Women and mood disorders. Menarche to menopause. Ann. Clin. Psychiatry 5, 249–254.
124. Stewart, D. E. (1988) Prophylactic lithium in postpartum affective psychosis. J Nerv. Ment. Dis. 176, 485–489.
125. Stewart, D. E., Klompenhouwer, J. L., Kendell, R. E., and van Hulst, A. M. (1991) Prophylactic lithium in puerperal psychosis. The experience of three centres. Br. J. Psychiatry 158, 393–397.

126. Austin, M. P. (1992) Puerperal affective psychosis: is there a case for lithium prophylaxis? Br. J. Psychiatry 161, 692–694.
127. Abou-Saleh, M. T. and Coppen, A. (1983) Puerperal affective disorders and response to lithium. Br. J. Psychiatry 142, 539.
128. van Gent, E. M. and Verhoeven, W. M. (1992) Bipolar illness, lithium prophylaxis, and pregnancy. Pharmacopsychiatry 25, 187–191.
129. Rohde, A. and Marneros, A. (1993) Postpartum psychoses: onset and long-term course. Psychopathology 26, 203–209.
130. Protheroe, C. (1969) Puerperal psychoses: a long term study 1927-1961. Br. J. Psychiatry 115, 9–30.
131. Videbech, P. and Gouliaev, G. (1995) First admission with puerperal psychosis: 7-14 years of follow-up. Acta Psychiatr Scand. 91, 167–173.
132. Wisner, K. L., Peindl, K., and Hanusa, B. H. (1994) Symptomatology of affective and psychotic illnesses related to childbearing. J. Affect. Disord. 30, 77–87.
133. Brokington, I. (1999) Infanticide Motherhood and Mental Health. New York: Oxford University Press, pp. 430–468.
134. d'Orban, P. T. (1979) Women who kill their children. Br. J. Psychiatry 134, 560–571.
135. Platz, C. and Kendell, R. E. (1988) A matched-control follow-up and family study of 'puerperal psychoses'. Br. J. Psychiatry 153, 90–94.
136. Whalley, L. J., Roberts, D. F., Wentzel, J., and Wright, A. F. (1982) Genetic factors in puerperal affective psychoses. Acta Psychiatr. Scand. 65, 180–193.
137. Jones, I. and Craddock, N. (2001) Familiality of the puerperal trigger in bipolar disorder: results of a family study. Am. J. Psychiatry 158, 913–917.
138. Coyle, N., Jones, I., Robertson, E., Lendon, C., and Craddock, N. (2000) Variation at the serotonin transporter gene influences susceptibility to bipolar affective puerperal psychosis. Lancet 356, 1490–1491.
139. Wisner, K. Prevention of postpartum episodes in bipolar women [abstract]. (1997) In: Syllabus and Proceedings Summary of the 151st Ann Meeting American Psychiatric Association (May 17–22) Toronto (ON). Washington, DC, American Psychiatric Association.
140. Viguera, A. C. and Cohen, L. S. (1998) The course and management of bipolar disorder during pregnancy. Psychopharmacol. Bull. 34, 339–346.
141. Burt, V. K., Suri, R., Altshuler, L., Stowe, Z., Hendrick, V. C., and Muntean, E. (2001) The use of psychotropic medications during breast-feeding. Am. J. Psychiatry 158, 1001–1009.
142. (2001) Transfer of drugs and other chemicals into human milk. Pediatrics 108, 776–789.
143. Ito, S. (2000) Drug therapy for breast-feeding women. N. Engl. J. Med. 343, 118–126.
144. Ernst, C. L. and Goldberg, J. F. (2002) The reproductive safety profile of mood stabilizers, atypical antipsychotics, and broad-spectrum psychotropics. J. Clin. Psychiatry 63 (Suppl. 4), 42–55.
145. Llewellyn, A., Stowe, Z. N., and Strader, J. R., Jr. (1998) The use of lithium and management of women with bipolar disorder during pregnancy and lactation. J. Clin. Psychiatry 59 (Suppl. 6), 57–64.
146. Targum, S. D., Davenport, Y. B., and Webster, M. J. (1979) Postpartum mania in bipolar manic-depressive patients withdrawn from lithium carbonate. J. Nerv. Ment. Dis. 167, 572–574.
147. Chaudron, L. H. and Jefferson, J. W. (2000) Mood stabilizers during breastfeeding: a review. J. Clin. Psychiatry 61, 79–90.

148. Leibenluft, E. (1997) Issues in the treatment of women with bipolar illness. *J* Clin. Psychiatry 58 (Suppl. 15), 5–11.

149. Physicians' Desk Reference (2001) Montvale, NJ: Medical Economics Company, Inc.

150. Holmes, L. B., Harvey, E. A., Coull, B. A., Huntington, K. B., Khoshbin, S., Hayes, A. M., and Ryan, L. M. (2001) The teratogenicity of anticonvulsant drugs. N. Engl. J. Med. 344, 1132–1138.

151. Wisner, K. L. and Perel, J. M. (1998) Serum levels of valproate and carbamazepine in breastfeeding mother-infant pairs. J. Clin. Psychopharmacol. 18, 167–169.

152. Stahl, M. M., Neiderud, J., and Vinge, E. (1997) Thrombocytopenic purpura and anemia in a breast-fed infant whose mother was treated with valproic acid. J. Pediatr. 130, 1001–1003.

153. Physicians' Desk Reference (2001). Montvale, NJ: Medical Economics Company, Inc.

154. Iqbal, M. M., Gundlapalli, S. P., Ryan, W. G., Ryals, T., and Passman, T. E. (2001) Effects of antimanic mood-stabilizing drugs on fetuses, neonates, and nursing infants. South. Med. J. 94, 304–322.

155. Kuhnz, W., Jager-Roman, E., Rating, D., Deichl, A., Kunze, J., Helge, H., and Nau, H. (1983) Carbamazepine and carbamazepine-10,11- epoxide during pregnancy and postnatal period in epileptic mother and their nursed infants: pharmacokinetics and clinical effects. Pediatr. Pharmacol. (New York) 3, 199–208.

156. Kaneko, S., Suzuki, K., Sato, T., et al. (1982) The problems of antiepileptic medication in the neonatal period: is breast-feeding advisable? In Janz, D., Dam, M., Richens, A., eds. Epilepsy, Pregnancy, and the Child. New York: Raven Press, pp. 343–348.

157. Niebyl, J. R., Blake, D. A., Freeman, J. M., and Luff, R. D. (1979) Carbamazepine levels in pregnancy and lactation. Obstet. Gynecol. 53, 139–140.

158. Tomson, T., Ohman, I., and Vitols, S. (1997) Lamotrigine in pregnancy and lactation: a case report. Epilepsia 38, 1039–1041.

159. Ohman, I., Tomson, T., and Vitols, S. (1998) Lamotrigine levels in plasma and breast milk in nursing women and their infants. Epilepsia 21(Suppl. 2), 39.

160. Sabers, A., Buchholt, J. M., Uldall, P., and Hansen, E. L. (2001) Lamotrigine plasma levels reduced by oral contraceptives. Epilepsy Res. 47, 151–154.

161. von Unruh, G. E., Froescher, W., Hoffmann, F., and Niesen, M. (1984) Valproic acid in breast milk: how much is really there? Ther. Drug Monit. 6, 272–276.

162. Malone, K., Papagni, K., Ramini, S., and Keltner, N. L. (2004) Antidepressants, antipsychotics, benzodiazepines, and the breastfeeding dyad. Perspect. Psychiatr. Care 40, 73–85.

163. Clozaril product information (2001) In: Physicians' Desk Reference. Montvale, NJ: Medical Economics Company, Inc., pp. 2155–2159.

164. Risperdal product information (2001) In: Physicians' Desk Reference. Montvale, NJ: Medical Economics Company, Inc., pp. 1580–1584.

165. Aripiprazole. Drugdex Drug Evaluations (1974–2003). Thomson MICROMEDEX, Healthcare Series (Vol. 117).

166. Yoshida, K., Smith, B., Craggs, M., and Kumar, R. (1998) Neuroleptic drugs in breast-milk: a study of pharmacokinetics and of possible adverse effects in breast-fed infants. Psychol. Med. 28, 81–91.

167. Zarate, C. A., Jr. (2000) Antipsychotic drug side effect issues in bipolar manic patients. J Clin. Psychiatry 61 (Suppl. 8), 52–61.

168. Goodwin, F. K. and Jamison, K. R. (1990) Manic depressive illness. In: Clinical Guidelines. New York: Oxford University Press, pp. 665–724.

169. (2002) Practice guideline for the treatment of patients with bipolar disorder (revision). Am. J. Psychiatry 159, 1–50.
170. Patrick, M. J., Tilstone, W. J., and Reavey, P. (1972) Diazepam and breast-feeding. Lancet 1, 542–543.
171. Iqbal, M. M., Sobhan, T., and Ryals, T. (2002) Effects of commonly used benzodiazepines on the fetus, the neonate, and the nursing infant. Psychiatr. Serv. 53, 39–49.
172. Darwish, M., Martin, P. T., Cevallos, W. H., Tse, S., Wheeler, S., and Troy, S. M. (1999) Rapid disappearance of zaleplon from breast milk after oral administration to lactating women. J. Clin. Pharmacol. 39, 670–674.
173. Miller, L. J. (2002) Postpartum depression. JAMA 287, 762–765.
174. McElroy, S. L. (2004) Bipolar disorders: special diagnostic and treatment considerations in women. CNS Spectr. 9, 5–18.
175. McElroy, S. L., Arnold, L. M., and Altshuler, L. L. (2005) Bipolarity in women: therapeutic issues. In: Akiskal, H. S., Tohen, M., ed. Bipolar Psychopharmacotherapy: Caring for the Patient. John Wiley & Sons, Ltd.

6

Schizophrenia During Pregnancy and the Postpartum Period

Mary V. Seeman

Summary

The aim of this chapter is to outline the reproductive care needs of women suffering from schizophrenia. After a brief introduction about the illness and the medications used to treat it, the chapter reviews antenatal needs, course of illness during pregnancy, risks to mother and fetus when illness goes untreated, the outcomes of pregnancy for women with schizophrenia, the postpartum course, later outcomes for offspring, the benefits and risks of antipsychotic medication during pregnancy and breast-feeding, and the general services that these women require. Optimal intervention during pregnancy and the postpartum period helps prevent psychiatric disability in the next generation.

Key Words: Schizophrenia; women; pregnancy; breast-feeding; postpartum.

1. INTRODUCTION

Schizophrenia is a complex brain disorder with similar prevalence across races, social strata, cultures, and environments. Worldwide, 1% of individuals are affected. It is a disorder of high heritability *(1)* with symptoms first emerging in men in late adolescence and somewhat later in women *(2)*. The symptoms can be debilitating: profound social withdrawal, mental disorganization, misinterpretation of reality, and misperceptions such as hallucinatory voices. Symptoms that exceed normal experience (e.g., seeing things that others cannot see) are called "positive" symptoms. Diminished experience (e.g., apathy, loss of motivation) is referred to as a "negative" symptom. Also present in schizophrenia are cognitive symptoms—difficulty in focusing attention, difficulty with abstract thinking, memory problems, problems maintaining a meaningful conversation—as well as affective symptoms—

From: *Current Clinical Practice: Psychiatric Disorders in Pregnancy and the Postpartum: Principles and Treatment*
Edited by: V. Hendrick © Humana Press, Totowa, NJ

Table 1
Schizophrenia Symptoms

- Hallucinations
- Delusions
- Motor and thought disorganization
- Social withdrawal, loss of interest and energy
- Mood instability
- Impaired attention (inability to focus/sustain attention)
- Impaired executive function (poor problem solving, reduced ability to learn from mistakes or feedback, reduced capacity to form new concepts)
- Impaired memory (encoding, consolidation, retrieval, and recognition)
- Impaired language processing

behavioral symptoms, and interpersonal symptoms (Table 1). Schizophrenia, untreated, interferes with most activities of everyday life.

On neuropsychological testing, patients with schizophrenia show a pattern of widespread dysfunction. Imaging studies reveal reductions in the size of many brain structures when compared with age and sex controls (3). Schizophrenia is considered to be a genetically determined neurodevelopmental disorder made more severe by environmental factors such as prenatal infections, birth complications, and brain injury. It is very likely that what we currently call schizophrenia will turn out to be a cluster of etiologically different illnesses with overlapping symptoms.

Interpersonal difficulties and the tendency toward isolation mean that individuals with schizophrenia rarely establish committed long-term relationships with the opposite sex. Women with schizophrenia, however, function better than men in the social domain; they do have romantic partners and they do become mothers. Currently, in Europe and North America, approx 60% of women with schizophrenia are mothers (4).

Although pharmacotherapy is only one part of a comprehensive biopsychosocial treatment plan for each individual patient, it is, nevertheless, an essential part. First-generation antipsychotics had many asociated side effects, including extrapyramidal symptoms (EPS) and tardive dyskinesia. In addition, they frequently led to sedation, cognitive impairment, weight gain, diabetes, hyperprolactinemia (associated with sexual and fertility problems), cardiac conduction problems, seizures, postural hypotension, and antimuscarinic effects such as dry mouth, constipation, and urinary retention (5). Second-generation antipsychotic agents, the "atypical" drugs, offer potentially broader symptom control and most clinical guidelines now recommend them as first-line treatments. Claims have been made that they control not only the positive

Table 2
Advantages of Second-Generation Over First-Generation Antipsychotic Drugs

- Improved therapeutic effect in some treatment-resistant patients
- Improved therapeutic effect on negative symptoms and neurocognitive deficits
- Reduced potential to cause acute EPS (akathisia, dystonia, parkinsonism)
- Reduced potential to cause longer-term EPS (e.g., tardive dystonia, tardive dyskinesia, tardive akathisia)
- For some of the newer drugs, reduced potential to elevate prolactin levels

EPS, extrapyramidal symptoms.

Table 3
Atypical Antipsychotic Drugs Used in Schizophrenia

- Risperidone
- Olanzapine
- Quetiapine
- Ziprasidone
- Aripiprazole
- Clozapine

symptoms but also the negative, cognitive, and affective symptoms. Their use brings with it fewer side effects such as EPS (*see* Table 2) and tardive dyskinesia. However, these newer agents have their own unwanted effects: insulin and leptin effects lead to obesity and an increased risk of diabetes (Table 3) *(6)*.

2. ANTENATAL NEEDS OF WOMEN WITH SCHIZOPHRENIA

Fertility is lower among women with schizophrenia than in the general population, but this may change with the widespread use of the newer antipsychotics that do not raise prolactin levels and, thus, do not interfere with conception *(7)*. In a recent publication from Finland that looked at fertility rates of 870,093 individuals born in that country in the 1950s, 1.3% was reported to be patients with schizophrenia. These individuals would still have been treated with first-generation drugs. The mean number of offspring among the patients was 0.83 for women and 0.44 for men, compared with 1.83 and 1.65 among women and men in the general population *(8)*.

In preparation for a healthy pregnancy and optimal mothering, women of childbearing age with a severe, ongoing illness such as schizophrenia require more than standard psychiatric care. They need support and training in many important areas often lacking in even the most comprehensive rehabilitation programs, such as health promotion, family planning, relationship issues, safety issues, and preparation for pregnancy (9,10).

Health promotion includes teaching nutrition and fitness, as well as provision of smoking- and substance-cessation programs. Self-care can be poor in schizophrenia. A pregnant mother needs to consume 2000–2800 calories a day and eat a well-balanced diet that includes vitamins and minerals. Would-be mothers should be prescribed folic acid supplements prior to getting pregnant. Women with schizophrenia have high rates of smoking and alcohol use (11), contributing to increased risks for neonates. Obesity is a major problem in schizophrenia, not only because of the drugs but also because of a relatively sedentary lifestyle and a lack of energy (12). Fast food diets, a result of poverty and lack of motivation and culinary skills, add to the problem. As a consequence, eclampsia and gestational diabetes are added risks of pregnancy (13).

For family planning to be effective in this population, one must take into consideration the cognitive impairments inherent in this illness as well as the vulnerability to uninvited sexual contact and the relative lack of assertiveness (14). Safety counseling is important because women with schizophrenia may be living on the street or in shelters or in unsafe neighborhoods and are consequently easy prey to sexual assault, injury, the transmission of disease, and unwanted pregnancy. Relationship counseling is equally important. Many women report a lack of voice in their relationships and have little experience in maintaining relationships or in ending relationships when they prove unsatisfactory.

Preparation for pregnancy classes or support groups for women with schizophrenia of childbearing age (15) require a focus on the importance of prenatal care should pregnancy occur, available options when the pregnancy is unwanted, education about child development, prepregnancy folate supplementation, explanation about the mandate and authority of child welfare agencies, information about obtaining appropriate family housing, and help with budgeting in preparation for the financial obligations of single parenting.

About half of pregnancies in women with schizophrenia are unplanned (4,16). This implies that these fetuses may well be exposed to nicotine, substances of abuse, and potentially high doses of medications during the first critical trimester of pregnancy.

3. COURSE OF ILLNESS IN PREGNANCY

Most pregnant women with schizophrenia are single and live in poverty, often in poor housing, often estranged from their immediate and extended families (16). Severity of illness over the course of pregnancy varies. It is not known whether changes associated with pregnancy and lactation significantly alter the course of schizophrenia symptoms. For women with chronic severe psychiatric illness across diagnoses, there is a slight but significant reduction in rates of contact with psychiatric services and admissions during pregnancy compared with periods before and after childbirth (17). Although many women experience a lessening of symptoms, some become more delusional, deny the pregnancy, and may try to harm the fetus (18). About 25% of pregnancies are electively terminated in this population (4).

4. RISKS OF UNTREATED ILLNESS TO MOTHER AND FETUS

Becoming a mother is important to most women with schizophrenia (19), and this may paradoxically lead to an abrupt discontinuation of medication, motivated by the wish to not harm the fetus. Subsequent exacerbation of illness may lead to poor self-care and a failure to stay involved with health care providers and family members.

Women with schizophrenia face the stigma associated with their diagnosis—their families, their caregivers, and their communities do not approve of them bearing children. Denial of pregnancy (18) may be a way for psychotic women to deal with that perception—a self-defeating strategy that deprives the pregnant woman of much-needed prenatal care.

5. PREGNANCY OUTCOMES

The available literature points to an increased risk of obstetrical complications in this population (20). A recent study examined nonoptimal pregnancy outcome in schizophrenia. The study sample was comprised of 2096 births by 1438 mothers diagnosed with schizophrenia and 1,555,975 births in the general population. Significantly increased risks for stillbirth, infant death, preterm delivery, low birthweight (LBW), and small-for-gestational-age were found among the offspring of women with schizophrenia. Women with an episode of schizophrenia during pregnancy had a fourfold increased risk of LBW and stillbirth. Controlling for a high incidence of smoking during pregnancy among these women (51 vs 24% in the general population) and other maternal factors (single motherhood, maternal age, parity, maternal education, mother's country of birth, and pregnancy-induced hypertensive diseases) in a multiple regression model reduced the risk estimates markedly. However, the risks for adverse pregnancy outcomes were still doubled for women with an episode of schizophrenia during pregnancy compared with women in the control group even after adjustments were made *(21)*.

An important outcome for these mothers is the loss of parental custody at birth *(22)*. Because of the stigma associated with this diagnosis, women with schizophrenia are frequently prejudged to be incapable of caring for their infant, and their children are apprehended at birth, exposing these women to lifelong experiences of loss and mourning.

6. COURSE OF ILLNESS POSTPARTUM

Of women with schizophrenia, 16% are hospitalized with a postpartum psychosis within 6 mo of giving birth *(4)*. The mechanism by which childbirth precipitates a psychosis may be related to the sudden drop of sex steroids following labor, but studies remain inconclusive. It has been suggested that dopaminergic transmission is increased by postpartum estrogen withdrawal *(23)*. This is an argument for raising the dose of antipsychotic medication after delivery, but the threat of custody loss can paradoxically make these women stay away from their health care providers and stop taking their medications, either because they are afraid they will not hear their infant crying at night or because they think medication use precludes breast-feeding. Strategies for the prevention and clinical management of postpartum exacerbations include early identification of women at risk; close monitoring throughout pregnancy, support and child-care assistance, prompt recognition of impending psychosis, and aggressive pharmacotherapy *(24)*.

If a woman develops a postpartum psychosis, she will generally require admission to the hospital, preferably to a mother and baby unit where she and the baby can be together. On such a unit, all contact between the mother and baby is supervised; as mother's mental health improves, she is encouraged to look after her infant on her own. Pharmacological treatment will depend on the clinical picture and on whether or not the mother is breast-feeding. Electroconvulsive therapy (ECT) can be used *(25)* but is usually reserved for medication resistance. The prognosis for the episode is good, but the effect of even a short acute illness during this critical time may have deleterious effects on the mother–child bond and may precipitate child apprehension by child protective services.

7. LATER OUTCOMES

Children of mothers with schizophrenia are a high-risk group for developing later psychopathology *(26)*. In the Swedish High-Risk Project, the offspring of mothers with schizophrenia ($n = 28$) showed a significantly increased frequency of *Diagnostic and Statistical Manual of Mental Disorders*, 3rd ed., revised, axis I and axis II disorders compared with offspring of controls ($n = 91$). In addition, these children were found to have poor global functioning, high symptom checklist-90 scores, and a history of mental health care and psychopharmacological medication use *(27)*. Some of the early psychopathology of these children may reflect their genetic predisposition to developing schizophrenia *(28)*. This is important to underscore because child protective services can attribute the child's slow development and psychopathology to bad mothering and can, on this basis, remove the child from the mother. This is unfair to a mother who is doing her best with a difficult child under difficult circumstances. It makes more sense to provide the mother with extra supports.

8. ANTIPSYCHOTIC MEDICATIONS IN PREGNANCY

An increase in body fat during pregnancy means greater storage of antipsychotic drugs, all of which are lipophilic *(29)*. Some cytochrome P-450 (CYP) enzymes such as 3A4, which breaks down quetiapine and clozapine, and 2D6, which metabolizes risperidone, are thought to be induced by sex hormones during pregnancy *(30–33)*. This would cause enhanced clearance and *lower* plasma levels for the parent compound. But some drugs, risperidone for example, have active metabolites. There is some evidence, on the other hand, that CYP1A2, the main metabolizing enzyme for olanzapine, is downregulated during pregnancy *(34)*. This would suggest *increased* plasma levels of this drug during pregnancy. Interindividual variations, however, are so great that results of studies in this area are often contradictory *(35,36)*. To add to the complexity, the maternal placenta produces CYP enzymes, as does the fetal liver, very early in fetal life *(37,38)*. This is a built-in safety mechanism to protect the fetal brain from potentially harmful effects of exogenous toxins, but it may paradoxically increase fetal levels of active drug metabolites.

Total protein is reduced during pregnancy, thereby decreasing drug binding and *increasing* the protein-free drug fraction that enters the brain. Glomerular filtration rates increase during pregnancy, speeding up the rate of clearance. Taken together, higher doses of medication are generally required in pregnancy than in the nonpregnant state in order to achieve therapeutic *serum* levels. On the other hand, progressively greater levels of estrogen augment dopamine receptor blockade in the brain so that, for many women with schizophrenia, actual doses needed in order to keep symptoms at bay during pregnancy may be *lower* than were required in the nonpregnant stage *(17)*.

With respect to side effects, in the second trimester of pregnancy there is a physiological drop in blood pressure, which may add to the orthostatic hypotension effects of some antipsychotic drugs (clozapine, quetiapine). Constipation, which is common in pregnancy, may be worsened by medications with anticholinergic side effects (olanzapine, clozapine). The sedation induced by some antipsychotics (olanzapine, quetiapine, clozapine) must also be taken into consideration, especially after childbirth *(39)*.

9. ANTIPSYCHOTIC EFFECTS ON PREGNANCY OUTCOMES

No medication regimen can be considered completely safe during pregnancy. By the same token, the added risk is often minimal and far smaller than the risk of the mother going untreated. Women with schizophrenia have been found to be at relatively increased risk for poor obstetrical outcomes, including preterm delivery, LBW, and neonates who are small for their gestational age *(40)*. This may, in part, be the effect of medications but is, to a large extent, attributable to these women's relative lack of prenatal care, poor nutrition, alcohol, nicotine, and drug use, higher body mass index, poverty, and general lack of self-care.

Teratogens affect those structures that are undergoing rapid change at the time of exposure. For the central nervous system, that means weeks 2–4 of pregnancy. The greater the dose of the teratogen, the greater is the effect. Teratogens can affect behavior as well as structure, and this may not be obvious at birth. The long-term effects of potential behavioral teratogens depend to a large extent on the quality of the postnatal environment and on the genetic makeup of the child. Not all fetuses are equally affected by identical exposure.

The consensus is that use of low-potency phenothiazines (coventional antipsychotics) during the first trimester increases the risk of congenital abnormalities by an additional 4 cases per 1000 (odds ratio = 1.21; $p = 0.04$) *(39)*. Not enough is known about the safety of the now more commonly used atypical drugs, but because of substantial weight gain *(41)*, a theoretical risk of neural tube defects has been raised *(42)*. Novartis has data on 200 cases of clozapine in pregnancy *(43)*. This indicates a 6% rate of malformations in infants, but the rate is probably artificially elevated because it represents only those pregnancy outcomes that were spontaneously reported to Novartis. The company recommends monitoring blood glucose and lipids during pregnancy, especially in women who are obese, glucose intolerant, or who have a family history of diabetes. The effect on the course of labor is uncertain; there has been one report of neonatal convulsions 8 d after birth and one report of floppy infant syndrome. There is the theoretical possibility of idiosyncratic drug-induced agranulocytosis in the fetus/neonate and not in the mother. There have been no reports of developmental delays, but the Company recommends low doses during pregnancy because the plasma concentration of clozapine is higher in the fetus than in the mother, and it also recommends against breast-feeding.

The Lilly Worldwide Pharmacovigilance Safety Database has outcomes available from 96 prospectively ascertained and 67 retrospectively ascertained olanzapine-exposed pregnancies. Spontaneous abortion occurred in 13%, stillbirth in 3%, major malformation in 1%, and prematurity in 2%—all within the range of normal historical control rates *(44)*. There are other case reports attesting to the safety of olanzapine *(45,46)*, of risperidone *(47)*, and of quetiapine in pregnancy *(48,49)*. It is likely that each drug demonstrates somewhat different pharmacokinetics during pregnancy and that the risks, such as they are, are different for each individual drug. The main message is that it is much safer for the baby when mothers are treated for their problems. Babies need healthy mothers.

10. BREAST-FEEDING

Postpartum, the doses of antipsychotics generally need to be raised in order to prevent postpartum exacerbation of illness. Antipsychotic drugs are lipid soluble but highly protein-bound, so that plasma:milk ratios are high. The amount of antipsychotics found in breast milk is usually less than 30% of that found in maternal plasma. Nonetheless, because infants have little body fat, reduced protein binding, and lower excretion rates, the effects of drugs absorbed through breast-feeding can affect the infant's central nervous system.

Delayed development at 12–18 mo of age has been reported for three infants exposed to a combination of the first-generation antipsychotics, haloperidol and chlorpromazine. Because only one of the three infants had detectable serum levels of the drug, this finding is hard to interpret *(50)*. One report indicates a low level of olanzapine in infant plasma (compared with mother) and a level during breast-feeding that was

undetectable *(51)*. No adverse effects attributable to olanzapine ingestion through breast-feeding were noted in three infants exposed both *in
utero* and through nursing *(44)*. Ilett and colleagues *(51)* recently studied
the transfer of risperidone and 9-hydroxyrisperidone into breast milk in
three women. Neither risperidone nor its active metabolite was detected
in the plasma of the breast-fed infants and no adverse effects were noted.
The relative infant dose was substantially lower than the arbitrary 10%
of putative therapeutic dose for an infant of similar size—the accepted
standard for threshold of concern *(52)*. To be safe, breast-feeding mothers are advised to take their daily antipsychotic medication in divided
doses right after breast-feeding at least until the infant matures (6 wk)
(53–55). It is recommended that all breast-fed infants of mothers with
schizophrenia be closely monitored by a pediatrician. Depending on
circumstance, a possible strategy is to alternate breast- and bottle-feeding
in order to minimize infant exposure for the first months of life (mother's
milk is expressed and discarded to ensure continuing lactation).

11. SERVICES REQUIRED FOR WOMEN WITH SCHIZOPHRENIA DURING CHILDBEARING YEARS

There is a need for integrated services that can provide antenatal,
pregnancy, and postpartum comprehensive care to women with schizophrenia. When the child is born, these women can benefit from home
visitors who focus on enhancing the mother's responsiveness to infant
cues (although home visitors are not always welcome) *(56)*. Parent
coaching teaches mothers how to play with their infants and helps them
to respond in a soothing way to an infant in distress. Such interventions
enhance a mother's feeling of effectiveness and demonstrate good infant
outcomes *(57)*. A multisystemic approach works well with high-risk
families *(58)*. This approach uses a variety of treatments, including family therapy, parent coaching, supportive therapy for the mother, social
skills training, and case management and advocacy. The first stage of
intervention includes an assessment of the risk, protective factors, and
identified needs of the family in order to choose the most suitable interventions. Ongoing monitoring and assessment is necessary to determine
whether any adjustments to the standard intervention are necessary for
a particular mother–infant dyad. Linkages with mother's mental health
providers and other community services are essential.

To help improve services for parents with psychotic disorders, a survey was conducted in three Australian treatment agencies. Of the 342
individuals who participated in the study, 124 were parents. Forty-eight
parents in the study had children under the age of 16, and 20 of these

parents (42%) had children living with them. Most parents in this study relied on relatives or friends for assistance with child care. Barriers to child-care services identified by the parents were inability to pay, lack of local services, and fear of losing custody *(59)*. Some important characteristics of needed services were identified as (a) a family-centered service in an easily accessible location that includes multiple supports, such as daycare, bus/cab fares, and case managers for parents and children and (b) a well-advertised single point of entry to mental health services that include psychoeducation, parent workshops and support groups, and shared care programs (liaison with family doctors, obstetricians, pediatricians). Therapeutic daycare programs for the infants are ideal to ensure proper nutrition, sensitive interactions, and safety.

12. CONCLUSION

Women with schizophrenia are a group for whom family education, pregnancy, and parenting services have not traditionally been regarded as necessary. As these women become integrated into community living, it is important to anticipate pregnancy and to provide the necessary education, support, and services to ensure successful parenting. In this way, the children of these disadvantaged mothers will not themselves become disadvantaged. Prevention of psychiatric disability is difficult because much of the toll is a result of inherited factors and chance occurrence. The most profitable area for prevention is early on, during the pregnancy of mentally ill mothers. The children born to these mothers are at high genetic risk and at high parenting risk. Knowledgeable intervention at the time of pregnancy is the most effective strategy available in the prevention of second-generation psychiatric disorder.

REFERENCES

1. Bramon, E. and Sham, P. C. (2001) The common genetic liability between schizophrenia and bipolar disorder: a review. Curr. Psychiatry Rep. 3, 332–337.
2. Cohen, R., Seeman, M. V., Gotowiec, A., et al. (1999) Earlier puberty as a predictor of later onset of schizophrenia in women. Am. J. Psychiatry 156, 1059–1064.
3. Javitt, D. C. and Coyle, J. T. (2004) Decoding schizophrenia. Sci. Am. (Jan.), 32–39.
4. Barkla, J., Byrne, L., Hearle, J., et al. (2000) Pregnancy in women with psychotic disorder. Arch. Women's Ment. Health 3, 23–26.
5. Lambert, T. J. and Castle, D. J. (2003) Pharmacological approaches to the management of schizophrenia. Med. J. Aust. 178 (Suppl.), S57–S61.
6. Sernyak, M. J., Leslie, D. L., Alarcon, R. D., et al. (2002) Association of diabetes mellitus with use of atypical neuroleptics in the treatment of schizophrenia. Am. J. Psychiatry 159, 561–566.

7. Howard, L. M., Kumar, C., Leese, M., et al. (2002) The general fertility rate in women with psychotic disorders. Am. J. Psychiatry 159, 991–997.

8. Haukka, J., Suvisaari, J., and Lonnqvist, J. (2003) Fertility of patients with schizophrenia, their siblings, and the general population: a cohort study from 1950 to 1959 in Finland. Am. J. Psychiatry 160, 460–463.

9. Korenbrot, C. C., Steinberg, A., Bender, C., et al. (2002) Preconception care: a systematic review. Matern. Child Health J. 6, 75–88.

10. Seeman, M. V. (2004) Schizophrenia and motherhood. In: Göpfert, M., Webster, J., and Seeman, M.V., eds. Parental Psychiatric Disorder: Distressed Parents and Their Families, 2nd ed. Cambridge: Cambridge University Press, pp. 161–171.

11. Vanable, P. A., Carey, M. P., Carey, K. B., et al. (2003) Smoking among psychiatric outpatients: relationship to substance use, diagnosis, and illness severity. Psychol. Addict. Behav. 17, 259–265.

12. Tardieu, S., Micallef, J., Gentile, S., et al. (2003)Weight gain profiles of new antipsychotics: public health consequences. Obes. Rev. 4, 129–138.

13. Bryson, C. L., Ioannou, G. N., Rulyak, S. J., et al. (2003) Association between gestational diabetes and pregnancy-induced hypertension. Am. J. Epidemiol. 158, 148–153.

14. Miller, L. J. and Finnerty, M. (1998) Family planning knowledge, attitudes and practices in women with schizophrenic spectrum disorders. J. Psychosom. Obstet. Gynaecol. 19, 210–217.

15. Huebner, C. E., Tyll, L., Luallen, J., et al. (2001) PrePare: a program of enhanced prenatal services within health-maintenance organization settings. Health Educ. Res. 16, 71–80.

16. Rudolph, B., Larson, G. I., Sweeney, S., et al. (1990) Hospitalized pregnant psychotic women: characteristics and treatment issues. Hosp. Comm. Psychiatry 41, 159–163.

17. Seeman, M. and Lang, M. (1990) The role of estrogens in schizophrenia gender differences. Schizophrenia Bull. 16, 185–194.

18. Miller, L. J. (1990) Psychotic denial of pregnancy: phenomenology and clinical management. Hosp.Comm. Psychiatry 41, 1233–1237.

19. Savvidou, I., Bozikas, V. P., Hatzigeleki, S., et al. (2003) Narratives about their children by mothers hospitalized on a psychiatric unit. Fam. Proc. 42, 391–402.

20. Sacker, A., Done, D. J. and Crow, T. J. (1996) Obstetric complications in children born to parents with schizophrenia: a meta-analysis of case-control studies. Psychol. Med. 26, 279–287.

21. Nilssonm, E., Lichtenstein, P., Cnattingius, S., et al. (2002) Women with schizophrenia: pregnancy outcome and infant death among their offspring. Schizophr. Res. 58, 221–229.

22. Homas, T. and Tori, C. D. (1999) Sequelae of abortion and relinquishment of child custody among women with major psychiatric disorders. Psychol. Rep. 84, 773–790.

23. Grigoriadis, S. and Seeman, M. V. (2002) The role of estrogen in schizophrenia: Implications for schizophrenia practice guidelines for women. Can. J. Psychiatry 47, 437–442.

24. Sharma, V. (2003) Pharmacotherapy of postpartum psychosis. Expert Opin. Pharmacother. 4, 1651–1658.

25. Reed, P., Sermin, N., Appleby, L., et al. (1999) A comparison of clinical response to electroconvulsive therapy in puerperal and non-puerperal psychoses. J. Affect. Disord. 54, 255–260.

26. Niemi, L. T., Suvisaari, J. M., Tuulio-Henriksson, A., et al. (2003) Childhood developmental abnormalities in schizophrenia: evidence from high-risk studies. Schizophr. Res. 60, 239–258.

27. Schubert, E. W. and McNeil, T. F. (2003) Prospective study of adult mental disturbance in offspring of women with psychosis. Arch. Gen. Psychiatry 60, 473–480.

28. Hans, S. L., Auerbach, J. G., Asarnow, J. R., et al. (2000) Social adjustment of adolescents at risk for schizophrenia: the Jerusalem Infant Development Study. J. Am. Acad. Child Adolesc. Psychiatry 39, 1406–1414.

29. Dawes, M. and Chowienczyk, P. J. (2001) Drugs in pregnancy. Pharmacokinetics in pregnancy. Best Pract. Res. Clin. Obstet. Gynaecol. 15, 819–826.

30. Schwartz, J. B. (2003) The influence of sex on pharmacokinetics. Clin. Pharmacokinet. 42, 107–121.

31. Meibohm, B., Beierle, I., and Derendorf, H. (2002) How important are gender differences in pharmacokinetics? Clin. Pharmacokinet. 41, 329–342.

32. Hagg, S., Spigset, O., and Dahlqvist, R. (2001) Influence of gender and oral contraceptives on CYP2D6 and CYP2C19 activity in healthy volunteers. Br. J. Clin. Pharmacol. 51, 169–173.

33. Wadelius, M., Darj, E., Frenne, G., et al. (1997) Induction of CYP2D6 in pregnancy. Clin. Pharmacol. Ther. 62, 400–407.

34. Zaigler, M., Rietbrock, S., Szymanski, J., et al. (2000) Variation of CYP1A2-dependent caffeine metabolism during menstrual cycle in healthy women. Int. J. Clin. Pharmacol. Ther. 38, 235–244.

35. McCune, J. S., Lindley, C., Decker, J. L., et al. (2001) Lack of gender differences and large intrasubject variability in cytochrome P450 activity measured by phenotyping with dextromethorphan. J. Clin. Pharmacol. 41, 723–731.

36. Lind, A. B., Wadelius, M., Darj, E., et al. (2003) Gene expression of cytochrome P450 1B1 and 2D6 in leukocytes in human pregnancy. Pharmacol. Toxicol. 92, 295–299.

37. Hakkola, J., Raunio, H., Purkunen, R., et al. (1996) Detection of cytochrome P450 gene expression in human placenta in first trimester of pregnancy. Biochem. Pharmacol. 52, 379–383.

38. de Wildt, S. N., Kearns, G. L., Leeder, J. S., et al. (1999) Cytochrome P450 3A: ontogeny and drug disposition. Clin. Pharmacokinet. 37, 485–505.

39. Pinkofsky, H. B. (2000) Effects of antipsychotics on the unborn child: what is known and how should this influence prescribing? Paediatr. Drugs 2, 83–90.

40. Patton, S. W., Misri, S., Corral, M. R., et al. (2002) Antipsychotic medication during pregnancy and lactation in women with schizophrenia: evaluating the risk. Can. J. Psychiatry 47, 959–965.

41. Meyer, J. M. (2001) Effects of atypical antipsychotics on weight and serum lipid levels. J. Clin. Psychiatry 62 (Suppl. 27), 27–34.

42. Koren, G., Cohn, T., Chitayat, D., et al. (2002) Use of atypical antipsychotics during pregnancy and the risk of neural tube defects in infants. Am. J. Psychiatry 159, 136–137.

43. Nguyen, H. N. and Lalonde, P. (2003) Clozapine and pregnancy. Encephale 29, 119–124.

44. Goldstein, D. J., Corbin, L. A., and Fung, M. C. (2000) Olanzapine-exposed pregnancies and lactation: early experience. J. Clin. Psychopharmacol. 20, 399–403.

45. Malek-Ahmadi, P. (2001) Olanzapine in pregnancy. Ann. Pharmacother. 35, 1294–1295.

46. Mendhekar, D. N., War, L., Sharma, J. B., et al. (2002) Olanzapine and pregnancy. Pharmacopsychiatry 35, 122–123.
47. Ratnayake, T. and Libretto, S. E. (2002) No complications with risperidone treatment before and throughout pregnancy and during the nursing period. J. Clin. Psychiatry 63, 76–77.
48. Taylor, T. M., O'Toole, M. S., Ohlsen, R. I., et al. (2003) Safety of quetiapine during pregnancy. Am. J. Psychiatry 160, 588–589.
49. Tenyi, T., Trixler, M., and Keresztes, Z. (2002) Quetiapine and pregnancy. Am. J. Psychiatry 159, 674.
50. Yoshida, K., Smith, B., Craggs, M., et al. (1998) Neuroleptic drugs in breast-milk: a study of pharmacokinetics and of possible adverse effects in breast-fed infants. Psychol. Med. 28, 81–91.
51. Ilett, K. F., Hackett, L. P., Kristensen, J. H., et al. (2004)Transfer of risperidone and 9-hydroxyrisperidone into human milk. Ann. Pharmacother. 38, 273–276.
52. Kirchheiner, J., Berghofer, A., and Bolk-Weischedel, D. (2000) Healthy outcome under olanzapine treatment in a pregnant woman. Pharmacopsychiatry 33, 78–80.
53. Arnon, J., Shechtman, S., and Ornoy, A. (2000) The use of psychiatric drugs in pregnancy and lactation. Isr. J. Psychiatry Relat. Sci. 37, 205–222.
54. Burt, V. K., Suri, R., Altshuler, L., et al. (2001) The use of psychotropic medications during breast-feeding. Am. J. Psychiatry 158, 1001–1009.
55. Ernst, C. L. and Goldberg, J. F. (2002) The reproductive safety profile of mood stabilizers, atypical antipsychotics, and broad-spectrum psychotropics. J. Clin. Psychiatry 63(Suppl. 4), 42–55.
56. Knott, M. and Latter, S. (1999) Help or hindrance? Single, unsupported mothers' perceptions of health visiting. J. Adv. Nurs. 30, 580–588.
57. Juffer, F., Hoksbergen, R. A. C., Riksen-Walraven, J. M., et al (1997) Early intervention in adoptive families. Supporting maternal sensitive responsiveness, infant-mother attachment and infant competence. J. Child Psychol. Psychiatry 18, 1039–1050.
58. Henggeler, S. W., Schoenwald, S. K,. and Pickrel, S. G. (1995) Multisystemic therapy: bridging the gap between university- and community-based treatment. J. Consult. Clin. Psychol. 63, 709–717.
59. Hearle, J., Plant, K., Jenner, L., et al. (1999) A survey of contact with offspring and assistance with child care among parents with psychotic disorders. Psychiatr. Serv. 50, 1354–1356.

7

Pregnancy and Substance Abuse

Karen A. Miotto, Elizabeth Suti,
Monique M. Hernandez,
and Phivan L. Pham

Summary

Knowledge of substance use disorders is essential for health care providers treating pregnant women. Early intervention is vital to improve the health and welfare of both the mother and child. This chapter provides an overview of the consequences and treatments of maternal substance use disorders during pregnancy and breast-feeding. Effective techniques for assessment and intervention are reviewed, as well as psychosocial problems that often accompany maternal substance abuse. Information about various illicit drugs is presented along with strategies for managing withdrawal symptoms. This chapter also outlines potential short- and long-term effects on the child from drug exposure during pregnancy and breast-feeding. Reporting and legal issues are addressed for cases of drug- and/or alcohol-dependent women who present late in pregnancy or who do not respond to available treatments before delivery.

Key Words: Women; substance abuse; pregnancy; breast-feeding.

1. INTRODUCTION

Pregnancy provides an important opportunity for health care providers to intervene with substance-using women. For some women, the thought of giving birth provides a powerful motivation to stop using substances or to seek addiction treatment. Intervention early in pregnancy optimizes the chance of a successful outcome.

Substance abuse ranges from occasional use to end-stage dependency. A woman may inadvertently engage in substance use before realizing she is pregnant. Women who are able to stop using once they are aware of their pregnancy may only need information about the possible fetal

From: *Current Clinical Practice: Psychiatric Disorders in Pregnancy and the Postpartum: Principles and Treatment*
Edited by: V. Hendrick © Humana Press, Totowa, NJ

effects of drugs and alcohol. Treating more advanced addictive disease requires multidisciplinary intervention and care. Key components include assessment, comprehensive obstetrical care, accessible substance abuse treatment, and ideally a continuum of follow-up treatment that supports women in their recovery and assists them with parenting issues. Substance-dependent pregnant women are best treated in specialized residential treatment facilities, when available.

The first part of this chapter provides information on the screening, assessment, and establishment of rapport with pregnant substance-using patients. The second part reviews information about the epidemiology of drug and alcohol use in pregnancy, patterns of use, and the consequences of maternal, fetal, and neonatal exposure to drugs and alcohol. In addition, legal aspects that arise in the treatment of the pregnant substance-dependent woman are addressed. The effects of cigarette smoking are beyond the scope of this chapter. However, cigarette smoking has been shown to produce adverse perinatal effects that confound studies of the maternal effects of drugs and alcohol.

The establishment of a therapeutic relationship with a pregnant substance user can be challenging for several reasons. Patients with severe addictive diseases often leave health care providers with a sense of frustration and hopelessness. Furthermore, pregnant addicts use drugs and alcohol at times with seemingly no regard for the fetus. It is important for clinicians to keep in mind that most pregnant women want to stop using drugs and alcohol, but many are unable to do so without the help of treatment. Addicted pregnant women experience guilt and shame because of their substance use, but, paradoxically, they sometimes continue to use substances to escape feelings of worthlessness and failure. The stigma and potential legal consequences of drug and alcohol use present an additional obstacle for women considering treatment. Finally, it is important to remember that many pregnant women with substance use disorders have been affected by a history of poor parenting and may be repeating maladaptive coping patterns.

2. ASSESSMENT AND SCREENING FOR SUBSTANCE ABUSE DURING PREGNANCY

Substance abuse assessment should be a routine part of prenatal care and is often best addressed while discussing other behavioral issues such as nutrition and exercise (1). It is important to inquire about the use of prescription and nonprescription drugs, as well as caffeine, tobacco, and alcohol. Noting the dosage, frequency, duration of use, and route of administration is an essential part of the history of illicit drug and alcohol use. A clinical assessment using addiction-screening instruments should be done with every pregnant patient, not just those in whom substance use is suspected. If possible, the health care provider who will have an ongoing relationship with the patient should perform the screening. Screening should continue throughout the pregnancy and may reveal more information on subsequent visits, as the patient's trust may increase with time. Obtaining a good substance use history is frequently dependent on the quality of the relationship the clinician is able to establish with the patient *(1)*. Inquiring about patterns of alcohol and drug use and providing education is an important part of routine care, even if the patient denies use *(2)*. It is critical to inquire about the substance use history of the woman's partner and to include the partner in the education process.

Brief interview-based screening methods are effective for obtaining patients' self-reports of substance use. However, a national survey of 856 primary care physicians and psychiatrists found that 32% did not routinely inquire about alcohol and drug consumption *(3)*. Reasons cited included the perceived lack of brief, well-validated screening tools for illicit drugs and alcohol and the lack of evidence of screening benefits. Many physicians are concerned that patients do not want to be asked about their drug use, or will not offer such information, despite reports that patients willingly disclose sensitive information to physicians *(3)*.

In fact, brief screening tools do exist. Examples of brief screening tools include the Five Ps questionnaire *(4)* and the Addiction Severity Index Pregnancy Status questionnaire(22 questions), which can be ordered from the National Clearinghouse for Alcohol and Drug Information (NCADI) *(5)*. The Five Ps questionnaire can be completed without considerable time expenditure:

1. Do you consider either of your parents to be an alcoholic or addict?
2. Does your partner have a problem with tobacco, alcohol, or other drugs? (Adding "his temper" to this list can help screen for domestic violence.)
3. What is your prior smoking history?
4. How much alcohol, drugs, or tobacco have you used in your past?
5. How much alcohol, tobacco, or other drugs have you used during this pregnancy?

Question 5 can be reframed by asking, "In the month before you knew you were pregnant, how much alcohol, tobacco, or other drugs did you use?" Physicians found more success when they did this. A response of "yes" to questions 3, 4, or 5 should be followed with further assessment *(4)*.

In addition to the clinical assessment, the following factors help identify patients at risk for substance abuse or dependence. These should alert the clinician to request further information. Although most of the following are not exclusive to substance abuse, they are likely to be present in serious psychiatric disorders, including addiction (6):

- History of previous or current substance use by pregnant woman and/or significant other
- Physical evidence (e.g., track marks, dilated pupils, poor weight gain, strange behavior)
- Noncompliance with prenatal care
- Symptoms of drug or alcohol withdrawal in the mother
- History of hepatitis B or C, HIV infection, or sexually transmitted disease
- Previous or current history of placental abruption or unexplained vaginal bleeding
- Previous child with fetal alcohol syndrome (FAS) or fetal alcohol effects (FAE)
- Preterm labor
- Intrauterine growth retardation (IUGR)
- History of significant mental illness
- Homelessness
- Domestic violence
- Child protective services involvement

In addition to clinical signs and symptoms, lab tests, such as drug-of-abuse screens, are helpful in making an objective diagnosis of addiction. However, such tests cannot distinguish between dependent and occasional users. Patients who dispute the results of an initial drug-of-abuse screen should be given the opportunity to have a test repeated as soon as possible. The sensitivity for detecting substance use depends on when the drug was last used. Marijuana can be detected in urine even after 14–30 d in daily users, but detection of cocaine, opiates, amphetamines, and barbiturates is possible only 2–4 d after use. Clinicians should be aware that drug users who wish to avoid drug detection may employ various techniques, including diluting or adulterating the sample, diuretic use, or the use of other substances to interfere with drug testing. A more detailed review of information about drug assessment during pregnancy is available on the Columbia University website (7).

3. EPIDEMIOLOGY OF SUBSTANCE ABUSE AND PREGNANCY

In 2002, the National Survey on Drug Use and Health (NSDUH) reported that pregnant women aged 15–25 yr were more likely to use illicit drugs and/or alcohol than pregnant women aged 26–44 (8). For example, the rate of past-month binge alcohol use among the younger group was 5% as compared with 2% in the older group. Drug use also varied by ethnic group, with approx 6% of black women, 4% of white women, and 2% of Hispanic women reporting using illicit drugs in the past month. The data were drawn from self-report surveys, which provide only a limited view of the extent of drug and alcohol use in pregnancy.

Treatment programs provide an additional source of epidemiological data. In the 2002 Drug and Alcohol Services Information System report, 4% of the 363,000 women of childbearing age (15–44 yr) who entered treatment were known to be pregnant at the time of admission *(9)*. Compared with their nonpregnant counterparts, pregnant women 15–44 yr of age were more likely to report cocaine/crack (22 vs 17%), amphetamines/methamphetamines (21 vs 13%), and marijuana (17 vs 13%) as their primary substance of abuse and less likely to report alcohol (18 vs 31%) *(9)*.

Although maternal substance abuse crosses all socioeconomic groups, many pregnant addicts encounter multiple socioenvironmental risk factors. Unstable home environments, exposure to violence, and the presence of co-occurring psychiatric disorders are not uncommon. Major risk factors for substance abuse in women include a history of childhood sexual or physical abuse, and/or a spouse or partner who abuses substances *(10,11)*. Another important risk factor is domestic violence; victims of violence are significantly more likely to abuse substances during pregnancy *(12,13)*.

4. MATERNAL ALCOHOL USE

4.1 Epidemiology of Fetal Alcohol Exposure

The 2001–2002 National Epidemiologic Survey on Alcohol and Related Conditions showed that the number of American adults who abuse alcohol increased from 13.8 million (7.41%) in 1991–1992 to 17.6 million (8.46%) in 2001–2002 (National Institute on Alcohol Abuse and Alcoholism) *(14)*. The accessibility of alcohol and its status as a legal substance is cause for concern because women who are unaware of their pregnancy may continue drinking. According to a cross-sectional study of 13,417 women, 45% reported consuming alcohol during the 3 mo before finding out they were pregnant, whereas 5% reported consuming six or more drinks per week *(15)*. Risk factors for frequent drinking during the periconceptional period included being one or more of the following: unmarried, a smoker, white non-Hispanic, 25 yr of age or older, or college-educated *(15)*. A role of health care providers is to educate women of childbearing age to consider the effects of drinking in cases of unknown pregnancy.

Efforts to decrease the level of alcohol consumption among pregnant women have included media campaigns and beverage warning labels. In the United States, Congress passed the Alcoholic Beverage Warning Label Act in 1988, requiring that warning labels be attached to all containers of alcoholic beverages. Several studies with select populations have determined that the media attention given to the hazardous effects of alcohol consumption on the fetus during pregnancy appear to have had a beneficial impact in both increasing awareness about the dangers and decreasing alcohol consumption during pregnancy *(16,17)*.

Despite the beverage warning labels, prenatal exposure to alcohol far exceeds exposure to illicit drugs. By one recent estimate, women give birth to more than 2.6 million infants exposed to alcohol each year *(18)*. Disorders associated with prenatal alcohol exposure include FAS, FAE, alcohol-related birth defects (ARBDs), and alcohol-related neurodevelopmental disorder. FAS is the most severe condition that affects the fetus when a woman drinks during pregnancy. It is a life-long, physically and mentally disabling condition. FAS is the most common cause of preventable mental retardation and birth defects *(19,20)*. FAS affects between 1.3 and 2.2 children per 1000 live births annually in North America *(18)*. Researchers estimate that cases of alcohol-related birth defects (ARBDs) exceed those of FAS by a ratio of 2:1 to 3:1 *(21)*.

4.2. FAS/FAE

The pattern of teratogenic malformations first observed by Jones et al. in 1973, linking "maternal alcoholism and aberrant morphogeneses in the offspring," was termed "fetal alcohol syndrome" *(20)*. The Fetal Alcohol Study Group of the Research Society on Alcoholism suggested that the diagnosis be made when there are visible markers in each of three categories *(22)*:

1. IUGR
2. Central nervous system (CNS) abnormality (neurological and intellectual impairments: retardation or intellectual delay)
3. At least two of the following craniofacial dysmorphologies:
   a. microcephaly
   b. micro-ophthalmia and/or short palpebral fissures
   c. poorly developed philtrum, thin upper lip, or flattening of the maxillary area

Other abnormalities associated with FAS include organ deformities such as heart defects, heart murmurs, genital malformations, and kidney and urinary defects. Skeletal deformities include deformed ribs and sternum, curved spine, and hip dislocations. Bent, fused, webbed, or missing fingers or toes have also been described.

High blood alcohol levels are believed to increase the risk for FAS. Alcohol can have detrimental effects on the fetus throughout gestation, but the greatest risks occur in the first trimester during the embryonic stage. Alcohol passes through the placenta to the fetus when a woman drinks. Even intermittent binge drinking can be dangerous to the fetus. Factors believed to be associated with the development of FAS include the following (23):

1. Frequency and quantity of maternal alcohol consumption during pregnancy
2. Timing of alcohol intake during gestation
3. Stage of development of the fetus at the time of its exposure to alcohol
4. Nutritional status of the mother and her intake of other drugs
5. Genetic background of the mother
6. Mother's overall state of health

FAS includes somatic and behavioral manifestations. Malformations of the head and face are the most common (20,23,24). In one study, the craniofacial characteristics found in children of heavy drinkers included bulged forehead, deep nasal bridge, upturned nose, indistinct cupid bow, thin upper lip, and retrognathia or recessed jaw (25). Behavioral effects commonly seen in FAS neonates include hyperactivity, hyperresponsiveness, hyperacusis, hypotonia, and tremulousness (26).

The effects of alcohol on a fetus fall on a continuum, and there is no precise distinction between FAS and FAE. Fetal alcohol effects describe a less severe pattern of damage that primarily affects behavior (27). The incidence rate of FAE is difficult to determine because the symptoms are not as specific as FAS. However, FAE is believed to occur more frequently than FAS (21).

4.3. Effects of Prenatal Exposure to Alcohol Throughout Life

The effects of FAS/FAE continue throughout the child's lifespan. Adolescents and adults diagnosed with FAS have lower than average intellectual functioning and are significantly more likely to need supplemental help in school (28). Arithmetic deficits appear to be one of the most characteristic academic disabilities of FAS (28).

Attention deficits, problems with judgment and comprehension, and conduct disorders are common characteristics of persons with FAS/FAE. People with FAS/FAE often have problems with memory functioning, making it difficult to fulfill obligations at school or work (29). Most children diagnosed with fetal alcohol-related problems are not identified at birth. They are identified when they reach school age and are referred to a counselor as a result of a learning disability or an attention deficit disorder. If clinicians can identify alcohol-related effects early, interventions can minimize their potential impact *(30)*.

4.4. Treatment for Alcohol Withdrawal Symptoms

Alcohol-dependent women who suddenly cease drinking may experience withdrawal symptoms that could be threatening to the mother, particularly if she has a history of withdrawal delirium or seizures. An additional concern is that alcohol withdrawal may also cause fetal distress. If a woman is experiencing alcohol withdrawal symptoms, inpatient detoxification is recommended. Most programs treat alcohol withdrawal in pregnant women with benzodiazepines. Benzodiazepines were previously thought to increase birth defects; however, recent studies have not supported this claim. Pooled data from cohort studies show no association between brief fetal exposure to benzodiazepines and the risk of major malformations or oral cleft *(31,32)*. However, benzodiazepines can cause neonatal hypotonia, hypothermia, and mild neonatal respiratory distress when taken in late pregnancy or around the time of delivery *(33)*.

4.5. Alcohol and Breast-Feeding

The effects on young children of exposure to moderate amounts of alcohol (about one standard drink or less a day) through breast milk are not clear. One study reported adverse effects on infants' sleep and gross motor development *(35)*, whereas another study did not identify motor deficits in exposed toddlers *(36)*. Nevertheless, women with substance and alcohol use disorders should be advised not to consume alcohol if nursing. An additional negative effect of maternal alcohol consumption is that it may slightly reduce milk production.

The concentration in breast milk parallels the mother's blood alcohol level *(34)*. A lactating woman who drinks can limit her infant's exposure to alcohol by refraining from nursing for several hours after drinking so the body can eliminate the alcohol *(36)*.

5. MATERNAL MARIJUANA USE

Most clinicians are familiar with marijuana, a leafy plant, also known by the following names: cannabis, pot, dope, weed, chronic, bud, ganja, and hashish. Marijuana may be either smoked or ingested. A "blunt" is the name for marijuana packed in cigar paper. A relatively new route of administration is the use of the cannabis "vaporizer," which is designed to let users inhale active cannabinoids by heating marijuana to a temperature just below the point of combustion where smoke is produced *(37)*. Vaporizer users may mistakenly believe that, because little or none of the carcinogenic tars and noxious gases found in marijuana smoke are emitted, it is therefore safe for use during pregnancy. Although the use of vaporizers may decrease some of the pulmonary toxicity, there is no evidence that their use is safe during pregnancy.

In recent years, the concentration of the major psychopharmacologically active component of cannabis, tetrahydrocannabinol (THC), has increased, as have reports of adverse effects. The increase in THC is a result of plant selection and cultivation changes *(38)*. Short-term adverse effects of marijuana use include memory and learning problems, distorted perception, and difficulty with problem solving. Psychiatric symptoms associated with marijuana use include anxiety, depression, paranoia, and psychosis *(39,40)*.

5.1. Epidemiology of Marijuana Use

Marijuana is the most frequently used illicit drug in the United States. Of the 6.8 million persons who are classified with either dependence or abuse of illicit drugs, 4.2 million are dependent on or abusing marijuana. This represents 1.8% of the total population 12 yr or older and 61.4% of all those classified with illicit drug dependence or abuse *(8)*. There is a strong association between the use of licit and illicit drugs among pregnant women. A 1992 survey conducted by the National Institute of Drug Abuse examined licit and illicit drug use in 2613 pregnant women and found that among women who drank alcohol and smoked cigarettes, 20.4% also used marijuana. Conversely, of those women who said they had not used cigarettes or alcohol, only 0.2% smoked marijuana *(42)*.

5.2. Fetal Effects of Marijuana

Endogenous cannabinoids appear to be involved in the regulation of human fertility and pregnancy. The first brain-derived endogenous cannabinoid identified was an arachidonylethanolamide, which was given the name anandamide. Cannabinoid receptors have been found in high abundance in the brain, the immune system, and the human uterine smooth muscle during pregnancy. Anandamide may have a role in the uterine tubes in delaying embryo development until the uterus is ready to receive the implanting blastocyst *(43)*. Anandamide is believed to also have a role in sustaining the embryo once it has been implanted *(43)*. Future studies of the cannabinoid system will most likely reveal details of its importance in reproduction and shed light on the effects of exogenous prenatal cannabinoid exposure.

Marijuana use during pregnancy can significantly affect the size of the neonate at birth. In the Avon Longitudinal Study of Pregnancy and Childhood, 12,000 pregnant women at 18–20 wk of gestation completed a questionnaire regarding their use of cannabis before and during pregnancy *(44)*. Although prenatal marijuana use was unrelated to the risk of perinatal death or the need for special neonatal care, babies of women who used marijuana at least once a week throughout pregnancy were 216 g lighter than those of nonusers. Furthermore, these infants had significantly shorter birth lengths and smaller head circumferences *(44)*. To date, studies with long-term follow-up have not found evidence of growth deficits or somatic teratogenicity as a result of prenatal marijuana exposure *(45–48)*. There are conflicting data suggesting that prenatal marijuana exposure is associated with adverse behavioral or cognitive effects beginning in the neonatal period. One small Jamaican study compared 20 neonates prenatally exposed to marijuana to 20 unexposed infants and found that the marijuana-exposed group displayed altered responses to visual stimuli, increased tremulousness, and a high-pitched cry *(49)*. However, another Jamaican study did not identify deficits or altered behaviors in prenatally exposed neonates at 3 d or 1 mo *(50)*. The Maternal Health Practices and Child Development Project, a longitudinal study of 580 children and their mothers, reported that prenatal exposure to marijuana negatively affected sleep and measures of intellectual development and behavior at older ages *(51)*. It is important to keep in mind, however, that multiple environmental factors influence children's development, including the quality of caregiver–child interactions. The impact of prenatal drug exposure on child development is therefore difficult to establish definitively.

5.3. Marijuana and Breast-Feeding

Little is known about the effects of postnatal marijuana exposure on the developing infant. When a nursing mother uses marijuana, THC is passed to the baby through her breast milk *(52)*. THC in the mother's milk appears in higher concentrations than in her blood *(52)*. A study involving 136 breast-fed infants reported that introducing the neonate to marijuana via the mother's milk was associated with a decrease in infant motor development at 1 yr of age *(52)*.

6. MATERNAL COCAINE USE

Cocaine is produced from the leaves of the coca plant. It may be taken intranasally or by injection, or it can be smoked. Cocaine's half-life is approx 1 h, and the drug's euphoria lasts 20–30 min *(53)*. Common street names include coke, snow, flake, blow, and crack. Crack refers to a smokeable form of cocaine made by processing cocaine hydrochloride with sodium bicarbonate and water, which is then heated to free the cocaine alkaloid (base) from the salt. This process allows the drug to burn efficiently. Smoking crack provides a rapid onset of effects comparable to intravenous administration. Cocaine is rapidly metabolized by pseudocholinesterases to benzoylecgonine, which is detected in a urine drug-of-abuse screen for cocaine. Cocaine usually makes the user feel euphoric and energetic. The rewarding effects of cocaine are mediated through the dopaminergic system. The adrenergic effects of cocaine are associated with an increase in heart rate and pulse. Common signs of use include rapid speech, fidgeting, and clenching of the jaw. Intranasal users may present with nasal ulcers or complaints of a frequent bloody nose. Intravenous users who share needles are at risk for hepatitis and HIV. Sexually transmitted diseases are common in women who engage in prostitution to support their drug habit. The physical effects of cocaine include dry mouth, sweating, loss of appetite, and insomnia. Frequent or heavy use can lead to psychotic symptoms, including agitation, delusions, bizarre behavior, and paranoia. These effects subside as the drug is eliminated from the body. Other major health risks include palpitations, heart attacks, respiratory failure, strokes, and seizures *(54)*.

6.1. Epidemiology of Cocaine Use

In 2002, the NSDUH estimated that 1.5 million Americans were dependent on or abusing cocaine, a decline from 5.7 million users in 1985 *(8)*. However, the rate of cocaine use among pregnant women in urban areas continues to be high *(55)*. In 2002, the Treatment Episode Data Set recorded more than 400,000 admissions of women 15–44 yr old to substance abuse treatment facilities and found that cocaine was the primary substance of abuse for 17% of admissions among pregnant women *(9)*.

6.2. Fetal Effects of Cocaine

It is difficult to isolate the fetal effects of cocaine from other confounding factors associated with pregnant substance use such as malnutrition, poor prenatal care, and multiple substance use. Furthermore, the dose and pattern of administration of cocaine varies among users. Some studies rely on maternal self-reported drug use or urine drug-of-abuse screens. Despite the limitations of these studies of maternal drug use, news media popularized the idea of "crack babies" born during the cocaine epidemic of the 1980s. These stories suggested that the babies were "born addicted" and would suffer lifelong problems. Unfortunately, such negative labels affected the way people perceived these infants and thereby shaped their expectations of the children's future. Some of the negative outcomes observed in children of cocaine users resulted from the poor quality of care provided during infancy, rather than from the direct effects of cocaine *in utero*.

Nonetheless, cocaine diffuses across the placenta and affects the blood supply to the fetus. Cocaine increases maternal and fetal blood pressure. Maternal hypertension may affect blood flow to the placenta, which can decrease oxygen to the fetus. Adverse fetal outcomes may result from cycles of relative ischemia, rebound vasodilation, and hyperperfusion that may develop from vasoconstrictive effects within the placenta *(55)*. Vasoconstriction is presumed to cause disruption of placental adherence to the uterine wall and thereby increases the risk of placental abruption. A meta-analysis of 33 epidemiological studies found that the risks of placental abruption and premature rupture of membranes were significantly associated with cocaine use *(56)*. In this analysis, the rates of major malformations, low birthweight (LBW), and prematurity among children of mothers who used cocaine prenatally were not higher than among children exposed prenatally to other drugs of abuse. However, the cocaine-exposed children were at significantly higher risk for major malformations than children of drug-free women *(56)*. Furthermore, in a prospective dose–response study, cocaine-exposed infants were at greater risk for IUGR and small head circumference *(57)*. Another study found that the duration of cocaine exposure during pregnancy correlated with a decrease in birthweight *(58)*.

Most studies have not identified a specific neonatal abstinence syndrome (NAS) associated with prenatal cocaine exposure. Hypertonicity and tremors in the neonatal period are more likely a manifestation of fetal cocaine exposure than signs of withdrawal. Neonates prenatally exposed to cocaine exhibit more irritability, insomnia, and crying than unexposed infants *(59)*. For the mothers, the signs and symptoms of cocaine withdrawal can include depression, insomnia or hypersomnia, increased appetite, and psychomotor agitation or retardation. There are no well-controlled studies using drugs to medically treat pregnant, cocaine-using women in withdrawal. In general, the pharmacological treatment for cocaine withdrawal is to treat significant symptoms such as agitation or insomnia. Inpatient treatment is ideal because of the high risk of relapse during early abstinence. Medical monitoring during withdrawal is ideally followed by a referral to ongoing drug treatment and relapse-prevention services.

Beyond the neonatal period, the effects of prenatal cocaine exposure are difficult to determine. Some studies report that infants exposed to prenatal cocaine use have exhibited depressed motor and interactive abilities as well as poor attentiveness as infants and toddlers. Many of these behaviors appear to diminish over time and can be treated with behavioral interventions *(60)*. A longitudinal study could not demonstrate a direct effect of prenatal cocaine exposure on preschool development *(61)*.

6.3. Cocaine and Breast-Feeding

Women using cocaine should be advised not to breast-feed because of the risk of passive intoxication of the infant, and ideally these infants should be cared for outside of the home until the mother is able to obtain treatment. Seizures can result from infant cocaine intoxication. However, maternal cocaine use is generally not reported, so that cocaine intoxication is usually unsuspected when an infant is brought in for a medical evaluation of a seizure. Another danger is if the mother smokes crack cocaine, neonates and infants in the area are at risk of intoxication because of passive inhalation *(59)*.

7. MATERNAL METHAMPHETAMINE USE

Methamphetamine is a derivative of amphetamine. It can be ingested, snorted, smoked, or used intravenously. Because its duration of action lasts 6–8 h, users tend to use it once or twice a day *(62)*. Common street names include speed, meth, tweek, chalk, ice, crystal, and glass. Methamphetamine is a potent stimulant, and its effects include increased confidence, wakefulness, and physical activity, as well as euphoria and decreased appetite. Other signs of use include pupil dilation, constant talking, tooth grinding, sweating, and irritability. Chronic, long-term use can cause insomnia, increased blood pressure, paranoia, psychosis, aggression, and mood lability. The toxic effects of methamphetamine include seizures, heart attacks, and strokes *(63)*. Health care providers should be aware that methamphetamine-dependent individuals report a high incidence of domestic and interpersonal violence, which may impact the welfare of the mother and the child *(64)*.

7.1. Epidemiology of Methamphetamine

The ease with which methamphetamine can be manufactured is a major factor contributing to its increased use across the country. The highest rates of usage occur among men and women between the ages of 18 and 23. According to the 2000 National Household Survey on Drug

Abuse, an estimated 8.8 million people (4% of the population) have tried methamphetamine at some time in their lives *(65)*. The recent rise in methamphetamine use across the nation has, of course, led to an increase in the number of pregnant women using methamphetamine. Unplanned pregnancy is a significant concern for this population. A study of female methamphetamine users found high levels of sexual risk behavior, including multiple partners, anonymous sex partners, and high rates of unprotected sex *(66)*. Women of childbearing age may be attracted to methamphetamine because of its appetite-suppressing effects.

7.2. Fetal Effects of Methamphetamine

There is a paucity of research on the fetal effects of maternal methamphetamine use. The available information associates prenatal methamphetamine use with an increased incidence of placental hemorrhages and premature deliveries. Methamphetamine-exposed infants are at greater risk for IUGR *(67)* and decreased head circumference *(68)*. Similar to cocaine, withdrawal from methamphetamine is not medically dangerous to the mother or the fetus. Nonetheless, nonspecific neonatal withdrawal symptoms requiring pharmacological interventions have been identified in a very small number of neonates *(67)*. Withdrawal symptoms in non-pregnant methamphetamine users include moderate levels of depression, anhedonia, irritability, sleep disturbance, and poor concentration, which resolve quickly for most individuals *(69)*.

Unusual behaviors, such as abnormal reflexes and excessive irritability, have been identified in methamphetamine-exposed neonates *(68)*. It is unclear if prenatal methamphetamine exposure is neurotoxic to the developing brain and to what extent a good psychosocial environment after birth can compensate for methamphetamine-associated deficits. A pilot study of 13 methamphetamine-exposed children indicated lower scores on measures of visual motor integration, attention, verbal memory, and long-term spatial memory and smaller subcortical volumes on magnetic resonance imaging *(70)*. As with cocaine, methamphetamine dependence in pregnant women is best managed in an inpatient treatment setting with follow-up substance abuse treatment.

7.3. Methamphetamine and Breast-Feeding

Methamphetamine passes into breast milk and may affect a nursing baby. One study of the therapeutic use of amphetamines found that the concentration of amphetamine was higher in breast milk than in maternal blood and small amounts of amphetamine were detected in the infant's urine sample *(71)*. Further studies are needed to assess the effects of postnatal exposure to methamphetamine.

8. MATERNAL OPIOID USE

Heroin is processed from morphine, a naturally occurring opiate extracted from poppy plants. It is sold illegally, often tied in the ends of small balloons. Common street names for heroin include smack, dope, "H," China white, black tar, and junk. Heroin can be smoked, sniffed, or injected intravenously or intramuscularly. After an injection, the user experiences euphoria, relaxation, warmth, and an absence of anxiety. Because the duration of action is 4–6 h *(72)*, users tend to use it two to three times a day. The signs of heroin use include drowsiness, itching, pinpoint pupils, loss of appetite, slowed breathing, and constipation. Death in chronic intravenous heroin users is often the result of overdose. Heroin users are also at risk for developing collapsed veins, endocarditis, abscesses, cellulitis, HIV, AIDS, and hepatitis *(73)*.

The hallmarks of opiate dependence are tolerance and withdrawal upon cessation. Some women use heroin in combination with prescription opioid medications to avoid symptoms of withdrawal. Other women use only prescription opioids. Assessment for pain disorders can give the health care professional additional information about potential substance abuse. Sources of prescription opiates include family members or friends, diverted sources purchased on the street, or "doctor shopping" to obtain the drug. Withdrawal symptoms from prescription opiates are the same as those from heroin. The onset and duration of the symptoms vary with the half-life of the drug. The addicted woman experiences medically distressing signs and symptoms such as severe anxiety, vomiting, chills, sweating, stomach cramps, body aches, runny nose, increased respiration rate, depression, and irritability *(73)*.

8.1. Epidemiology of Opioid Use

In 2002, the Drug Enforcement Administration reported that approx 1.2% of the population in the United States reported heroin use at least once in their lifetime. Heroin is among the four most frequently mentioned drugs reported in drug-related death cases in 2002 *(74)*. There is limited information available on maternal prescription opioid use, although prescription opiate use is increasing across the United States *(75)*.

8.2. Fetal Effects of Opioid Use

Maternal heroin use can cause significant perinatal complications. These can be compounded by the presence of bloodborne infections, which are not uncommon in intravenous users. Heroin-associated complications in pregnancy include toxemia, IUGR, miscarriage, premature rupture of membranes, infections, breech presentation, and preterm labor. Adverse outcomes reported in the neonates include LBW, prematurity, neonatal abstinence syndrome, stillbirth, and sudden infant death syndrome (6).

8.3. Methadone Treatment

Methadone maintenance has been the primary treatment for opioid dependence in pregnancy for the past 30 yr, and evidence exists that treatment with methadone, combined with comprehensive prenatal care, can significantly reduce the incidence of obstetric and fetal complications and neonatal morbidity and mortality.

The Center for Substance Abuse and Treatment TIP 2 guidelines indicate that methadone maintenance provides many advantages for pregnant opioid-dependent women (76). Methadone prevents the onset of opioid withdrawal for 24 h, reduces drug craving, and blocks the euphoric effects when additional opioids are taken. Methadone maintenance therapy also prevents erratic maternal opioid levels and protects the fetus from repeated episodes of withdrawal that may cause signs of fetal distress. Studies of methadone-maintained pregnant women show an improvement in maternal nutrition and neonatal weights. Methadone maintenance decreases the woman's risk of HIV infection, hepatitis, and sexually transmitted diseases and reduces behaviors often associated with drug-seeking such as prostitution. In combination with psychosocial treatment, it improves the woman's ability to participate in prenatal care, prepare for the birth of the infant, and provide a stable home (6). Methadone is a synthetic opioid that cannot be prescribed by a physician for the treatment of opioid addiction, but rather is dispensed from licensed clinics that are generally located in urban areas (77).

As pregnancy progresses, some methadone-maintained women require elevations of the dose to maintain the same plasma level. Higher doses of methadone in the third trimester have been associated with improved fetal growth and longer duration of gestation; therefore, more liberal methadone dosing in pregnancy may improve initial and long-term neonatal outcome. Of opiate-exposed infants, 60–90% develop NAS. Generally, methadone-exposed infants are reported to have a higher incidence of abstinence and more prolonged duration of abstinence than those whose mothers used heroin. However, maternal dosage does not appear to correlate with neonatal withdrawal, and maternal benefits of effective methadone dosing are not offset by neonatal harm (78). Therefore, it is not necessary to lower the methadone doses during pregnancy. Doing so may promote illicit drug use and increase the risk to the fetus (79).

NAS is characterized by CNS, gastrointestinal, and respiratory dysfunction. If pharmacological treatment is indicated, neonatal abstinence syndrome is treated with tapering doses of diluted opium or morphine solutions. Signs and symptoms of NAS include muscle spasms, irritability, high-pitched crying, diarrhea, disturbed sleep and feeding, vomiting, hiccups, stuffy nose, sneezing, and breathing problems. The duration of these symptoms is typically 1–2 wk. NAS associated with methadone typically lasts longer than heroin-associated NAS. NAS can be treated safely in the hospital after birth *(78)*.

8.4. Methadone and Breast-Feeding

Mothers who are treated with methadone and are abstinent from substance use should not be discouraged from breast-feeding. Negligible amounts of methadone appear to be transmitted in breast milk *(80)*, and recent guidelines have maintained that, regardless of the mother's dose, nursing is unlikely to adversely affect the infant. The amount of methadone transmitted to an infant from breast milk is not enough to prevent NAS. Breast-feeding fosters maternal attachment and is valuable for both the mother and infant. However, mothers may become discouraged as they try to nurse an infant undergoing NAS because the infant's symptoms may interfere with nursing. These problems can be addressed by a lactation consultant working with the substance abuse and medical treatment staff *(80)*.

8.5. Buprenorphine Treatment

In 2002, the US Food and Drug Administration approved the use of buprenorphine as an alternative to methadone for opioid addiction treatment. Buprenorphine is a partial μ-opioid agonist with a good safety profile. As indicated, methadone is only available from licensed clinics and this limits the availability of treatment. Buprenorphine has a greater geographical reach because primary care physicians can prescribe it from their offices *(81)*. The safety of buprenorphine in pregnancy has not been established towing to the lack of adequately controlled prospective studies. However, recent studies of pregnant women have shown positive results. Overall, buprenorphine treatment during pregnancy has had effects comparable to methadone but, notably, has been associated with lower incidences of NAS *(82–84)*. In one study, infants of mothers treated with buprenorphine required no pharmacological treatment for NAS *(83)*. Buprenorphine treatment may provide a promising alternative to improve maternal and infant outcomes. At present there are no clinical data on the safety of buprenorphine during breast-feeding, so its use is not recommended in nursing mothers *(85)*.

8.6. Behavioral Effects of Heroin Use on the Child

Little is known about lifetime cognitive and behavioral effects on children of women using heroin during pregnancy. The studies that identify deficits cannot rule out the contribution of psychosocial factors such as impaired parenting. Some authors have reported that prenatal heroin exposure is associated with adjustment problems and psycholinguistic and other deficits through 6 yr of age (86). To date, research into long-term effects of heroin has been inconclusive, suggesting that if there are long-term effects, they may be subtle or may take years to appear. Prenatal drug exposure may lead to sensitization, resulting in a greater vulnerability to substance use disorders in later life. Isolating the neurobiological vulnerabilities from the genetic and environmental risk factors is a challenge for research in this area.

9. LEGAL ISSUES SURROUNDING PREGNANT SUBSTANCE-ABUSING WOMEN

It is important for health care providers caring for pregnant substance-dependent women to know about the regulations and laws regarding child welfare. These change periodically and vary considerably from state to state in their scope and approach to maternal substance use. An excellent review of this subject indicates that longstanding decisions of the Supreme Court have prohibited criminalizing of an illness, and no state except South Carolina has adopted specific legislation criminalizing pregnant women who abuse substances (86). However, many states have modified their civil child protection laws by mandating reports to child welfare authorities or defining child neglect to encompass cases in which a newborn is physically dependent, tests positive for, or has been harmed by substances of abuse. In some states, a positive toxicology screen for alcohol or drugs of abuse at the time of delivery is automatic grounds for removal of the child from the home (87).

Twenty-five states have adopted a less punitive approach, with the goal of encouraging, not deterring, prenatal health care. In these states, cases of maternal drug or alcohol use are referred to the hospital social worker, who evaluates and determines whether it is safe for the child to be taken home (88,89). If the mother's drug use provides an unsafe home environment for her child, the social worker will file a suspected child abuse report. Following the report, an assessment is made whether to remove the child from the home. Identifying and reporting newborns exposed to maternal substance abuse can lead to positive changes in the care of the infant and successful rehabilitation opportunities for the mothers *(90)*. Ideally, a mother will be referred to a residential treatment facility that provides care for the mother and her child. However, such resources are not often available.

The best outcome for a mother with an addictive disorder is to have integrated substance treatment and psychosocial services, for example, when child protective services is involved. The National Center on Substance Abuse and Child Welfare (NCSACW) was formed to implement collaboration among substance abuse, child welfare, and family judicial systems *(91)*. NCSACW recognizes the detrimental effects of criminalizing substance-using women and is providing education, assistance, and resources to destigmatize addiction and implement treatment. The impact of maternal substance use on the foster care system is enormous. Studies by the Child Welfare League of America found that, in most states, child maltreatment and neglect as a result of parental substance abuse was one of the most common reasons for foster care placement *(92)*. Research shows that 80% of children in foster care are at risk for an array of physical and developmental problems because of prenatal exposure to maternal substance abuse *(93)*. As during the cocaine epidemic in the 1980s, there is now an increasing rate of foster care placements resulting from the increase in methamphetamine addiction. For many mothers whose infants are placed in foster care, the goal of reunification becomes a powerful motivation to participate in substance abuse treatment.

10. CONCLUSION

Health care providers play a pivotal role in identifying substance abuse during pregnancy by recognizing the signs and symptoms and administering routine assessments and drug-of-abuse screening. Substance abuse in pregnant women is a condition that requires immediate medical attention. Prenatal exposure to legal and illicit substances has been shown to have negative effects on the developing fetus, as well as on the growing child. The stigma associated with substance use in pregnancy and the threat of criminalization deter many women from seeking prenatal care and substance abuse treatment and from revealing their substance use history to physicians. Establishing rapport with substance-using pregnant women is vital for intervention.

Despite limited data on the extent of substance abuse in pregnant women, available information indicates that use spans all socioeconomic and racial backgrounds. Reports indicate that Caucasian women are more likely to consume alcohol, whereas minority women are more frequently reported to use illicit drugs during pregnancy. Women who smoke are more likely to use licit and illicit substances during pregnancy.

In addition, pregnant substance-using women often have a history of multiple psychosocial disadvantages.

Clinical data on the effects of maternal alcohol consumption on the fetus are the most widely researched and understood compared to other substances of abuse. *In utero* exposure to alcohol is associated with a range of disorders from physical malformation to cognitive deficits. Prevention efforts begin with health care providers advising women to take appropriate measures to avoid unintentional pregnancy if they are consuming alcohol.

The teratogenic effects of maternal use of illicit drugs are not as clear as the effects of alcohol. However, several studies suggest that, among other risks, an adverse outcome associated with marijuana and heroin is LBW, whereas stimulant use has been associated with placental abruption and hemorrhage. The effects of maternal drug use are difficult to assess because of confounding psychosocial factors that obscure the understanding of causal relationships. Deficits associated with maternal drug use can be compounded in unstable environments and ameliorated in nurturing ones.

Ideally, pregnant women withdrawing from drugs and alcohol can be treated in an in-patient or residential facility because of the high risk of relapse in early abstinence. Severe symptoms of withdrawal from alcohol warrant treatment with benzodiazepines. Opiate-dependent patients should be referred to methadone treatment programs, whereas stimulant withdrawal generally does not require pharmacological treatment. The distressing symptoms of withdrawal provide a window of opportunity to engage the patient in substance abuse treatment. Matching the severity of the problem with the appropriate level of care is necessary to help women begin the process of abstinence and recovery. It is important to maintain a list of local resources and provide women with options. Studies have shown that people who are given choices are more successful in treatment. Treatment resources include maternity support services, county substance abuse services, hospital treatment programs, residential treatment programs, outpatient treatment programs, mental health clinics, and 12-step and other self-help programs

Addiction is a treatable but chronic relapsing illness. Pregnancy may provide an important window of opportunity to engage women in substance abuse treatment. In some cases, a woman may be in denial about her illness, and the severity of her addiction may endanger the child. For the best interest of the child and mother, child protective services involvement may be necessary. The loss of a child to foster care and the goal of reunification may motivate a woman to seek treatment. In recent years substance abuse research has focused on women and gender differences in drug and alcohol use. An understanding of gender differences may help to prevent initiation of substance use and better understand the antecedents and consequences of drug and alcohol use in women. Studies are also needed to better understand the impact of drug use on pregnancy and maternal functioning, as well as the effects on the newborn and the behavioral, cognitive, and social development of children prenatally exposed to drugs and alcohol.

REFERENCES

1. Archie, C. (2002) Substance abuse in pregnancy. In: Pregler, J. P. and DeCherney, A. H., eds. Women's Health: Principles and Clinical Practice. Hamilton, Ontario: BC Decker Inc., pp. 206–217.
2. Substance abuse during pregnancy: guidelines for screening (2002) Retrieved March 25, 2005, from Washington State Department of Health website: http://www.doh.wa.gov/cfh/mch/documents/screening_guidelines.pdf
3. Friedmann, P. D., McCullough, D., and Saitz, R. (2001) Screening and intervention for illicit drug abuse: a national survey of primary care physicians and psychiatrists. Arch. Intern. Med. 161, 248–251.
4. Foster, K. (2003) Protecting fetal neurons. Retrieved April 14, 2005, from Sonoma Medicine website: http://www.scma.org/magazine/scp/Fall03/foster.html
5. ASI Pregnancy Status National Clearinghouse for Alcohol and Drug Information, P.O. Box 2345, Rockville, MD 20852. 1-800-729-6686.
6. Pregnant, substance-using women: treatment improvement protocol (TIP) series. (1993) Retrieved April 19, 2005, from Substance Abuse and Mental Health Services Administration. Center for Substance Abuse Treatment website: http://www.ncbi.nlm.nih.gov/books/bv.fcgi?rid=hstat5.section.22581
7. Guide to clinical preventive services, 2nd ed. Mental disorders and substance abuse: screening for drug abuse. (1996) Retrieved April 5, 2005, from website: http://cpmcnet.columbia.edu/texts/gcps/gcps0063.html
8. The National Survey on Drug Use and Health Report. (2004) Pregnancy and substance use. Retrieved March 27, 2005, from website: http://www.drugabusestatistics.samhsa.gov/2k3/pregnancy/pregnancy.htm
9. The DASIS report: Pregnant Women in Substance Abuse Treatment (2002). Retrieved March 21, 2005, from website: http://www.drugabusestatistics.samhsa.gov/2k4/pregTX/pregTX.htm
10. Goldberg, M. E. (1995) Substance-abusing women: false stereotypes and real needs. Soc. Work 40, 789–798.
11. Wilsnack, S. C., Vogeltanz, N. D., Klassen, A. D. and Harris, T. R. (1997) Childhood sexual abuse and women's substance abuse: national survey findings. J. Stud. Alcohol 58, 264–271.
12. Martin, S. L., English, K. T., Clark, K. A., et al. (1996) Violence and substance use among North Carolina pregnant women. Am. J. Psychiatry 86, 991–998.
13. Martin, S. L., Beaumont, J. L.K., and Kupper, L. L. (2003) Substance use before and during pregnancy: links to intimate partner violence. Am. J. Drug Alcohol Abuse 29, 599–617.
14. National Institute on Alcohol Abuse and Alcoholism (2005) Retrieved April 28, 2005 from website: http://www.niaaa.nih.gov/press/2005/Recovery.htm.

15. Floyd, R. L., Decoufle, P., and Hungerford, D. W. (1999) Alcohol use prior to pregnancy recognition. Am. J. Prev. Med. 17, 101–107.

16. Dufour, M. C., Williams, G. D., Campbell, K. E., et al. (1994) Knowledge of FAS and the risks of heavy drinking during pregnancy, 1985 and 1990. In: Fetal Alcohol Syndrome Prevention Research (Hankin, J. R., August 2002). Retrieved April 9, 2005, from NIDA website: http://www.niaaa.nih.gov/publications/arh26-1/58-65.htm

17. Preventing alcohol-exposed pregnancies: increasing public awareness of the risks of alcohol use during pregnancy through targeted media campaigns. (August 2004) Retrieved April 9, 2005, from website: http://www.cdc.gov/ncbddd/fas/pubawarenss.htm

18. Gomby, D. and Shiono, P. (1991) Estimating the number of substance-exposed infants. In: Hot Topic: Drug-Exposed Children. Retrieved April 1, 2005, from the National Adoption Information Clearinghouse website: www.nurtureadopt.org/af/adoptionarticles/drug-exposedchildren.htm

19. Kvigne, V. L., Leonardson, G. R., Neff-Smith, M., et al. (2004) Characteristics of children who have full or incomplete fetal alcohol syndrome. J. Pediatr. 145, 635–640.

20. Jones, K. L., Smith, D. W., Ulleland, C. N., and Streissguth, P. (1973) Pattern of malformation in offspring of chronic alcoholic mothers. Lancet 1, 1267–1271.

21. Weiner, L. and Morse, B. A. (1988) FAS: clinical perspectives and prevention. In: Chasnoff, I. J., ed. Drugs, Alcohol, Pregnancy and Parenting. Hingham, MA: Kluwer Academic Publishers.

22. Sokol, R. J. and Clarren, S. K. (1989) Guidelines for use of terminology describing the impact of prenatal alcohol on the offspring. Alcohol Clin. Exp. Res. 13, 597–598.

23. Michaelis, E. K. and Michaelis, M. L. (2001) Cellular [W1] and molecular bases of alcohol's teratogenic effects. Retrieved March 23, 2005, from website: http://www.fetalalcohol.com/articles/docs/Cellmolecular.rtf

24. Coles, C. (2001) Critical periods for prenatal alcohol exposure: evidence from animal and human studies. Retrieved March 25, 2005, from website: http://www.fetalalcohol.com/articles/docs/CritPeriod.rtf

25. Rostand, A., Kaminski, M., Lelong, N., et al. (1990) Alcohol use in pregnancy, craniofacial features, and fetal growth. J. Epidemiol. Comm. Health 44, 302–306.

26. Danis, R. P., Newton, N., and Keith, L. (1981) Pregnancy and alcohol. Curr. Probl. Obstet. Gynecol. 4, 2–48.

27. Caruso, K. and Bensel, R. (1993) Fetal alcohol syndrome and fetal alcohol effects. J. Clin. Health Aff. 76, 25–29.

28. Streissguth, A. P., Aase, J. M., Clarren, S. K., et al. (1991) Fetal alcohol syndrome in adolescents and adults. JAMA 265, 1961–1967.

29. Connor, P. D. and Streissguth, A. P. (2001) Effect of prenatal exposure to alcohol across the life span. NIAAA. Retrieved March 10, 2005, from website: http://www.fetalalcohol.com/articles/docs/PrenatalExposure.rtf

30. National Center on Birth Defects and Developmental Disabilities (NCBDDD) and Centers for Disease Control and Prevention. Fetal Alcohol Information. Retrieved November 23, 2005, from website: http://www.cdc.gov/ncbddd/fas/fasask.htm

31. Dolovich, L. R., Addis, A., Vaillancourt, J. M. R., et al. (1998) Benzodiazepine use in pregnancy and major malformations or oral cleft: meta-analysis of cohort and case-control studies. Br. Med. J. 317, 839–843.

32. Ormond, K. and Pergament, E. (1998) Update: Benzodiazepines in pregnancy. Illinois teratogen information services (IT IS) newsletter. Retrieved March 5, 2005, from website: http://www.fetal-exposure.org/BENZOUPDATE.html

33. Ashton, H. (1995) Toxicity and adverse consequences of benzodiazepine use. Retrieved April 28, 2005, from website: http://www.benzo.org.uk/ashtox.htm.
34. Gunzerath, L., Faden, V., Zakhari, S., et al. (2004) National Institute on Alcohol Abuse and Alcoholism report on moderate drinking. [editorial] Alcohol. Clin. Exp. Res. 28, 829–847
35. Mennella, J. (2001) Alcohol's effect on lactation. Alcohol Res. Health 25, 230–234.
36. Little R.E., Northstone, K., and Golding, J. (ALSPAC Study Team). (2002) Alcohol, breast-feeding, and development at 18 months. Pediatrics 109, E72.
37. National Organization for the Reform of Marijuana Laws (NORML). (2001) Multidisciplinary Association for Psychedelic Studies (MAPS) Study shows vaporizers reduce toxins in marijuana smoke. (January 2001) Retrieved April 9, 2005, from website: http://www.canorml.org/healthfacts/vaporizerstudy1.html
38. U.S. Drug Enforcement Administration. Cannabis. Retrieved April 9, 2005, from the DEA website: http://www.usdoj.gov/dea/pubs/abuse/7-pot.htm
39. Leweke, F. M., Gerth C. W., and Klosterkotter, J. (2004) Cannabis-associated psychosis: current status of research. CNS Drugs 18, 895–910.
40. Verdoux, H., Sorbara, F., Gindre, C., et al. (2003) Cannabis use and dimensions of psychosis in a nonclinical population of female subjects. Schizophr. Res. 59, 77–84.
41. National Survey on Drug Use and Health: pregnancy and substance use (2004) Retrieved on April 21, 2005, from Substance Abuse and Mental Health Services Administration (SAMHSA) website: http://www.oas.samhsa.gov/2k3/pregnancy/pregnancy.pdf
42. Mathias, R. (January/February 1995) NIDA Survey provides first national data on drug use during pregnancy. Nida Notes 10(1). Retrieved April 9, 2005, from website: http://www.drugabuse.gov/NIDA_Notes/NNVol10N1/NIDASurvey.html
43. Stocker, S. (March 2000) Marijuana-like compound in womb may influence early pregnancy. Nida Notes 15(1). Retrieved April 9, 2005, from website: http://www.drugabuse.gov/NIDA_Notes/NNVol15N1/Marijuana.html
44. Fergusson, D. M., Horwood, L. J., and Northstone, K. (2002) Maternal use of cannabis and pregnancy outcome. BJOG Int. J. Obstet. Gynaecol.109, 21–27.
45. Fried, P. and Watkinson, B. (1988) 12- and 24-month neurobehavioral follow-up of children prenatally exposed to marijuana, cigarettes and alcohol. Neurotoxicol. Teratol. 10, 305–313.
46. Day, N., Sambamoorthi, U., Taylor, P., et al. (1991) Prenatal marijuana use and neonatal outcome. Neurotoxicol. Teratol. 13, 329–334.
47. Day, N., Cornelius, M., Goldschmidt, L., et al. (1992) The effects of prenatal tobacco and marijuana use on offspring growth from birth through three years of age. Neurotoxicol. Teratol. 14, 407–414.
48. Astley, S. J., Clarren, S. K., Little, R. E., et al. (1992) Analysis of facial shape in children gestationally exposed to marijuana, alcohol, and/or cocaine. Pediatrics 89, 67–77.
49. Lester, B. M. and Dreher, M. (1989) Effects of marijuana use during pregnancy on newborn cry. Child. Dev. 60, 765–771.
50. Dreher, M. C., Nugent, K. and Hudgins, R. (1994) Prenatal marijuana exposure and neonatal outcomes in Jamaica: an ethnographic study. Pediatrics 93, 254–260.
51. Day, N. L. and Richardson, G. A. (2001) Comparative teratogenicity of alcohol and other drugs. Retrieved March 20, 2005, from website: http://www.fetalalcohol.com/articles/docs/CompTerat.rtf

52. Astley, S. J. and Little, R. E. (1990) Maternal marijuana use during lactation and infant development at one year. Neurotoxicol. Teratol. 12(2), 161–188.
53. Zickler, P. (September 1999) Methamphetamine, cocaine abusers have different patterns of drug use, suffer different cognitive impairments. NIDA Notes 16(5). Retrieved April 15, 2005, from website: http://www.drugabuse.gov/NIDA_Notes/NNVol16N5/Meth_Coc.html
54. NIDA info facts: crack and cocaine (2005). Retrieved April 9, 2005, from website: http://www.nida.nih.gov/Infofax/Cocaine.html
55. Pauli, R. M. (December 1996) In depth: cocaine, pregnancy and risk of intrauterine death. Newslett. Wisconsin Stillbirth Service Program 3(4). Retrieved March 7, 2005, from website: http://www.wisc.edu/wissp/wisspers/dec97001.htm
56. Addis, A., Moretti, M. E., Ahmed, S. F., et al. (2001) Fetal effects of cocaine: an updated meta-analysis. Reprod. Toxicol. 15, 341–369.
57. Chiriboga, C. A., Brust, J. C., Bateman, D., et al. (1999) Dose-response effect of fetal cocaine exposure on newborn neurologic function. Pediatrics 103, 79–85
58. Coles, C. D., Platzman, K. A., Smith, I., et al. (1992) Effects of cocaine and alcohol use in pregnancy on neonatal growth and neurobehavioral status. Neurotoxicol. Teratol. 14, 23–33.
59. Chiriboga, C. M. (2003) Fetal alcohol and drug effects. Neurologist 9, 267–279.
60. Zickler, P. (September 1999) NIDA studies clarify developmental effects of prenatal cocaine exposure. NIDA Notes 14(3). Retrieved March 15, 2005, from website: http://www.drugabuse.gov/NIDA_Notes/NNVol14N3/Prenatal.html
61. Behnke, M., Eyler, F. D., Warner, T. D., et al. (2005) Outcome from a prospective, longitudinal study of prenatal cocaine use: preschool development at 3 years of age. J. Pediatr. Psychol. E-publication.
62. Methamphetamine/amphetamine. Retrieved April 25, 2005, from the Indiana State Department of Toxicology website: http://isdt.iusm.iu.edu/METHAMPHETAMINE.htm
63. NIDA research report series — methamphetamine abuse and addiction: what are the immediate effects of methamphetamine abuse? (2005) Retrieved April 12, 2005, from website: http://www.drugabuse.gov/ResearchReports/methamph/methamph3.html#short
64. Cohen, J. B., Dickow, A., Horner, K., et al. (2003) Abuse and violence history of men and women in treatment for methamphetamine dependence. Am. J. Addict. 12, 377–385.
65. NIDA research report series — methamphetamine abuse and addiction: what is the scope of methamphetamine abuse in the United States? Retrieved April 12, 2005, from website: http://www.drugabuse.gov/ResearchReports/Methamph/methamph2.html#scope
66. Semple, S. J., Grant, I., and Patterson, T. L. (2004) Female methamphetamine users: social characteristics and sexual risk behavior. Women Health 40, 35–50.
67. Smith, L., Yonekura, M. L., Wallace, T., et al (2003) Effects of prenatal methamphetamine exposure on fetal growth and drug withdrawal symptoms in infants born at term. J. Dev. Behav. Pediatr. 24, 17–23.
68. Mackenzie, R. G. and Heischober, B. (1997) Methamphetamine. Pediatr. Rev. 18, 305–309.
69. Newton, T. F., Kalechstein, A. D., Duran, S., et al. (2004) Methamphetamine abstinence syndrome: preliminary findings. Am. J. Addict. 13, 248–255.
70. Chang, L., Smith, L. M., LoPresti, C., et al. (2004) Smaller subcortical volumes and cognitive deficits in children with prenatal methamphetamine exposure. Psychiatry Res. 132, 95–106.

71. Steiner, E., Villen, T., Hallberg, M., and Rane, A. (1984) Amphetamine secretion in breast milk. Eur. J. Clin. Pharmacol. 27, 123–124.
72. Pharmacodynamics. Retrieved April 1, 2005, from website: http://www.druglibrary. org/schaffer/heroin/ase/chap_2_1.htm
73. NIDA info facts: heroin (2004) Retrieved April 9, 2005, from website: http:// www.drugabuse.gov/PDF/Infofacts/Heroin.pdf
74. U.S. Drug Enforcement Administration. Heroin. Retrieved April 9, 2005, from the DEA website: http://www.dea.gov/concern/heroin_factsheet.html#2
75. Leshner, A. I. (June 2001) Continuing concern over imported pharmaceuticals. Hearing before the Subcommittee on Oversight and Investigations, Committee on Energy and Commerce, U.S. House of Representatives. Retrieved on March 16, 2005, from the NIDA website: http://www.nida.nih.gov/Testimony/6-7-01Testimony.html
76. Alcohol and other drug treatment guidelines for pregnant substance-using women: guideline 4-opioid stabilization. In: Marion, I. J., chair. Pregnant, Substance-Using Women: Treatment Improvement Protocol (TIP) DHHS publication; Series 2 (1993), 18–21.
77. Broekhuysen, E. S. (April 2000) Methadone. Retrieved March 22, 2005, from the Office of National Drug Control Policy (ONDCP) website: http://www. whitehousedrugpolicy.gov/publications/factsht/methadone/
78. Berghella, V., Lim, P. J., Hill, M. K., et al. (2003) Maternal methadone dose and neonatal withdrawal. Am. J. Obstet. Gynecol. 189, 312–317.
79. Finnegan, L. P. and Kandall, S. R. (1997) Maternal and neonatal effects of alcohol and drugs. In:. Lowinson, H. L., Ruiz, P., Milman, R. B., and Langrod, J. G., eds. Substance Abuse: A Comprehensive Textbook. Baltimore: Williams and Wilkins, pp. 513–534.
80. Jansson, L. M., Velez, M., and Harrow, C. (2004) Methadone maintenance and lactation: a review of the literature and current management guidelines. J. Hum. Lactation 20, 62–71.
81. The Medical Letter on Drugs and Therapeutics (February 2003) Retrieved April 28, 2005, from website: http://www.medletter.com/freedocs/buprenorphine.pdf
82. Johnson, R. E., Jones, H. E., and Fischer, G. (2003) Use of buprenorphine in pregnancy: patient management and effects on the neonate. Drug Alcohol Depend. 70, S87–S101.
83. Johnson, R. E., Jones, H. E., Jasinski, D. R., et al (2001) Buprenorphine treatment of pregnant opioid-dependent women: maternal and neonatal outcomes. Drug Alcohol Depend. 63, 97–103.
84. Fischer, G., Johnson, R. E., Eder, H., et al. (2004) Treatment of opioid-dependent pregnant women with buprenorphine. Addiction 95, 239–244.
85. Clinical guidelines for the use of buprenorphine in pregnancy. (2003) Retrieved April 25, 2005, from website: http://www.turningpoint.org.au/library/CTG_Bup_ Pregnancy_060104.pdf
86. Brady, J. P., Posner, M., Lang, C., and Rosati, M. J. (1994) Risk and reality: the implications of prenatal exposure to alcohol and other drugs. The Education Development Center, Inc. Retrieved, March 21, 2005, from Risk and Reality, a joint project of the U.S. Department of Health and Human Services (DHHS) and the U.S. Department of Education (ED) website: http://www.aspe.hhs.gov/hsp/cyp/ drugkids.htm
87. Harris, L. H. and Paltrow, A. A. L. (2003) The status of pregnant women and fetuses in US criminal law. JAMA 289, 1697–1699. Retrieved March 28, 2005, from website: http://jama.ama-assn.org/cgi/content/full/289/13/1697#REF-JMS0402-3-1-21

88. Dailard, C. and Nash, E. (December 2000) State responses to substance abuse among pregnant women. The Guttmacher Report on Public Policy 3(6) Retrieved March 23, 2005, from website: http://www.guttmacher.org/pubs/tgr/03/6/gr030603.html

89. Dailard, C. and Nash, E. (2000) State responses to pregnant substance abuse among women. The Guttmacher Report on Public Policy 3(6) (see table: Laws Pertaining to Pregnant Women Who Use Drugs). Retrieved March 23, 2005, from website: http://www.guttmacher.org/tables/gr030603t.html

90. MacMahon J. R. (1997) Perinatal substance abuse: the impact of reporting infants to child protective services. Pediatrics 100(5), E1.

91. About Us. (2003) National Center on Substance Abuse and Child Welfare. Retrieved March 15, 2005, from SAMHSA website: www.ncsacw.samhsa.gov/aboutus.asp

92. The Impact of Substance Abuse on Foster Care. (February 1999) Retrieved April 25, 2005, from website: http://www.connectforkids.org/articles/substance_abuse_foster_care#theories

93. Substance Abuse and Child Welfare. Retrieved April 22, 2005, from Children's Home Society website: http://www.chs-wa.org/2_advsubstanceabuseBACK.htm

8

Eating Disorders in Pregnancy and the Postpartum

Empirically Informed Treatment Guidelines

Debra L. Franko

Summary

Eating disorders are most often diagnosed during the childbearing years. Pregnancy and postpartum issues for women with eating disorders are discussed with regard to symptoms, complications, course of pregnancy, delivery, breast-feeding, and postpartum depression (PPD). Research findings indicate that women with eating disorders during pregnancy may be at risk for a variety of pregnancy and obstetric complications. Moreover, there appears to be an association between eating-disorder symptoms and low birthweight as well as premature delivery. PPD is higher in women with eating disorders, and feeding issues have been documented. Assessment and treatment guidelines are presented to assist health care providers in caring for pregnant patients with eating disorders.

Key Words: Pregnancy; eating disorders; complications; maternal weight gain; low birthweight; premature delivery; breast-feeding; postpartum depression.

1. INTRODUCTION

Eating disorders primarily affect women in the childbearing years. As such, many women with past or current eating disorders will experience pregnancy. Clinicians and researchers have explored the interactions between pregnancy and eating disorders in both office practice settings and empirical studies. This chapter summarizes the empirical literature and offers research-informed assessment and treatment strategies for

From: *Current Clinical Practice: Psychiatric Disorders in Pregnancy and the Postpartum: Principles and Treatment*
Edited by: V. Hendrick © Humana Press, Totowa, NJ

addressing the clinical needs of pregnant women with a past or current eating disorder.

2. EATING DISORDERS: DEFINITIONS

Two eating disorders are recognized by the American Psychiatric Association in the *Diagnostic and Statistical Manual of Mental Disorders (1)*. Anorexia nervosa (AN) is characterized by (a) refusal to maintain a normal body weight and weight that is 85% or lower than expected for age and height; (b) intense fear of gaining weight or becoming fat, even when underweight; (c) disturbance in the way in which one's body weight or shape is experienced, extreme influence of body weight or shape on self-evaluation, or denial of the seriousness of the current low body weight; and (d) loss of menses for 3 mo or never getting menses. AN has two subtypes—restricting type and binge-eating/purging type—defined by the absence or presence of binge eating and compensatory purging behaviors, such as vomiting or laxative use. Bulimia nervosa (BN) is defined by (a) recurrent episodes of binge eating twice weekly for 3 mo with loss of control, (b) recurrent inappropriate compensatory behavior (e.g., vomiting, excessively exercising) in order to prevent weight gain, and (c) self-evaluation that is influenced too much by body shape and weight. BN also occurs in one of two subtypes: the purging subtype is characterized by the use of vomiting, laxatives, or diuretics to compensate for binge eating; the nonpurging subtype refers to the use of excessive exercise or fasting to deal with caloric intake.

Because the symptom picture of each of these disorders involves behaviors and attitudes related to food and weight, it is not surprising that pregnancy, with increased caloric needs and body weight, might be problematic for women diagnosed with eating disorders. Eating disorders are associated with nutritional, metabolic, endocrine, and psychological changes that have the potential to have negative effects on fetal development *(2)*. Early case histories supported this contention *(3)*, with reports of miscarriage, fetal abnormalities, and low birthweights (LBW; *4,5*). In the past decade, a number of larger scale studies have confirmed the findings of these earlier case reports.

Although a relatively small literature exists detailing the effects of eating disorders on pregnancy, the available evidence suggests that there are potentially detrimental consequences for both mother and fetus when a pregnant woman has an eating disorder. The goals of this chapter are to (a) highlight relevant literature on the potential interactions between pregnancy and eating disorders, (b) alert professionals to warning signs of an eating disorder and offer suggestions for accurate and straightforward assessment strategies, (c) provide treatment guidelines for health care professionals working with a pregnant woman with an eating disorder, and (d) address important issues in the postpartum.

3. IMPACT OF PREGNANCY ON EATING-DISORDER SYMPTOMS

Several studies have examined the effect of pregnancy on eating-disorder symptoms. In one of the few prospective studies to examine the impact and outcome of pregnancy, Blais et al. *(6)* interviewed 54 eating-disordered women before, during, and after pregnancy. Although pregnancy outcome was not related to any clinical variables, the live birth rate was 10% lower than the expected population rate. Eating-disorder symptoms were found to decrease from 3 mo prepregnancy to conception and from prepregnancy to 3 mo postpartum for both anorexic and bulimic patients *(6)*. However, for women diagnosed with AN, symptom levels returned to prepregnancy levels within 6 mo following delivery. For women with a previous history of BN who were not symptomatic at conception, there was no return of bulimic symptoms through 9 mo postpartum. Morgan and colleagues *(7)* reported similar findings in a study of 94 women diagnosed with BN who, overall, improved throughout pregnancy. After delivery, however, 57% had worse symptoms than prior to conception, although 34% were symptom-free. Relapse to bulimic symptoms was predicted by the severity and duration of BN, a history of gestational diabetes, and a pregnancy that was unplanned. These two studies, as well as several others *(8–10)*, appear to suggest that improvement in symptoms may be limited to the pregnancy period and perhaps for a brief time postpartum, but that a significant portion of women return to eating-disorder symptoms after giving birth. It should be noted that some women remain symptomatic throughout the 9 mo of pregnancy as well. Unfortunately, there is no way to predict whether symptoms will remit or continue during pregnancy. In light of this, several authors *(6,7,13)* have suggested that women with eating disorders consider gaining symptom control before becoming pregnant in order to increase the likelihood of a positive pregnancy.

4. IMPACT OF EATING DISORDERS ON PREGNANCY COURSE AND OUTCOME

The empirical literature summarizing the effects of anorexic and bulimic symptoms during pregnancy is somewhat limited because many published studies are primarily retrospective and have been conducted with relatively small sample sizes. The most often cited complications of pregnancy in anorexic and bulimic women include inadequate or excessive weight gain, miscarriage, and hyperemesis *(11,12)*. There have also been case reports of vaginal bleeding, hypertension, and postepisiotomy suture damage in pregnant women with eating disorders *(13)*. The most frequently described obstetric and delivery complications include premature delivery, LBW, and low Apgar scores *(14)*. Reports detailing prenatal mortality, fetal abnormalities, stillbirth, breech delivery, and cleft palate have also been recorded in women with eating disorders *(15,16)*.

Several well-documented obstetric and fetal complications are of particular concern, including miscarriage, hyperemesis, premature delivery, LBW, and delivery by cesarean section. The information available on each is now briefly reviewed.

The rate of miscarriage has been found to be higher in women with eating disorders than in normal healthy control women *(12,17)*. Abraham *(17)* reported that 10 of 43 patients had suffered at least one miscarriage, compared with 15% in the community sample. In a controlled study, Bulik and colleagues *(12)* reported that significantly more women with AN had miscarriages (38%) than in the age-matched control group (16%). However, in a study of 82 pregnancies in eating-disordered women, 11 (13%) ended in miscarriage, a proportion close to the national average *(6)*. The reasons for this apparent discrepancy across studies are not known; however, most authors suggest that compromised health status and/or nutritional deficits may account for miscarriages when they occur. The general conclusion in the literature is that women with eating disorders may be at greater risk than non-eating-disordered women for a pregnancy to end in miscarriage.

Hyperemesis gravidarum (HG) has been found to be more common in women with eating disorders than in control women. Abraham *(17)* reported that although the community prevalence of HG is 1 in 1000 pregnant women, nearly 10% of 25 actively bulimic women had experienced this symptom during their pregnancy. This finding was consistent with Stewart *(18)*, who reported that HG occurred more frequently in eating-disordered women (relative to controls) who had ovulation induced in response to infertility. It is possible that the greater frequency of HG in women with BN may be related to fear of weight gain and may provide "permission" for bulimic symptoms. Because women with BN regularly use self-induced vomiting as a means of weight control and caloric compensation, the pregnant bulimic woman may see HG as an acceptable way to manage weight during pregnancy. In a sense, HG might allow her to continue her symptomatic behavior by hiding it under the pretense of a medical consequence of pregnancy.

The well-documented and important relationship between pregnancy weight gain and birthweight *(19)* poses a challenge in pregnant eating-disordered patients. It has been reported that such patients gain less weight, have smaller babies than healthy women, and may have a higher risk of premature delivery *(11,12,17)*. In the largest prospective study to date *(20)*, women with a history of hospitalization for an eating disorder prior to pregnancy (n = 302) were twice as likely to have LBW infants relative to controls (n = 900). Furthermore, women with eating disorders were 70% more likely to have a premature delivery and 80% more likely to have a small-for-gestational-age baby than control mothers. The authors speculate that weight-controlling behaviors (e.g., dieting, vomiting) and compromised maternal blood flow of nutrients to the fetus may have contributed to impaired fetal growth. Moreover, undernourishment and/ or the use of laxatives and appetite suppressants may also have negatively affected birthweight, size, and timing of delivery.

It should be noted that even women with problematic eating behaviors (short of clinical eating disorders) appear to be at some risk. In a study with an innovative design, Conti et al. *(21)* investigated the association between pregnancy outcome and eating behaviors in 88 women who delivered LBW babies. The group was divided into 34 mothers who delivered small-for-gestational-age infants at term and 54 mothers who delivered premature infants (<37 wk). Women who delivered small babies at term reported more disturbed eating behaviors before and during pregnancy as well as postdelivery. In this study, the unique predictors of having a small-for-gestational-age infant included low prepregnancy weight, smoking, low maternal weekly weight gain, and an elevated score on a self-report bulimia screening questionnaire. Factors that predicted a premature birth were lower occupational status, vomiting during pregnancy, and lower dietary restraint. The authors concluded that growth retardation in the small-for-gestational-age infant could be partly determined by maternal eating behaviors and patterns of disturbed eating before and during pregnancy.

Two studies suggest that delivery by cesarean section may occur more frequently in women with eating disorders than in controls. Bulik et al. *(12)* reported a rate of 16% in anorexic women (compared with 3% in controls), whereas Franko and colleagues *(22)* found a rate of 24% in both anorexic and bulimic women. It is possible that women with eating disorders are viewed as higher risk by the obstetrician, which may increase the possibility of cesarean section. Alternatively, the symptomatic behaviors of anorexic and bulimic women may lead to complications in labor and delivery, which may result in a nonvaginal delivery. The available data do not provide information that clarifies why cesarean sections appear to be more common in this population, but a high frequency of cesarean section was found in two relatively large samples

(66 and 54 women) of eating-disordered women, suggests that they are at risk for nonvaginal deliveries.

It is of note, however, that one prospective study of 54 pregnancies in women with eating disorders *(22)* reported relatively positive results. Specifically, the majority of eating-disordered women in this sample had average-length pregnancies that resulted in normal-birthweight babies with good Apgar scores *(22)*. Although 8% of the sample reported birth defects, by and large there were minimal obstetric or fetal complications. However, as noted earlier, the rate of birth by cesarean section (24%) was higher than expected. Moreover, a number of clinically significant differences was found between women who were symptomatic at the time of pregnancy compared with those who were not. Symptomatic women reported more obstetric and fetal complications, a higher rate of complicated deliveries, and more postpartum depression (PPD) than the nonsymptomatic group.

Taken together, the studies published to date indicate that both a history of an eating disorder as well as current symptomatology pose substantial risks to pregnancy course and outcome. As such, it is important for health providers to become aware of the risks and potential consequences as well as assessment and treatment strategies for pregnant women with eating disorders.

5. DETECTION AND ASSESSMENT OF EATING DISORDERS

There is evidence that women with AN or BN are reluctant to reveal their symptoms and behaviors to health care professionals. In fact, eating disorders are frequently undisclosed to clinicians and may be undetected in clinical settings up to 50% of the time *(23,24)*. An early study by Martin and Wollitzer *(25)* conducted in a family practice clinic found that 21% of female patients had a confirmed history of purging, and of these 58% had never told anyone about their purging and only 2% had discussed it with a family physician. Available data suggest that suboptimal recognition may be attributed to a variety of factors, including a lack of patient disclosure of symptoms *(26)*, a low index of clinical suspicion for these disorders *(23)*, and the clinical stereotyping of eating disorders as primarily affecting non-Hispanic, white girls and women *(27)*. Only two studies have examined disclosure patterns in reproductive health settings. In a small case study, women were found to be reluctant to volunteer their eating disorder history information during their pregnancies *(28)*, and in a series of 66 consecutive women presenting for infertility, 17% were diagnosed with an eating disorder, none of whom disclosed the eating disorder to the health care providers *(24)*.

These studies suggest that it is unlikely that a woman with either a current or past eating disorder will disclose this information spontaneously to a health care provider. As such, it is incumbent on providers to be familiar with warning signs and assessment strategies for eating disorders in order to diagnose accurately and quickly, particularly when a woman is suspected to be or planning to become pregnant.

Because every patient does not require a full assessment for an eating disorder, three warning signs have been proposed for detecting the need for further assessment of an eating disorder in a pregnant woman *(29)*. They are (a) positive history of an eating disorder, (b) lack of weight gain in two consecutive visits in the second trimester, and (c) HG. These warning signs have been discussed *(13)*, with an additional suggestion that a woman who reports the use of any weight-loss medication (e.g., diet pills) should be further assessed for an eating disorder.

Brinch and colleagues *(11)* reported that simply having a history of an eating disorder can pose significant risk for pregnancy outcome, based on findings that although 36 of the 50 mothers in their study had recovered from AN prior to conception, the data still indicated significantly elevated rates of both infant mortality and LBW for this group. Inadequate weight gain, particularly in the second trimester, is a clear indication that something is amiss and should be investigated thoroughly from both the medical and psychological perspectives. Finally, several authors have suggested that the presence of an eating disorder should be considered whenever hyperemesis is present, and there are data that support this relationship *(30)*.

If an eating disorder is suspected, careful and thorough questioning is indicated to determine the type and severity of symptoms. If confirmed, it is essential that the patient be referred to a mental health and nutrition professional experienced in working with eating disorders or, at the very least, that the patient's clinician obtain a consultation from an expert. The focus here is on how to assess patients whom a provider suspects may have an eating disorder.

6. ASSESSING THE SUSPECTED PRESENCE OF AN EATING DISORDER

Because there are no reliable laboratory indicators for the signs of eating disorders, detection depends on careful questioning and vigilance on the part of the provider. High levels of shame and secrecy are common in eating disorders, making it important that questions are asked in an open-ended and nonjudgmental manner in order to maximize the chance of honest responses. Particular questions may be more likely to yield disclosure. For example, Freund et al. *(31)*, in a primary care setting, found that the two questions "Do you ever eat in secret?" and "Are you satisfied with your eating patterns?" had high sensitivity and specificity in identifying patients with BN. It has recently been suggested that questions asked sensitively at the time of weight taking, such as "How are you feeling about the weight you've gained so far?," might encourage additional discussion about eating issues *(13)*. Questions that specifically inquire about weight history, satisfaction with weight and body image, dieting history, and lowest and highest postadolescent weight may provide an entrée into discussion about past or present disordered eating behaviors.

In addition, a number of screening tools are available that assess eating-disorder symptomatology. The most reliable and valid instruments include the Questionnaire for Eating Disorder Diagnoses (Q-EDD) *(32)* and the Eating Disorder Examination questionnaire *(33)*. Both are relatively short and provide diagnoses of AN and BN. Studies have found that both have good discriminant validity, internal consistency, and concurrent validity (for a review of the reliability and validity studies for these tools, *see* refs. *32* and *34*).

The Q-EDD *(32)* is a reliable and valid measure used to determine eating-disorder status. The Q-EDD is a 50-item self-report questionnaire, which takes 5–10 min to complete. Psychometric data support the use of the Q-EDD to differentiate between (a) eating-disordered and non-eating-disordered individuals, (b) eating-disordered, at-risk, and asymptomatic individuals, and (c) between anorexic and bulimic individuals. The Eating Disorder Examination questionnaire *(33)* includes four subscales (restraint, shape concern, weight concern, and eating concern), as well as frequency ratings of the key behaviors comprising the diagnostic criteria such as binge eating, vomiting, laxative abuse, and excessive exercise. Each of the four subscales consists of very specific questions assessing behaviors and beliefs that are associated with eating disorders, but are not required for diagnosis. Because the items are so specific, they are often a good "backdoor" assessment strategy when a patient is denying the more overt symptoms *(29)*.

The use of either of these brief questionnaires may be helpful in confirming a suspected diagnosis or providing a venue by which a patient can "tell" a health care provider about a past or current eating disorder. Careful follow-up discussion should be carried out with compassion and concern if the questionnaire responses indicate eating-disorder pathology.

7. TREATMENT GUIDELINES

Treatment for eating disorders is most effective with a multidisciplinary team approach that includes medical, mental health, and nutrition professionals *(35)*. When an eating-disordered patient is pregnant, the importance of communication among the obstetrician, mental health professionals, and dietitian cannot be overemphasized, and the patient's agreement with this collaboration must be sought. The mental health clinician coordinates the treatment team and makes appropriate additional referrals. The most important role of the obstetrician is to support the patient and to encourage her to remain in treatment with the team. Several authors *(8,15)* have reported positive results with an actively bulimic patient who was treated by a multidisciplinary team throughout her pregnancy.

Although the medical staff will not be the provider of psychological treatment for the eating-disordered patient, it may be useful for physicians, nurses, and midwives to have the following general treatment guidelines in mind to increase the likelihood of positive pregnancy outcome. Obstetrical staff should be aware of the tactics that may be used by patients with eating disorders to undermine treatment. Because such patients generally have significant fears about weight gain, at each visit the identified eating-disorder patient should be weighed in a hospital gown or scant clothing, as it is known that anorexic patients may try to conceal their true weight by adding articles of clothing or heavy objects in their pockets. It is appropriate to ask the patient whether or not she wants to know her weight. A patient with an eating disorder may prefer not to know her weight, a request that should be respected unless the patient is not gaining adequately. If this is the case, she should be told in a concerned and noncritical manner about the need for weight gain, without the use of scare tactics. An explanation of the size, anatomical development, and gestational age of the fetus can provide information to the patient that may help her to eat "for the baby," with less focus on her own increasing weight. Information provided by the dietician concerning the importance of healthy nutrition for fetal growth and good pregnancy outcome is recommended.

Ongoing communication among members of the patient's treatment team is essential in the overall care of the pregnant patient with an eating disorder. In some cases, patients with eating disorders may try to "split" the treatment team, by misrepresenting what others have said or by telling important information to one, but not all team members. If the team communicates on a regular basis, this potential problem can most often be avoided. It is also common that patients with eating disorders can express very positive feelings toward one of their health care providers and disparage the rest of the team, often in an attempt to undermine the treatment. Agreement among team members on important issues such as how much weight the patient needs to gain each month (or each week in the last month of pregnancy) will help the patient to achieve her goals. Clear explanations as to the potential consequences of inadequate weight gain should be communicated to the patient in an atmosphere of care and concern. Patients may need to be seen more frequently than non-eating-disordered patients by the treatment team or may need to be hospitalized in order to ensure appropriate weight gain. Eating disorders can represent a chronic condition that require ongoing psychological, nutritional, and, in some cases, pharmacological treatment (35).

8. COURSE OF PREGNANCY FOR WOMEN WITH EATING DISORDERS

There are no studies investigating the course of pregnancy in women with eating disorders. Based on clinical accounts (28), several issues appear to be relevant with regard to the course of pregnancy in a woman with an eating disorder. These include issues specific to the three trimesters and center around weight gain, eating-disorder symptom change throughout and beyond pregnancy, and preparation for parenthood. The goals of the clinician (whether mental health or medical) are to help and support the patient to eat adequately throughout pregnancy; decrease or eliminate anorexic or bulimic behaviors; and explore feelings about pregnancy, childbirth, and parenting in a caring and empathic way. These issues surface in various ways over the course of pregnancy.

8.1. First Trimester

The first trimester is quite difficult for a number of reasons. Weight gain often begins to occur before the patient has made her pregnancy known to others; she is likely to experience anxiety that her weight gain will be attributed by others to being out of control and getting fat. Consider that many women with eating disorders have spent a substantial part of their adolescent and young adult lives trying to control their weight and now, early on in pregnancy, weight is increasing at a substantial rate. In addition, controlling one's appetite is often a primary goal for women with eating disorders (36), and in pregnancy it is normative and essential for a woman's appetite to be greater than usual. Furthermore, there is a substantial increase in fatigue during the first 3 mo of pregnancy. For the eating-disordered woman who often ignores or denies her own needs, this increase in hunger and fatigue can be terrifying and lead to feelings of being out of control. These negative affective states can trigger eating-disorder behavior such as restrictive dieting or binge eating. Both mental health and obstetric providers can help the patient by encouraging her to talk about these feelings rather than acting on them.

Two related issues figure prominently during the first 3 mo, although they are likely to be of concern throughout the pregnancy as well. The first is a fear of harming the baby as a result of eating-disorder behaviors, and the second is the experience of loss of control. The patient's fears must be explored as completely as possible, and this is best done in psychotherapy. Therapy is often the only place that a patient feels free to talk about the fears related to her symptoms vis-à-vis her pregnancy. The patient may be afraid that the baby is not being properly nourished and thus may not grow adequately. The patient may also worry that behaviors such as purging may actually be harming the baby in some way, particularly in light of medical complications that she herself may have experienced or feared over the years.

Loss of control is a major theme that is likely to be a focus from conception all the way through the early parenting years. Routines, schedules, rituals, and diets are typical for patients with eating disorders and are undertaken in an effort to fight an inner sense of chaos. They often serve as an attempt to gain control over appetites, needs, and life circumstances, particularly during times when the patient feels she is not in control. It is normative to experience pregnancy as a time when one's body is out of control, growing enormously in a relatively short period of time. The woman loses the ability to control the shape and size of her body, particularly her breasts and abdomen. Issues related to intimacy, sexuality, and closeness, particularly in the context of a larger body, can be extremely anxiety provoking for a woman with an eating disorder (37). These changes in body shape and size, as well as a more "sexual" body, can be terrifying for the anorexic or bulimic patient who has often struggled much of her life to keep her body thin and fit and for whom sexuality may be highly conflictual.

8.2. Second Trimester

The second trimester is one of relative calm, and women generally report this as the easiest 3 mo of the pregnancy. If the eating-disordered patient continues in psychotherapy, which is recommended, this period can serve as a time to examine a number of psychological issues that may emerge when the pregnant patient is feeling more energetic and capable of doing some exploratory work in therapy.

Looking back on one's own experience of being parented in anticipation of becoming a parent is a common theme. The patient may grapple with feelings of anger, sadness, and disappointment over the parenting she received as a child, which may have been experienced as inadequate or conflict-ridden. In this context, the patient with an eating disorder may struggle to determine how not to replicate that experience with her own child. This can be a time of tremendous growth and learning and offers a psychotherapist and other providers the opportunity for modeling and teaching of appropriate and warm parenting behaviors.

Becoming a parent may stimulate issues of separation, autonomy, and maintaining appropriate boundaries. Helping the patient to learn to separate her own needs from the needs of first the fetus and then the child is an important issue to explore during this time. Meeting both her own and her child's needs has implications in terms of the physical and the psychological well being of mother and child.

Issues related to identity are often prominent for the eating-disordered patient and may emerge during this period of pregnancy. It is during this trimester that the pregnancy often becomes very real for the patient, with the first movement of the fetus and beginning to "show" the pregnancy. During this period, the mother-to-be often begins to see herself in this parental context. As such, questions about new roles and responsibilities surface as the woman begins to think about taking on the care of another. For the patient whose identity may have been defined by outward appearance, external achievements, and pleasing others, the shift to caring for someone else may present challenges that can be talked through with professionals.

8.3. Third Trimester

The third trimester can be a very trying time for the pregnant patient. She has gained weight and may be anticipating how to lose it quickly after delivery. The last month of pregnancy often involves a substantial increase in appetite at a time when the patient is likely already feeling overwhelmed with her pregnancy weight gain. She may experience the increased appetite as further evidence of loss of control and may resort to using purgatives or restricting her intake as a means to compensate, at a time when healthy nutrition is so vital.

Body image issues, although present throughout pregnancy, tend to be especially problematic during this time. The eating-disordered patient is generally not able to accurately estimate her body size, even when she is thin or of normal weight. Her perception of her pregnant body is likely to be even more distorted. In seeing herself as bigger than she really is, her tendency may be to revert to minimizing her intake to keep herself from getting larger. The patient's increased weight in pregnancy may bring back memories of her pubescent weight gain, which may have been when her eating disorder started. Feelings of self-loathing, fears of spiraling out of control, and memories of being teased may all be brought up as painful reminders of an earlier time. The patient's response may be to gain control in the only way she has learned how, by restricting or compensating for whatever food she takes into her body.

9. HELPFUL STRATEGIES

Together with exploring or supporting these issues with the patient, there are several more pragmatic strategies that the clinician can use to help the patient through this often difficult 9 mo. Involvement with the spouse or partner is very important. It is well known that many women will choose not to tell their spouse about the eating disorder (37). During pregnancy, however, it is perhaps more important than ever before that the woman with an eating disorder makes her partner aware of her struggles with food and that the partner be enlisted for support. This may be the time for couples therapy, either with the woman's primary therapist or with someone new who is knowledgeable about eating disorders. Support will be needed not only during pregnancy, but also thereafter, in dealing with postpartum issues and caring for a newborn. In one of the prospective studies discussed earlier, the factor most strongly associated with positive pregnancy outcome was marital status (6). The authors speculated that the presence of a marital partner would likely mean the availability of social, financial, and emotional support. Encouraging the pregnant eating-disordered woman to confide in and obtain support from her partner is an important role for the health care team.

In order to help the pregnant eating-disordered patient take care of herself (and thereby take care of the baby), it is critical to make the fetus as real as possible throughout the pregnancy. A discussion of the importance of nutrition for the developing fetus might offer the woman an incentive to eat. Encouraging the patient to read materials that connect her nutritional intake with the growth of the fetus can be very useful (38). An explanation of the size, anatomical development, and gestational age of the fetus can provide information to the woman that might help her eat "for the baby" with less focus on her own increasing weight. This can be done early in the pregnancy through the use of visual materials such as the book *A Child Is Born (39)*, as well as throughout the pregnancy. It is helpful to sensitively inform the patient of the potential harmful effects that eating-disorder behaviors can have on the fetus, but to do so cautiously so as not to add to the burden of guilt the patient is likely to already bear.

Although the recommendations put forth here are based on the available research, it is important to note that only two prospective longitudinal

studies of pregnancy and eating disorders have been published to date
(20,22). However, given the accumulating evidence of serious potential
risk in patients with a history of or a current eating disorder, health care
professionals should consider these proposed guidelines for adequate
assessment and care when treating a pregnant patient with an eating
disorder.

10. POSTPARTUM ISSUES

The period after delivery is most often experienced as stressful as well
as joyful for most new mothers. For the patient with an eating disorder,
the added stresses of her symptoms, pregnancy weight gain, and new
feeding demands may pose particular challenges in the postpartum
period.

One issue of great concern is PPD *(40)*. The prevalence of clinical
depression in the postpartum period in the general population is estimated to be approx 12% *(41)*. Franko et al. *(22)* reported more than three
times that rate (35%), an elevation that is consistent with the findings of
earlier studies *(7,17)*. In this prospective study a higher frequency of
PPD was found in the group of women who were symptomatic with
eating-disorder symptoms during pregnancy *(22)*. Nearly half of the
symptomatic group reported PPD, which may have been a function of
previous affective disorder and/or the physiological and psychological
stresses of having an active eating disorder during pregnancy. Similarly,
Morgan et al. *(7)* found one-third of a sample of 94 bulimic women to
have PPD. It is noteworthy that in the bulimic women with a history of
AN, two-thirds were diagnosed with PPD. Abraham *(17)* reported that
9 of 26 women with BN were treated for PPD, with 7 of those 9 having
had eating-disorder symptoms during pregnancy. More recently,
Abraham et al. *(42)* reported on 181 women who were assessed for PPD
and anxiety in the week after delivery. Of these, 19 had a restricting
eating disorder and 10 had a binge–purge eating disorder. Higher distress during the postpartum period was associated with fear of weight
gain before and during pregnancy as well as frequency of vomiting
during the first 3–4 mo of pregnancy. Women who binged and purged
showed more distress than women who restricted.

We can speculate that patients with eating disorders have stresses that
may not be present in healthy women, such as body image issues, extreme
weight concerns, anxiety, and symptomatic behaviors, which may make
them more vulnerable to depression in the postpartum period. In addition, approx 40% of women with eating disorders have a history of
affective disorder *(43)*, which also puts them at risk for PPD *(44)*. Fur-

thermore, the vulnerability to PPD may be increased by the medical complications of eating disorders (e.g., dehydration and electrolyte instability), as well as by environmental factors such as poor social support *(42)*. It is extremely important to assess for depression in the postpartum period and provide appropriate psychological and, if necessary, pharmacological treatment.

10.1. Weight Loss in the Postpartum Period

Weight loss is another area of concern in the postpartum period. The risk of resuming eating-disordered behaviors during this time should be considered to be quite high, as patients are generally anxious to return to prepregnancy weights. Data supports this contention, as several studies have found substantial return of symptoms after delivery *(6,7)*. Working with a registered dietician who can suggest appropriate weight loss strategies may be helpful in the first few postpartum months. Similarly, encouraging the patient to join a once-weekly exercise class for new mothers can aid in both losing weight sensibly and decreasing social isolation. Monitoring the rate of weight loss is very important because too rapid a loss may serve as a trigger for the return of binge eating and purging.

10.2. Breast-Feeding and Feeding Issues

As the new mother struggles in her efforts to lose weight, she may also have difficulties in feeding her baby. To date, there are seven studies of four samples of eating-disordered mothers and their offspring *(45–51)*. In summary, these studies find that, compared with controls, the children of women with eating disorders weigh less at infancy and at 1 yr, have more difficulty with breast-feeding and bottle-weaning, and have more emotional difficulties and eating behavior disturbances (inhibited, secretive, or overeating). During mealtime, interactions are characterized by more conflict in eating-disorder dyads, and mothers were found to make fewer positive comments during mealtimes. One study *(49)* found that 20% of the variance in weight at 1 yr was accounted for by conflict during mealtime. The eating-disordered mothers reported more negative affectivity in their children and more concern for their daughter's weight and preferred thinner babies. A recent review of this literature concluded that "children of mothers with eating disorders are themselves at increased risk of disturbance in a variety of domains" *(52)*.

These data suggest that encouraging the new mother to talk to her pediatrician and nurse practitioner about appropriate feeding schedules and infant weight gain will be useful. It may also be helpful to include the pediatrician in the treatment team. Therapeutic issues that arise may include the patient's struggle to nourish both herself and her baby, to separate and meet both sets of physical and psychological needs, and to work to not recreate the conflicts around food in her new family.

11. CONCLUSION

Consistent with the recommendations of others *(7,12,17)*, close observation throughout pregnancy by obstetric and mental health providers is vital for patients with active eating disorders. Given the accumulating evidence of serious potential risk in patients with a history of or a current eating disorder, it is suggested that health care professionals routinely screen and assess for eating disorders in women and inquire carefully when a pregnant woman has a history of an eating disorder. The proposed treatment guidelines may provide assistance to both mental health and obstetric health care providers in optimizing maternal and fetal outcome.

REFERENCES

1. American Psychiatric Association. (1994) Diagnostic and Statistical Manual of Mental Disorders. Washington, DC: APA Press
2. Fairburn, C. G. and Harrison, P. J. (2003) Eating disorders. Lancet 361, 407–416.
3. Milner, G. and O'Leary, M. M. (1988) Anorexia nervosa occurring in pregnancy. Acta Psychiatr. Scand. 77, 491–492.
4. Willis, D. C. and Rand, C. S. W. (1988) Pregnancy in bulimic women. Obstet. Gynecol. 71, 708-710.
5. Lacey, J. H. and Smith, G. (1987) Bulimia nervosa: the impact on mother and baby. Br. J. Psych. 150, 777–781.
6. Blais, M. A., Becker, A. E., Burwell, R. A., et al. (2000) Pregnancy: outcome and impact in a cohort of eating disordered women. Int. J. Eat. Disord. 27, 140–149.
7. Morgan, J. F., Lacey, J. H., and Sedgwick, P. M. (1999) Impact of pregnancy on bulimia nervosa. Br. J. Psych. 174, 135–140.
8. Conrad, R., Schablewski, J., Schilling, G., and Liedtke, R. (2003) Worsening of symptoms of bulimia nervosa during pregnancy. Psychosomatics 44, 76–78.
9. Mitchell, J. E., Seim, H. C., Glotter, D., Soll, E. A., and Pyle, R. L. (1991) A retrospective study of pregnancy in bulimia nervosa. Int. J. Eat. Disord. 10, 209–214.
10. Lemberg, R. and Phillips, J. (1989) The impact of pregnancy on anorexia nervosa and bulimia. Int. J. Eat. Disord. 8, 285–295.
11. Brinch, M., Isager, T., and Tolstrup, K. (1988) Anorexia nervosa and motherhood: Reproduction pattern and mothering behavior of 50 women. Acta Psychiatr. Scand. 77, 98–104
12. Bulik, C. M., Sullivan, P. F., Fear, J. L., Pickering, A., Dawn, A., and McCullin, M. (1999) Fertility and reproduction in women with anorexia nervosa: a controlled study. J. Clin. Psych. 60, 130–135.
13. Mitchell-Gieleghem, A., Mittelstaedt, M. E., and Bulik, C. M. (2002) Eating disorders and childbearing: concealment and consequences. Birth 29, 182–191.

14. James, D. C. (2001) Eating disorders, fertility, and pregnancy: relationships and complications. J. Perinat. Neonatal Nurs. 15, 36–48.
15. Feingold, M., Kaminer, Y., Lyons, K., Chaudhury, A., Costigan, K., and Cetrulo, C. (1988) Bulimia nervosa in pregnancy: a case report. Obstet. Gynecol. 71, 1025–1027.
16. Stewart, D. E., Raskin, J., Garfinkel, P. E., MacDonald, O. L., and Robinson, G. E. (1987) Anorexia nervosa, bulimia, and pregnancy. Am. J. Obstet. Gynecol. 157, 1194–1198.
17. Abraham, S. (1998) Sexuality and reproduction in bulimia nervosa patients over 10 years. J. Psychosom. Res. 44, 491–502.
18. Stewart, D. E. (1992) Reproductive functions in eating disorders. Ann. Med. 24, 287–291.
19. Muscati, S. K., Gray-Donald, K., and Koski, K. G. (1996) Timing of weight gain during pregnancy: promoting fetal growth and minimizing maternal weight retention. Int. J. Obes. Relat. Metab. Disord. 20, 526–532.
20. Sollid, C. P., Wisborg, K., Hjort, J., and Secher, N. J. (2004) Eating disorder that was diagnosed before pregnancy and pregnancy outcome. Am. J. Obstet. Gynecol. 190, 206–210.
21. Conti, J., Abraham, S., and Taylor. A. (1998) Eating behavior and pregnancy outcome. J. Psychosom. Res. 44, 465–477.
22. Franko, D. F., Blais, M. A., Becker, A. E., et al. (2001) Pregnancy complications and neonatal outcome in eating disordered women. Am. J. Psych. 158, 1461–1466.
23. King, M. B. (1991) The natural history of eating pathology in attenders to primary medical care. Int. J. Eat. Disord. 10, 379–387.
24. Stewart, D. E., Robinson, E., Goldbloom, D. S., and Wright, C. (1990) Infertility and eating disorders. Am. J. Obstet. Gynecol. 163, 2196–2199.
25. Martin, J. R. and Wollitzer, A. O. (1988) The prevalence, secrecy, and psychology of purging in a family practice setting. Int. J. Eat. Disord. 7, 515–519.
26. Becker, A. E., Grinspoon, S. K., Klibanski, A., and Herzog, D. B. (1999) Eating disorders. N. Engl. J. Med. 340, 1092–1098.
27. Becker, A. E., Franko, D. L., Nussbaum, K., and Herzog, D. B. (2003) Secondary prevention for eating disorders. Int. J. Eat. Disord. 35, 179–189.
28. Hollifield, J. and Hobdy, J. (1990) The course of pregnancy complicated by bulimia. Psychotherapy 27, 249–255.
29. Franko, D. L. and Spurrell, E. B. (2000) Detection and management of eating disorders during pregnancy. Obstet. Gynecol.. 95, 942–946.
30. Lingam, R. and McCluskey, S. (1996) Eating disorders associated with hyperemesis gravidarum. J. Psychosom. Res. 40, 231–234.
31. Freund, K. M., Graham, S. M., Lesky, L. G., and Moskowitz, M. A. (1993) Detection of bulimia in a primary care setting. J. Gen. Intern. Med. 8, 236–242.
32. Mintz, L. B., O'Halloran, S. M., Mulholland, A. M., and Schneider, P. A. (1997) Questionnaire for eating disorder diagnoses: reliability and validity of operationalizing DSM-IV criteria into a self-report format. J. Counsel. Psych. 44, 63–79.
33. Fairburn, C. G., and Cooper, Z. (1993) The Eating Disorder Examination, 12th ed. In: Fairburn, C.G. and Wilson, G.T., eds. Binge Eating: Nature, Assessment, and Treatment. New York: Guilford Press.
34. Williamson, D. A., Anderson, D. A., Jackman, L. P., and Jackson, S. R. (1995) Assessment of eating disordered thoughts, feelings, and behaviors. In: Allison, D. B., ed. Handbook of Assessment Methods for Eating Behaviors and Weight Related Problems: Measures, Theory and Research, pp. 347–386.

35. American Psychiatric Association Work Group on Eating Disorders (2000) Practice guidelines for the treatment of patients with eating disorders (revision). Am. J. Psych. 157 (1 Suppl.), 1–39.
36. Knapp, C. (2003) Appetites. New York: Counterpoint Press.
37. Woodside D. B., Lackstrom, J. B., and Shekter-Wolfson, L. (2000) Marriage in eating disorders: comparisons between patients and spouses and changes over the course of treatment. J. Psychosom. Res. 49, 165–168.
38. Ward, E. M. (1998) Pregnancy Nutrition: Good Health for You and Your Baby. New York: Wiley.
39. Nilsson, L. (2003) A Child Is Born (4th ed.). New York: Delacorte Press.
40. Franko, D. L. and Hilsinger, E. (1995) Depression and bulimia in a pregnant woman. Harv. Rev. Psych. 2, 282–287.
41. Gotlib, I. H. (1998) Postpartum depression. In: Blechman, E. A.and Brownell, K. D., eds. Behavioral Medicine and Women: A Comprehensive Handbook. New York: Guilford Press, pp. 489–494.
42. Abraham, S., Taylor, A., and Conti, J. (2001) Postnatal depression, eating, exercise, and vomiting before and during pregnancy. Int. J. Eat. Disord. 29, 482–487.
43. Wonderlich, S. A.and Mitchell, J. E. (1997) Eating disorders and comorbidity: empirical, conceptual, and clinical implications. Eat. Disord. Res. 33, 381–388.
44. O'Hara, M. W., Schlechte, J. A., Lewis, D. A., and Wright, E. J. (1991) Prospective study of postpartum blues: Biologic and psychosocial factors. Arch. Gen. Psych. 48, 801–806.
45. Agras, S., Hammer, L., and McNicholas, F. (1999) A prospective study of the influence of eating-disordered mothers on their children. Int. J. Eat. Disord. 25, 253–262.
46. Evans, J. and le Grange, D. (1995) Body size and parenting in eating disorders: A comparative study of the attitudes of mothers towards their children. Int. J. Eat. Disord. 18, 39–48.
47. Stein, A., Woolley, H., Cooper, S. D., and Fairburn, C. G. (1994) An observational study of mothers with eating disorders and their infants. J. Child Psychol. Psych. 35, 733–748.
48. Stein, A., Murray, L, Cooper, P., and Fairburn, C. G. (1996) Infant growth in the context of maternal eating disorders and maternal depression: a comparative study. Psych. Med. 26, 569–574.
49. Stein, A., Woolley, H., and McPherson, K. (1999). Conflict between mothers with eating disorders and their infants during mealtimes. Br. J. Psych. 175, 455–461.
50. Stice, E., Agras, W. S., and Hammer, L. (1999) Risk factors for the emergence of childhood eating disturbances: a five-year prospective study. Int. J. Eat. Disord. 25, 375–387.
51. Waugh, E. and Bulik, C. M. (1999) Offspring of women with eating disorders. Int. J. Eat. Disord. 25, 123–133.
52. Park, R. J., Senior, R., and Stein, A. (2003) The offspring of mothers with eating disorders. Eur. Child Adolesc. Psych. 12 (Suppl. 1), i110–i119.

9

Children of Parents With Mental Illness

Outcomes and Interventions

Mary F. Brunette and Teresa Jacobsen

Summary

Many psychiatrically ill women bear and raise children. An extensive literature has documented the potential effects on children resulting from exposure to parental mental illness. Negative outcomes may also result from children's genetic vulnerabilities, exposure to environmental stressors, and maladaptive parenting styles. Parents' psychiatric symptoms can affect their parenting behavior and interfere with their awareness of their children's needs. This chapter reviews the effects of parental mental illness on children and discusses various interventions that can help minimize adverse outcomes. It also addresses ethical and legal issues that arise when working with mentally ill parents.

Key Words: Parenting; children; infants; mental illness; development.

1. INTRODUCTION

Approximately half of the 12 million Americans with major mood or psychotic disorders *(1)* are parents *(2)*. Mental illnesses often develop during the years of childbearing and childrearing, although adults often have children before any mental illness becomes prominent *(2,3)*. Additionally, women who have already developed a mental illness are just as likely to give birth and to parent children as women who have not developed a mental illness. Although clinicians often presume the contrary, even women with severe mental illnesses are usually sexually active *(4–6)*. Furthermore, women with mental illness, more often than men,

From: *Current Clinical Practice: Psychiatric Disorders in Pregnancy and the Postpartum: Principles and Treatment*
Edited by: V. Hendrick © Humana Press, Totowa, NJ

end up raising their children (70% of women vs 30% of men) *(3)*. Given that parenting is a central part of the lives of most women who have a mental illness, it is important for physicians and other health care providers to understand the effects of maternal mental illness on both parenting and children.

This chapter focuses on the outcomes of children of parents with mental illness. It begins by reviewing a model for understanding the impact of parental mental illness on child outcomes. Next, the literature on the different factors that impact child outcomes in families with parental mental illness—the parents, the environment, and the child—are reviewed. Case examples of how children at different phases of development may respond to maternal mental illness are then presented, followed by a discussion of interventions to improve parenting and the family environment for high-risk families. The final section of the chapter addresses ethical and legal issues relevant to clinicians working with high-risk families.

Much of the research on parents with mental illness has focused on parents with depression, probably because depression is a common mental illness. Less research has been completed related to parents with other mental illnesses, including anxiety, psychotic, and bipolar disorders. Research in this area is also hampered by methodological shortcomings, including small numbers, lack of or inadequate comparison groups, measurement problems, inadequate attention to confounding factors, inattention to issues of co-morbidity, and overlap between definitions of parental illness symptoms and parenting behaviors. Studies with fewer shortcomings are highlighted.

Most of the studies that have assessed parenting have focused on mothers rather than fathers, despite the reality that fathers may impact children as much as or more than mothers. For this reason, we use "she" to refer to the parent, and we specify when research focused on fathers. We use the term "mental illness" to refer to a large group of mental illnesses, including schizophrenia, major depression, bipolar disorder, and other illnesses, each of which may present very differently and have different impacts on any particular parent. When possible, we refer to specific mental illnesses rather than use the general term.

2. DETERMINANTS OF CHILD OUTCOMES

Figure 1 presents a model, modified from models previously presented in the literature, of the major determinants of child outcomes *(7–11)*. The factors determining outcomes include parental influences, including genetic risk and parenting behavior; environmental factors;

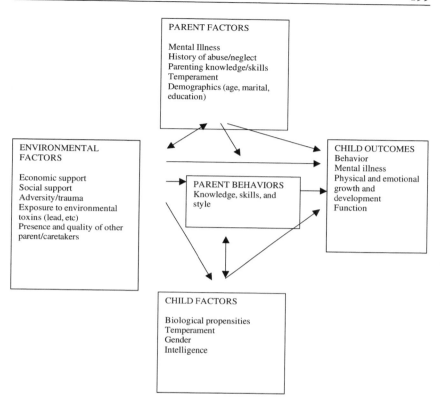

Fig 1. Factors affecting child outcomes.

and child factors, such as temperament and child cognitive functioning. Environmental and parent factors impact children directly as well as indirectly via their influence on parenting behavior, and categories of factors may interact with each other. Children with one type of temperament, for instance, may respond differently to mood changes in a mother than do children with other types of temperaments, thereby eliciting particular parenting behaviors *(12,13)*. In the next sections, the research related to each set of factors—parent, environment, and child—are reviewed.

2.1. Parent Factors Impacting Child Outcomes

2.1.1. HERITABILITY OF MENTAL ILLNESS

A developing body of research points to the importance of genetic factors in a child's liability to develop psychiatric disorders over his or

Table 1
Heritability of Major Mental Illnesses: Child's Lifetime Risk of Becoming Ill

	General population rates if neither parent is ill (%)	Risk if one parent is ill (%)	Risk if two parents are ill (%)	Risk for other monozygotic twin if one twin is ill (%)	Risk for dizygotic twin if one twin is ill (%)
Schizophrenia	1.5	10	40	18–60	15
Major depression	10	20–25	30–50	50–60	20
Bipolar disorder	1	5–10	—	40–70	10–20

her lifetime (14). Environmental context is also important in the etiology of psychiatric disorders, and the expression of a child's genetic liability appears to be impacted by and interact with the environmental context (15,16). The stress–vulnerability model, for instance, proposes that vulnerability, determined by a combination of genetic and early environmental events, interacts with later environmental stress to either precipitate the onset of a psychiatric disorder or to trigger a relapse of illness symptoms. For example, loss of an important relationship in a vulnerable child can constitute a stress that may precipitate or exacerbate a major depressive episode.

Genetic, twin, and family studies indicate that children born to parents with major mental illnesses are at higher risk to develop the same and other psychiatric illnesses than children whose parents do not have the illness. Table 1 shows the risks for children of parents with schizophrenia, major depression, and bipolar disorder. The heritability of schizophrenia is high, between 60 and 81%, and multiple genetic loci are thought to be involved (16–18). The heritability for major depression is estimated to be in the 10–45% range (19,20). The genetic heritability of bipolar disorders (with mania and depression) is higher than for unipolar depression (21). When a psychiatric disorder is present in both parents or in a parent and a grandparent, children may be more likely to develop the disorder than if only one parent expresses the disorder (22,23).

Even mental illnesses that appear to have a biological basis may develop in children in the absence of overt parental mental illness. One study, for instance, reported that 13% of adolescents with no family history of depression developed a depressive disorder (22). In such cases, the susceptibility to behavioral disorders may be conferred in part via environmental stresses, such as exposure to neonatal or childhood injury or toxins (e.g., lead), situational adversities or trauma (e.g., loss of a parent), or maladaptive parenting practices. In fact, the liability for conduct disorder and antisocial personality disorder, common externalizing disorders, appears to be heavily influenced by harsh parenting style *(15)*. For concerned women with a personal or family history of mental illness who are considering pregnancy, referral to genetic counseling to obtain information about the potential risk to their children for inheriting major mental illness can be helpful.

2.1.2. MENTAL ILLNESS SYMPTOMS AND PARENTING

Parental mental illness symptoms can influence child outcomes, with more severe or persistent symptoms generally being more problematic than milder or transient symptoms *(24,25)*. Symptoms may affect parenting behavior (e.g., psychosis may lead to misinterpretation of cues and inappropriate behavior or mania may lead to intrusiveness or overinvolvement). Mental illness symptoms of all types may interfere with a parent's understanding of a child's emotional and physical needs. In addition, mental illness symptoms can distract a parent from being able to attend to and respond to a child *(26–28)*.

Research suggests that parental psychiatric symptoms can be associated with child abuse or neglect, and in some cases mental illness symptoms may lead to safety concerns *(29–34)*. Women with psychotic symptoms, for instance, may experience delusions about their children, accompanied by thoughts or impulses to harm their children or themselves *(25)*. Impulses to harm that are based on delusions may lead to violence toward children, which has been reported in several studies to occur in 1–12.8% of severely ill women *(30,31)*. On the other hand, impulses to harm that are experienced as obsessive, intrusive, and incongruent with reality, such as those that may occur in women with postpartum depression, might lead to checking or avoidance behaviors (e.g., repetitive checking to ensure that the child is safe) rather than harmful behaviors *(35)*. Symptoms and related impulses to harm are usually time-limited and responsive to treatment, however, and therefore not indicative of overall parenting abilities *(32)*. Parents with good insight into their mental illness appear to be at less risk for harming their children than parents who lack insight into their illness *(36)*.

2.1.3. PARENTING STYLES

A large literature has documented that parenting styles affect child behavior and mental health. Problematic parenting styles in parents with mental illness (e.g., hostility or criticism toward a child) can increase the child's risk for problems, while adequate parenting styles (e.g., warmth, acceptance, and consistent limit-setting) appear to confer some protection to at-risk children (11,37,38). Parenting styles are believed to result from genetically influenced parental temperament, from attitudes and behaviors that the parent learned from her past and current environment, and from interactions with children (12). Large population-based studies have found that young parent age, poverty, and marital status (e.g., low social support) were associated with maladaptive parenting styles (39–42). Many parents who have a mental illness were poorly parented or experienced abuse or neglect themselves as children (43,44). Although these experiences may contribute to the development of early attachment problems and later psychiatric disorders, research is mixed as to whether a parent's history of being poorly parented will lead to later maladaptive parenting in adult–child relationships (45–48). Some research suggests that roughly one-third of these parents may exhibit maladaptive parenting attitudes and behaviors when raising their own children, thus repeating their own abuse history (39,41,42,49). However, many parents purposefully "try to do it differently" and work toward parenting their own children in a healthier way (50). Most studies of parenting behavior in parents with mental illness do not control for the parent's history of abuse or neglect.

Similar to women in the general population, women with mental illness exhibit a wide variety of parenting styles and skills. Studies utilizing direct observations comparing parents with mental illness and their children with matched controls have reported mixed findings regarding parenting. Some of these studies found no differences or very few differences between groups of women with mental illness and matched controls (51–54). Most published studies, however, suggest that women with mental illness are more likely than women without mental illness to exhibit problematic parenting behaviors, such as lower levels of attentiveness or higher levels of tension, intrusiveness, or criticism (6,55–63). Lovejoy and colleagues (64) conducted a review and meta-analysis of studies of parenting behavior in women with depressive disorders. They found that between one-fourth and one-half of studies reported a small to moderate effect in the expected direction for increased negative and disengaged maternal behaviors as well as reduced positive maternal behaviors with children. The effects were larger in mothers of infants than in mothers of preschoolers and school-aged children.

Although most research on parenting skills and mental illness has been conducted among women with depressive disorders (for reviews, see refs. 8,64–66), similar findings have been documented in mothers with other mood disorders, psychotic disorders *(6,52,56,59,62)*, and eating disorders (*see* ref. *67* for a review). Other research suggests that when a mother's illness is severe and chronic, parenting may be more seriously impaired than when the illness is less severe or responds rapidly to treatment *(68,69)* and can result in relinquishment or loss of child custody either temporarily or permanently *(70,71)*. Some mothers who give up or lose custody are still able to provide intermittent parenting over the course of their children's development *(72)*, although frequent changes in custody arrangements can in some cases be disruptive to child development *(63,73)*.

Of considerable importance, research suggests that maladaptive parenting styles, rather than parental psychiatric disorders, may be a particularly important pathway to poor child outcomes *(74–79)*. For example, Johnson and colleagues conducted a longitudinal study of 593 families in which parental psychiatric disorders appeared to increase their children's risk for psychiatric disorders *(75)*. However, the magnitude of the association between parent's and children's psychiatric disorders was significantly reduced (from 0.41 to 0.23) when analyses controlled for parenting styles *(75)*. Furthermore, rates of psychiatric disorders were higher in children of parents with maladaptive parenting styles regardless of whether or not the parent had a mental illness. In other words, the children's risk for psychiatric disorder was related to their parents' maladaptive parenting. Findings from studies of smaller groups of families also have suggested that parenting style mediates the relationship between parental mental illness and negative child outcomes, including psychiatric disorders. For example, maternal hostility *(77,78)*, criticism *(80,81)*, and lack of responsiveness *(82)* have been found to contribute in part to the relationship between maternal depression or anxiety and negative child outcomes.

3. ENVIRONMENTAL FACTORS IMPACTING CHILD OUTCOMES

Low maternal socioeconomic status (SES; *9,83–86*), low social support *(39,83,84,87)*, parental conflict *(52,89–95)*, and trauma *(94,95–97)* are important environmental risk factors that have been associated with poor child outcomes. Some of these factors may be related to negative outcomes because of their association with ineffective parenting styles, increased exposure to violence and poor role models, and reduced opportunities for support *(7,39,85,98)* or via their association with other risk factors, such as poor prenatal care and exposure to poor nutrition or environmental toxins *(88)*.

The other parent figure and the relationship between parent figures can also affect child outcomes. The other parent may provide support to the mother, parent the child, and also pass on some level of biological risk to the child (*see* ref. *99* for a review and meta-analysis of the association between paternal and maternal psychopathology and child outcomes). When the parenting provided by the other parent figure (usually the father) is positive *(100)*, outcomes may be good *(38)*. Likewise, other parenting figures such as grandparents or child-care providers can provide positive parenting and potentially improve children's outcomes, although little research has thus far tested the logical hypothesis that healthy relationships with other caregivers can protect children who are at risk due to other factors *(38)*. Research has consistently shown that early childhood intervention in the form of preschool is associated with improved childhood outcomes (e.g., refs. *101* and *102*). In contrast, additional risk may be conferred on a child when the other parent or caregiver has a mental illness or a maladaptive parenting style *(103)*.

Discord between parental figures has been associated with ineffective parenting styles *(53,61,93)* and with poor child outcomes in families with mental illness *(52,89–93)*. Marital problems have been found to mediate the relationship between maternal depression and toddler's behavior problems *(104)* and between maternal depression and children's internalizing symptoms *(90)*.

Other negative events or traumatic experiences in a child's environment have been associated with adverse outcomes in children *(105)*, including the development of internalizing and externalizing symptoms, psychiatric disorders, cognitive problems, and interpersonal problems (*see* ref. *97* for a review). Of note, separation from a parent or parent figure, even one with symptoms or parenting deficits, may be experienced as traumatic *(106)*. Children react to trauma with great variability, and factors other than trauma may mediate and moderate children's reactions to trauma *(96)*. Notably, although exposure to trauma may increase the risk for the development of problematic outcomes, most traumatized children do not appear to develop overt psychiatric disorders in childhood. Adversity may interact with maternal mental illness to negatively impact children, although some research suggests that negative life events are less likely to account for symptoms or problems in children of mothers with psychiatric problems than in children of parents who do not have psychiatric problems *(93,105)*.

Recent studies have shown that demographic and environmental risk factors may interact with parental mental illness to predict or account for maladaptive parenting behaviors or poor child outcomes *(24,89,92,107–110)*.

For example, low SES or single parenthood has been associated with low birthweight (LBW) and slower development in infants of parents with psychosis or depression *(24,110)*. Moreover, the effects of maternal mental illness on child outcome have been found to be different depending on the mother's SES and background. Research on high-risk depressed women (e.g., low SES, education, and support) has generally found that maternal mental illness was associated with more parenting problems and poor child outcomes (e.g., refs. *57* and *111*), whereas studies of low-risk depressed women (e.g., middle income, educated, married women) did not confirm these associations (e.g., refs. *53* and *54*). In a meta-analysis of 46 observational studies of maternal depression and parenting, the effect sizes for parenting behavior among socioeconomically disadvantaged women were moderate, whereas the effect sizes were not different from zero among women who were not disadvantaged *(64)*, indicating that socioeconomic hardship by itself or in conjunction with other factors may be an important predictor of maladaptive parenting.

4. CHILD FACTORS ASSOCIATED WITH POOR CHILD OUTCOMES

Early on, LBW, prematurity, and other perinatal complications may lead to delays or deficits in a child's cognitive and motor development *(110,112,113)*. Very LBW, in particular, is associated with increased risk for cognitive and behavioral problems, such as attention deficit disorder, as well as other medical problems (for review, *see* ref. *114*). Children who are premature or who have lower cognitive capacities appear to be at higher risk for being exposed to maladaptive parenting *(45,115,116)*, whereas high intelligence may be a protective factor *(117)*.

A child's temperament is another important factor impacting outcomes. Children with easygoing and outgoing temperaments may do better than children who are temperamentally more sensitive, shy, or difficult, perhaps because difficult children may be more likely to elicit insensitive or harsh caregiving from adults *(37,118–122)*, which may contribute to the development of problems over time. For example, children's reactive styles to their parents were studied in a large, population-based sample in Finland. The 12-yr-old children who reported high levels of psychiatric symptoms tended to respond to parental low mood with the most negative emotional reactions and in turn reported that they had experienced less effective parenting *(13)*. Children who reacted with other styles (such as ignoring) had lower levels of psychiatric symptoms. This study suggests that child characteristics may interact with parental mental illness to influence parenting quality.

Children of parents with mental illness may inherit a similar mental illness (*see* Section 2.2.1.), which can manifest itself with mood or behavior changes and skill deficits in infancy or childhood *(105)*. Whether these are caused by exposure to parental symptoms and/or maladaptive parenting, by inherited biological and temperamental propensities, or by both is unclear. Certainly, the cognitive and social skills deficits in vulnerable children can create more challenging parenting situations *(13)*. Supporting the notion of interactions between child and parent characteristics, population-based research has found that children with disabilities, including behavioral disorders, or with challenging temperaments were more likely to have experienced maltreatment by their caregivers *(86,95)*.

5. WHAT CAN HAPPEN TO CHILDREN OF PARENTS WITH MENTAL ILLNESS?

Overall, research suggests that the presence of maternal mental illness is associated with higher risk for problematic outcomes in their children, including the children's capacity for relationships or attachment, motor and cognitive growth and development, and behavioral problems and psychiatric disorders. As noted previously, research in this area is hampered by many methodological shortcomings and should be interpreted cautiously. Although many studies have found results in the expected direction (e.g., maternal mental illness is associated with worse child outcomes), the findings tend to be small and present for some but not all of the measures in each study. Furthermore, the statistical significance of the findings is often borderline.

5.1. Effects on Attachment Relationships

Infants born to mothers with serious mental disorders may be at heightened risk for developing insecure or disorganized attachment relationships *(49,57,58,61,92,123,124)* and for interpersonal difficulties *(125,126)*. Infants who have developed attachment problems may then be more likely than infants without attachment problems to go on to exhibit behavior problems and psychiatric disorders later in childhood *(79,116,127,128)*.

5.2. Effects on Motor and Cognitive Development

Maternal mental illness can exert a negative impact on infant growth, development, and cognition, especially if a mother is withdrawn or unavailable to provide the infant with stimulation *(82)*. The research on cognitive outcomes of children of depressed mothers *(see* ref. *66* for a review) and children of mothers with psychotic disorders *(129)* is mixed, and most of the studies are small or have other methodological difficulties. Smaller studies have nonetheless found that approx 20% of infants of mothers with mental illness exhibited cognitive or motor delays on some measures *(111,130,131)* and that maternal mental illness was associated with delays in child development *(126,132)*. In contrast, a large population-based study that controlled for maternal education, SES, and gender found no differences in cognitive development between babies of depressed mothers compared to babies of nondepressed mothers *(109)*. Another study found that the severity and chronicity of maternal depression was related to slower child vocabulary development *(103)*, but this study and others have found that the child's male gender, low parental SES, low parental education, and low parental intelligence accounted for most of the variation in children's cognitive development *(109,110,133)*. These demographic factors may be associated with parenting characteristics that impair cognitive development. For example, Milgrom and colleagues demonstrated that lower maternal responsiveness and stimulation explained the lower IQ found in young children of depressed mothers *(82)*.

5.3. Effects on Behavior and Mental Health

Children of parents with mental illness may be more likely to exhibit behavioral problems or psychiatric disorders than children of parents who do not have a psychiatric disorder *(22,76,93,126,134–139)*, although the majority of these children do not develop problems or disorders. Research suggests that exposure to maternal mental illness or associated ineffective parenting in the early years of development may be more detrimental than exposure in later years *(64)*.

Some research suggests that, like children whose parents do not have mental illness *(140)*, children who begin to exhibit problems early continue to demonstrate problems over time *(141)*. For example, preschoolers who had disturbed attachment as infants or who showed aggressive behavior as toddlers showed ongoing behavior problems at age 5 *(79)*. Murray and colleagues *(142)* found striking continuity between the behavior of children of depressed mothers at both 5 and 10 yr old.

The few existing longitudinal studies of children of mothers with major mental illness provide mixed findings on children's long-term outcomes. Bagedahl-Strindlund et al. *(143)* followed children of psychiatrically ill mothers over 22 yr and found that their development, academic achievement, and family situation was not different from those of matched controls. The authors linked the positive outcomes in part to the high level of social support provided for these families in Sweden. Other studies have found that, as they develop, children of mothers with major mental illness continue to be at increased risk for interpersonal difficulties *(105,144)* and psychopathology *(145)*. Rutter and Quinton *(146)* found that roughly one-third of the offspring of parents with psychiatric illness exhibited a persistent disorder themselves in adolescence, one-third show transient psychiatric difficulties, and one-third show no emotional or behavioral disturbance.

6. RISK IS CUMULATIVE

Research suggests that the impact of risk factors on child outcomes is cumulative: more risk factors (including risks related to the parents, the child, and the environment) leads to a higher likelihood of poor child outcomes *(86,96,147,148)*. For example, Nomura and colleagues found that children of parents with depression were more likely to develop mental illness themselves if they experienced abuse or neglect or if they witnessed conflict between their parents *(93)*. Some research has found this cumulative effect especially in younger children *(86,147)*. The observation that risk is cumulative has implications for clinical and public health interventions in that it suggests that a reduction in the number of risk factors can help a child and that not all risk factors need to be removed to improve a child's trajectory in life.

7. EXAMPLES OF CHILDREN OF MOTHERS WITH MENTAL ILLNESS

In this section we present vignettes where maternal mental illness has negatively affected children during infancy, during toddlerhood and the preschool years, and over the long term to illustrate the range and type of effects that maternal mental illness may have on a child.

7.1. Infants and Toddlers

Lisa felt slightly overwhelmed with mothering Mae, her healthy, full-term baby, but she also delighted in Mae's health and beauty. At 6 wk, Mae lit up and wriggled vigorously whenever she saw her mother. Her mother, however, was becoming seriously depressed. She lost interest in Mae and became easily irritated when she cried, and found herself speaking harshly to the baby. She was exhausted because, after feed-

ing Mae in the middle of the night, she lay awake worrying. To Lisa it seemed that Mae cried all the time and was not easily consoled. Lisa did not pursue treatment for her depression and continued to sleep poorly and to be easily irritated and frequently tearful. One year later, Lisa reported that Mae's negativity persisted. For instance, when Mae was angry or upset, she withdrew from her mother and refused to interact.

Lisa and Mae's story typifies how severe depression in the postpartum period can impact infant well-being and development. A mother in this situation may lose interest in her baby, perceive the baby as bothersome, or misinterpret the infant's cues. She may then handle the infant roughly, disengage from the infant, or engage the infant in negative interactions. Because the mother is often the infant's primary environment, her parenting behavior may have a significant impact on the infant, although the short-term outcome for mothers with postpartum disorders and their infants can be quite good, especially if a mother responds to treatment and gets support *(149)*.

If a mother's psychiatric disorder is more severe, affects her behavior, persists over time, and is present with other risk factors, it can exert a negative impact on infant relational, motor, and language development. Some infants and toddlers growing up with these experiences may express negative or flat affect with the mother, or they may be difficult to console *(112,150)*. Others may withdraw from interactions *(92)*. If these patterns persist, some children may develop an insecure attachment bond to the mother and have difficulties in seeking proximity, closeness, and comfort when it is needed. Infants who are understimulated are also at risk for delays in cognitive and motor development. Unless the problems are addressed and corrected, affected infants may continue on an unhealthy developmental pathway.

7.2. Preschool Children

Joan experienced her first episode of mania when her child, Lila, was born 4 yr ago. At that time, the child's father left the state. Since then, Joan experienced intermittent, profound depression, during which time she threatened to kill herself. Joan could not tolerate seeing sadness in Lila, as it reminded her of her own depression. When Lila was 2, Joan had difficulty responding to her tantrums and sleep problems. When Lila was 3, Joan pushed the child to toilet train and spanked her for accidents. The now 4-yr-old girl was outwardly cheerful, but hyper-alert to her mother's moods, always ready to obey her mother's requests.

In this example, the increasing severity and chronicity of Joan's symptoms and problematic parenting style was mirrored by the development of symptoms in her daughter, including sleep problems, tantrums, and difficulties in toilet training. Recent research also shows this correlation between severity and chronicity of maternal symptoms with more child symptoms in the preschool years, even when demographic risk factors were controlled for (e.g., ref. *133*). Preschool-aged children may exhibit behaviors that mirror the ill parent's symptoms, including lethargy or anxiety, which may be expressed as phobias and fears. Additionally, if the child's environment (including mother and other caregivers) has not provided enough cognitive stimulation *(57)*, preschool-aged children may demonstrate cognitive and motor delays *(89,113)*.

In terms of their attachment, preschool-aged children of mothers with psychiatric disorders may begin to show parentified caretaking behavior *(151)*. Others may show compulsive compliant behavior, a pattern characterized by hypervigilance, wariness, and overly compliant behavior toward the parent *(152,153)*. Children who have been removed from the parent's care and have experienced multiple caregivers may exhibit attachment disorders *(73)*.

7.3. School-Aged Children

Elana was diagnosed with schizophrenia when she was 26 and thereafter relied on disability payments. She had a son, Rico, with a man who was later diagnosed with bipolar disorder and who drank alcohol and used drugs. The parents lived in neighboring rural towns but raised their son together with the help of the father's extended family, who doted on Rico. Elana was a gentle and concerned parent. Throughout his schooling, Rico required extra help. He was diagnosed with a learning disability and later with mild depression. At age 12, he became embarrassed by his mother's frequent, lengthy letters and concerned phone calls to his school as well as by her persistent belief that she was inhabited by ghosts. At age 15, he began smoking marijuana regularly with his friends and failed most of his classes. He did not complete high school. He did not develop schizophrenia or bipolar disorder, but he smoked marijuana daily throughout his 20s. He maintained employment at a local manufacturing plant and lived with his girlfriend and his mother until she died.

As in Rico's case, older children develop more of an awareness of their parents' mental illness and may have a variety of reactions to the parent. Children may feel unsure or worried about their relationship with the parent. If a parent has acute symptoms, they may become upset and worried about their parent's well-being and safety. Although many experience a great deal of emotional pain and inner turmoil, they may keep their feelings to themselves, viewing outsiders with suspicion or mistrust *(154)*. Without supports, education, and functional parenting, older children of moderately to severely ill parents may become involved in parental symptoms, either by adopting a parent's depressive or delusional state or by becoming the object of psychotic or depressed behavior *(155,156)*. More commonly, children may adopt a parent's coping style. For example, children of depressed parents exhibit depressive cognitions under situations of stress *(78)*. Children of parents who abuse substances may start to do the same as teenagers *(157)*.

Many older children worry that they themselves will become ill and would benefit from concrete information and reassurance. Others may get involved in taking care of an ill parent. If extreme, "parentification" of children can have negative consequences for children's sense of self and their long-term development *(106)*. Some research, however, suggests that milder forms of helping may be protective. Solantaus-Simula and colleagues *(13)* found, for instance, that children who reacted to their parents' low moods with empathy had lower levels of symptoms than children who reacted with negative emotions.

8. INTERVENTIONS TO HELP MOTHERS WITH MENTAL ILLNESS AND THEIR CHILDREN

Given that children of parents with mental illness are more likely to develop mental health or behavioral problems than other children (*see* previous discussion), their families are important targets for prevention and treatment interventions. Prior to intervention regarding parenting, a comprehensive family evaluation should identify specific areas of family need that are to be addressed in the intervention *(158)*. To maximize success, interventions should occur as early as possible and be designed and delivered with cultural sensitivity *(159)*.

All mothers with mental illness will require competent treatment of the mental illness and education regarding its impact on their maternal role and family life. Partners and family members benefit from this type of education as well. The American Academy of Child and Adolescent Psychiatry (AACAP) points out that the following are helpful to children in these families: simple information about the cause and symptoms of their parent's illness, help and support from family members, a stable home environment, a sense of being loved by the ill parent, a strong relationship with another healthy adult, and positive peer relationships *(160)*. The AACAP also notes that children who have interests and successes in outside activities, including school, and who are able to develop good coping strategies and positive self-esteem tend to do well. If any of these areas are deficient, they can be potential targets for intervention.

Older children with significant mental illness symptoms or behavioral disturbances will need interventions specific to them (e.g., children with severe withdrawal caused by depression or with bizarre behavior as a result of psychotic symptoms will need medication and other therapeutic interventions) *(161)*. Many interventions for school-aged children have been developed and shown to be effective (*see* ref. *162*), but child interventions are not reviewed here. Some research suggests that interventions with the parents of older children with problems may be more effective and longer lasting than child-only interventions (e.g., ref. *163*). Because younger children spend most of their time with and are completely reliant on their parents, they require interventions that include their parents and the home environment. Medications or child-only psychotherapies do not change the many powerful influences (including parenting style) that can impact them. In this section we examine interventions that focus on the child's parent and home environment, including treatment of the parent's mental illness, parent training, and family support interventions.

8.1. Perinatal and Postpartum Treatment of Maternal Mental Illness

In the first few years after delivery of a child, women are at increased risk for new or recurrent mental illness *(164,165)*. Overall, women with mood disorders are at higher risk for postpartum exacerbation than women with psychotic disorders (*see* previous chapters) *(164)*. Aggressive treatment of psychiatric illness immediately after delivery, during the postpartum period, and over the course of childrearing can maximize maternal functioning and childrearing abilities. Psychosocial treatments, including cognitive-behavioral therapy, interpersonal therapy, supportive therapy, and case management to link parents with appropriate supports are helpful. Medications are also necessary to help most mothers with mental illness maintain stability. Effective medications are available to control the psychiatric symptoms of all the major mental illnesses. Education about the impact of the maternal mental illness on the mother, her parenting, and family interactions helps families function better *(166)* and is an important component of the treatment of the mental illness. Parents may benefit from assistance in talking with their children about their illness in an age-appropriate manner.

8.2. Parent Training and Family Support
With High-Risk Families

Interventions for high-risk families may focus on the parents, or they may include the parents and child(ren) as well as the environment. For families with adequate financial, social, and other environmental resources as well as limited or moderate mental illness symptoms in the parent and/or the child, parent skills training alone may improve parent and child functioning (162,167–169). For families with significant marital distress, interventions with the couple may be warranted (166). For families with additional environmental risk factors (e.g., low social support or poverty), a broader intervention, such as maternal–child home visiting to address the environment, parent, and child (170–175), may be warranted. A wide variety of programs have been developed specifically for parents with serious mental illness (176–180), but only a few have been studied to establish their effectiveness. These studies that do exist have been limited by methodological problems, including lack of comparison group (181,182), nonrandom comparison groups (57), small numbers (181,183), high dropout rates (184–186), and poor or unspecified assessment of parenting skills (55).

Maternal–child home visiting is a widely studied, effective model of preventive care for high-risk families. Home visiting typically involves working with new mothers in their homes to assist with postpartum care, to provide parent education and skills training, and to link families to other needed services (187). Although the research is mixed (e.g., refs. 188,189), most studies of maternal–child home visitation for mothers without mental illness have demonstrated improvements in the lives of participants as well as better child outcomes up to 15 yr later (170–172,190,191).

Seven controlled studies have examined the impact of maternal–child home visitation for at-risk women in the general population who are similar to women with significant mental illness. The interventions offered (a) a supportive relationship with a home visitor; (b) education and training about child development and parenting skills; (c) modeling and feedback for parent skills, such as the detailed infant program shown to be effective by Horowitz and colleagues (192); and (d) linkage to other services and supports. In three of the studies, mothers who received the services improved their interactions with their children compared with mothers who received the control interventions (183–185). A fourth home visitation program for depressed mothers prevented deterioration in mother–child interactions compared to mother–child interactions of those receiving the control intervention

(186). A fifth showed that the children of treated mothers improved *(57)*. The more time-limited interventions in two other studies did not improve parenting behavior in participants more than the control interventions *(193,194)*. These findings are consistent with studies of home visitation in the general population *(191)*, which suggest that participation in longer term interventions was more effective, and other research showing that positive outcomes were related to the cumulative amount of time spent in home visits *(195)*.

A promising parent–child home visiting program has been developed to meet the needs of parents with severe mental illness in community mental health treatment settings *(181)*. Preliminary work has suggested that this adaptation of maternal–child home visiting results in high rates of engagement into the program and improved parent skills. The clinicians in this program worked with the multidisciplinary mental health teams to coordinate and integrate services for the families. They provided home-based parent training, child support, and linkage to other community services. The parent skills training was modified to be more supportive, concrete, and repetitious to accommodate the learning difficulties of parents in this population. This and other research suggests that parent skills training in combination with a variety of other family supports may be an effective way to improve parent skills in mothers with severe mental illness *(55,57,181)*.

The availability of parent support programs can vary greatly from community to community. Community mental health centers may offer programs that include individual and group therapy for parents, parent skills training, coordination with and referral to community supports and services, and daycare. However, most public mental health settings do not provide services designed to support parents with mental illness *(196)*. There is thus an urgent need for public mental health, public health, and child protection administrations to coordinate in order to develop and fund parent support services to prevent maltreatment and improve outcomes for high-risk families.

9. ETHICAL AND LEGAL ISSUES

Clinicians may find themselves in the dual roles of monitoring deficient or at-risk parenting while also supporting parents and teaching them parent skills. When a clinician has evidence that abuse or neglect has occurred, he or she is required by law to report the problem to child welfare authorities. State laws vary, and clinicians should review the laws in their state. Clinicians need to inform parents of this reporting requirement with a focus on maintaining the therapeutic alliance because most parents are afraid of losing custody of their children *(159)*. Because violence between parents increases the likelihood of violence towards the children in the family *(187)*, families in which parental violence occurs should be closely monitored to prevent violence toward children.

The dual role of helper and reporter can be difficult to navigate *(198)*, but in most cases making a report to child welfare can be done therapeutically and need not disrupt the clinician's alliance with the parent *(199)*. Prior to reporting, the clinician should consult with peers and supervisors about the need to report and the approach to take. The clinician should then talk with the parent about her concerns and the reporting requirement. Some parents prefer to make the call themselves with their clinician present. Others prefer that the clinician make the report while they listen. The need to report can and should be used as a therapeutic tool to help patients improve parenting skills and the home environment for the family.

Active contacts with child protective service workers, who may be unfamiliar with mental illness, may smooth the process of reporting women or helping women who were reported by others for suspected abuse or neglect of their children *(200)*. Mental health providers, for instance, can remind child welfare workers that most mental illnesses have a waxing and waning course. Symptoms that impair parenting abilities often remit completely with adequate treatment, and thus parenting deficits may be transient. Other barriers to parenting (e.g., housing problems and parenting skills) may also be short lived because they improve with appropriate interventions. Clinicians can encourage parents to utilize appropriate family and community supports to help in caring for their children. In some cases engaging supports that improve the child's environment is all that is needed to help a parent maintain custody.

Clinicians are required to report potential child abuse or neglect. The decision to investigate a question of abuse or neglect and whether removal of the child is necessary is decided by child welfare departments and the legal system. The AACAP *(201)* recommends that the legal assessment of a parent's capacity to parent should be completed by an independent evaluator who is not in a therapeutic relationship with the family. In each family's situation, a full assessment should investigate the adequacy of the child's environment, the parents' abilities, and all other resources and supports for the child *(202–205)*. The legal system will then weigh the risks and benefits: there may be risks in staying with a psychotic or severely depressed mother, but there are also risks inherent in placing a child in an unknown environment *(206,207)*.

10. CONCLUSIONS

Most women with mental illness bear and raise children. Pregnancy and postpartum are times of high risk for illness exacerbation during which mental illness should be carefully treated. Children of these parents may be at higher risk for negative outcomes than children whose parents do not have a mental illness because of their biological vulnerability to mental illness, the presence of environmental stressors, and their parent's style of parenting. Outcomes may be improved by (a) assertive treatment of maternal mental illness, (b) supports and services to improve the familial environment and to address the child's specific needs, and (c) parent skills training for parents with maladaptive parenting styles. Interventions should be selected to target the needs of each individual family. Because adaptive parenting protects vulnerable children, parent skills training is a critical area of intervention to prevent problems from developing and persisting in at-risk children.

REFERENCES

1. Narrow, W. E., Rae, D. S., Robins, L. N. and Regier, D. A. (2002) Revised prevalence estimates of mental disorders in the United States.Using a clinical significance criterion to reconcile 2 surveys estimates. Arch. Gen. Psychiatry 59, 115–123.
2. Nicholson, J., Biebel, K., Katz-Leavy, J. and Williams, V.F. (2002) The prevalence of parenthood in adults with mental illness: implications for state and federal policy makers, programs, and providers. In: Manderscheid, R.W. and Henderson, M.J., eds. Mental Health, United States, 2002. Rockville, MD: U.S. Department of Health and Human Services, Substance Abuse and Mental Health Services Administration, Center for Mental Health Services.
3. Caton, C., Cournos, F., and Dominguez, B. (1999) Parenting and adjustment in schizophrenia. Psychiatr. Serv. 50, 239–243.
4. Brunette, M., Mercer, C., Rosenberg, S., and Carlson, K. (2000) HIV risk in persons with severe mental illness: practice in New Hampshire community mental health. J. Behav. Health Serv. Res. 27, 347–353.
5. McEvoy, J. P., Hatcher, A., Appelbaum, P. S., and Abernethy, V. (1983) Chronic schizophrenic women's attitudes toward sex, pregnancy, birth control, and childrearing. Hosp. Commun. Psychiatry 34, 536–539.
6. Weinberg, M. K. and Tronick, E. Z. (1998) The impact of maternal psychiatric illness on infant development. J. Clin. Psychiatry 59(2), 53–61.
7. Belsky, J. (1984) The determinants of parenting: a process model. Child Development 55, 83–96.
8. Goodman, S. H. and Gotlib, I. H. (1999) Risk for psychopathology in the children of depressed mothers: a developmental model for understanding mechanisms of transmission. Psychol. Rev. 106, 458–490.
9. Masten, A. S. and Coatsworth, J. D. (1998) The development of competence in favorable and unfavorable environments: lessons from research on successful children. Am. Psychol. 53, 205–220.

10. Seifer, R. and Dickstein, S. (1993) Parental mental illness and infant development. In: Zeanah, C. H., Jr., ed. Handbook of Infant Mental Health. New York: The Guilford Press, pp. 120–142.
11. Wyman, P. A., Cowen, E. L., Work, W. C., and Parker, G. R. (1999) Caregiving and developmental factors differentiating young at-risk urban children showing resilient versus stress-affected outcomes: a replication and extension. Child Development 70, 645–659.
12. Kendler, K. S. (1996) Parenting: a genetic-epidemiologic perspective. Am. J. Psychiatry 153, 11–20.
13. Solantaus-Simula, T., Punamaki, R., and Beardslee, W. R. (2002) Children's responses to low parental mood. II: associations with family perceptions of parenting styles and child distress. J. Am. Acad. Child Adolesc. Psychiatry 41, 287–295.
14. Rutter, M. and Plomin, R. (1997) Opportunities for psychiatry from genetic findings. Br. J. Psychiatry 171, 209–219.
15. Kendler, K. S., Prescott, C. A., Myers, J., and Neale, M. C. (2003) The structure of genetic and environmental risk factors for common psychiatric and substance use disorders in men and women. Arch. Gen. Psychiatry 60, 929–937.
16. Sullivan, P. F., Kendler, K. S., and Neale, M. C. (2003) Schizophrenia as a complex trait: evidence from a meta-analysis of twin studies. Arch. Gen. Psychiatry 60, 1187–1192.
17. Faroane, S. V., Taylor, L., and Tsuang, M. T. (2002) The molecular genetics of schizophrenia: an emerging consensus. In: Expert Reviews in Molecular Medicine. Cambridge: Cambridge University Press.
18. Waterworth, D. M., Bassett, A. S., and Brzustowicz, L. M. (2002) Recent advances in the genetics of schizophrenia. Cell. Mol. Life Sci. 59, 331–348.
19. Kendler, K. S., Neale, M. C., Kessler, R. C., Heath, A. C., and Eaves, L. J. (1993) A longitudinal twin study of personality and major depression in women. Arch. Gen. Psychiatry 50, 853–862.
20. Sullivan, P. F., Neale, M. C., and Kendler, K. S. (2000) Genetic epidemiology of major depression: review and meta-analysis. Am. J. Psychiatry 157(10), 1552–1562.
21. Craddock, N. and Jones, I. (1999) Genetics of bipolar disorder. J. Med. Genet. 36, 585–594.
22. Lieb, R., Isensee, B., Hsfler, M., Pfister, H. and Wittchen, H. (2002) Parental major depression and the risk of depression and other mental disorders in offspring. Arch. Gen. Psychiatry 59, 365–374.
23. Warner, V., Weissman, M. M., Mufson, L., and Wickramaratne, P. (1999) Grandparents, parents, and grandchildren at high risk for depression: a three generation study. J. Am. Acad. Child Adolesc. Psychiatry 38, 289–296.
24. Goodman, S. H. and Emery, E. K. (1992) Perinatal complications in births to low socioeconomic statues schizophrenia and depressed women. J. Abnorm. Psychol. 101, 225–229.
25. Kumar, R., Marks, M., Platz, C., and Yoshida, K. (1995) Clinical survey of a psychiatric mother and baby unit: characteristics of 100 consecutive admissions. J. Affect. Disord. 33, 11–22.
26. Campbell, S. B., Pierce, E. W., March, C. L., and Ewing, L. J. (1991) Noncompliant behavior, overactivity, and family stress as predictors of negative maternal control with preschool children. Dev. Psychopathol. 3, 175–190.
27. Hipwell, A. E., Goossens, F. A., Melhuish, E. C., and Kumar, R. (2000) Severe maternal psychopathology and infant-mother attachment. Dev. Psychopathol. 12, 157–175.

28. Murray, L. and Cooper, P. (1997) Postpartum depression and child development. Psychol. Med. 27, 253–260.
29. de Bellis, M. D., Broussard, E. R., Herring, D. J., Wexler, S., Moritz, G., and Benitez, J. G. (2001) Psychiatric co-morbidity in caregivers and children involved in maltreatment: a pilot research study with policy implications. Child Abuse Negl. 25, 923–944.
30. DaSilva, L. and Johnstone, E. C. (1981) A follow-up study of severe puerperal psychiatric illness. Br. J. Psychiatry 139, 346–354.
31. Davidson, J. and Robertson, E. (1985) A follow-up study of post partum illness, 1946-1978. Acta Psychiatr. Scand. 71, 451–457.
32. Jacobsen, T. and Miller, L. J. (1998) Mentally ill mothers who have killed: three cases addressing the issue of future parenting capability. Psychiatr. Serv. 49, 650–657.
33. Sidebotham, P., Golding, J., and Team, T. A. S. (2001) Child maltreatment in the "children of the nineties." Child Abuse Negl. 25, 1177–1200.
34. Rohde, A. and Marneros, A. (1993) Postpartum psychoses: onset and long-term course. Psychopathology 26, 203–209.
35. Wisner, K. L., Peindl, K. S., Gigliott, T., and Hanusa, B. H. (1999) Obsessions and compulsions in women with postpartum depression. J. Clin. Psychiatry 60, 176–180.
36. Mullick, M., Miller, L. J., and Jacobsen, T. (2001) Insight into mental illness and child maltreatment risk among mothers with major psychiatric disorders. Psychiatr. Serv. 52, 488–492.
37. Beckwith, L., Rozga, A., and Sigman, M. (2002) Maternal sensitivity and attachment in atypical groups. Adv. Child Dev. Behav. 30, 231–274.
38. Brennan, P. A., Brocque, R. L., and Hammen, C. (2003) Maternal depression, parent-child relationships, and resilient outcomes in adolescence. J. Am. Acad. Child Adolesc. Psychiatry 42, 1469–1477.
39. Dodge, K. A., Pettit, G. S., and Bates, J. E. (1994) Socialization mediators of the relation between socioeconomic status and child conduct problems. Child Development 65, 649–655.
40. Fox, R. A., Platz, D. L., and Bentley, K. S. (1995) Maternal factors related to parenting practices, developmental expectations, and perceptions of child behavior problems. J. Genet. Psychol. 156, 431–441.
41. Gara, M. A., Allen, L. A., Herzog, E. P., and Woolfolk, R. L. (2000) The abused child as parent: the structure and content of physically abused mothers' perceptions of their babies. Child Abuse Negl. 24, 627–639.
42. Newcomb, M. D. and Locke, T. F. (2001) Intergenerational cycle of maltreatment: a popular concept obscured by methodological limitations. Child Abuse Negl. 25, 1219–1240.
43. Brunette, M. F. and Drake, R. E. (1997) Gender differences in patients with schizophrenia and substance abuse. Compr. Psychiatry 38, 109–116.
44. Goodman, L. A., Dutton, M. S., and Harris, M. (1995) Episodially homeless women with serious mental illness: prevalence of physical and sexual assault. Am. J. Orthopsychiatry 65, 468–478.
45. Bugental, D. B. and Happaney, K. (2004) Predicting infant maltreatment in low-income families: the interactive effects of maternal attributions and child status at birth. Dev. Psychol. 40, 234–243.
46. Buist, A. and Janson, H. (2001) Childhood sexual abuse, parenting and postpartum depression —a 3-year follow-up study. Child Abuse Negl. 25, 909–921.

47. Leon, K., Jacobvitz, D. B., and Hazen, N. L. (2004) Maternal resolution of loss and abuse: associations with adjustment to the transition to parenthood. Infant Ment. Health J. 25, 130–148.

48. Ruscio, A.M. (2001) Predicting the child-rearing practices of mothers sexually abused in childhood. Child Abuse Negl. 25, 369-387.

49. Lyons-Ruth, K. (1996) Attachment relationships among children with aggressive behavior problems: The role of disorganized early attachment patterns. J. Consult. Clin. Psychol. 64, 64-73.

50. Egeland, B., Bosquet, M., and Levy-Chung, A. (2002) Continuities and discontinuities in the intergenerational transmission of child maltreatment: implications for breaking the cycle of abuse. Child Development 73, 528–543.

51. Campbell, S. B., Cohn, J. F., and Meyers, T. (1995) Depression in first-time mothers: mother-infant interaction and depression chronicity. Dev. Psychol. 31, 349–357.

52. Cox, A. D., Puckering, C., Pound, A., and Mills, M. (1987) The impact of maternal depression in young children. J. Child Psychol. Psychiatry 28, 917–928.

53. Hops, H., Biglan, A., Sherman, L., Arthur, J., Friedman, L., and Osteen, V. (1987) Home observations of family interactions of depressed women. J. Consult. Clin. Psychol. 55(3), 341–346.

54. Righetti-Veltema, M., Bousquet, A., and Manzano, J. (2003) Impact of postpartum depressive symptoms on mother and her 18-month infant. Eur. Child Adolesc. Psychiatry 12, 75–83.

55. Cohler, B. J. and Musick, J. S. (1983) Psychopathology of parenthood: Implications for mental health of children. Infant Ment. Health J. 4, 140–164.

56. Klehr, K. B., Cohler, B. J., and Musick, J. S. (1983) Character and behavior in the mentally ill and well mother. Infant Ment. Health J. 4, 250–271.

57. Lyons-Ruth, K., Connell, D. B., Grunegaum, H., and Botein, S. (1990) Infants at social risk: maternal depression and family support services as mediators of infant development and security of attachment. Child Development 61, 85–98.

58. Naslund, B., Persson-Blennow, I. McNeil, T. F., Kaij, L., and Malmquist-Larsson, A. (1984) Deviations on exploration, attachment, and fear of strangers in high-risk and control infants at one year of age. Am. J. Orthopsychiatry 54, 569–577.

59. Persson-Blennow, I., Naslund, B., McNeil, T. F., and Kaig, L. (1986) Offspring of women with nonorganic psychosis: mother-infant interaction at one year of age. Acta Psychiatr. Scand. 73, 207–213.

60. Naslund, B., Persson-Blennow, I., McNeil, T. F., and Kaij, L. (1985) Offspring of women with nonorganic psychosis: mother-infant interaction at three and six weeks of age. Acta Psychiatr. Scand. 71, 441–450.

61. Stein, A., Gath, D. H., Bucher, J., Bond, A., Day, A. and Cooper, P. J. (1991) The relationship between post-natal depression and mother-child interaction. Br. J. Psychiatry 158, 46–52.

62. Walker, E. and Emory, E. (1983) Infants at risk for psychopathology: offspring of schizophrenic parents. Child Development 54, 1269–1285.

63. White, C. and Barrowclough, C. (1998) Depressed and non depressed mothers with problematic preschoolers: attributions for child behaviours. Br. J. Clin. Psychol. 37, 385–398.

64. Lovejoy, M. C., Graczyk, P. A., O'Hara, E., and Neuman, G. (2000) Maternal Depression and parenting behavior: a meta-analytic review. Clin. Psychol. Rev. 20, 561–592.

65. Beardslee, W. R., Versage, E. M., and Gladstone, T. R. G. (1998) Children of affectively ill parents: a review of the past 10 years. J. Am. Acad. Child Adolesc. Psychiatry 37, 1134–1141.
66. Grace, S. L., Evindar, A., and Stewart, D. E. (2003) The effect of postpartum depression on child cognitive development and behavior: A review and critical analysis of the literature. Arch. Women's Ment. Health 6, 263–274.
67. Park, R. J., Senior, R., and Stein, A. (2003) The offspring of mothers with eating disorders. Eur. Child Adolesc. Psychiatry 12, 110–119.
68. Sameroff, A. J., Seifer, R., and Zax, M. (1982) Early development of children at risk for emotional disorder. Monogr. Soc. Res. Child Dev. 47, 7.
69. Uddenberg, N. and Engelsson, I. (1978) Prognosis of post partum mental disturbance: A prospective study of primiparous women and their 4 1/2 year old children. Acta Psychiatr. Scand. 48, 201–212.
70. Coverdale, J. H. and Aruffo, J.A. (1989) Family planning needs of female chronic psychiatric outpatients. Am. J. Psychiatry 146, 1489–1491.
71. Miller, L. J. and Finnerty, M. (1996) Sexuality, pregnancy, and childrearing among women with schizophrenia-spectrum disorders. Psychiatr. Serv. 4, 502–506.
72. Caton, C. I. M., Cournos, F., Felix, A., and Wyatt, R. J. (1998) Childhood experiences and current adjustment of offspring of indigent patients with schizophrenia. Psychiatr. Serv. 49, 86–90.
73. Jacobsen, T. and Miller, L. J. (1999) The caregiving contexts of young children who have been removed from the care of a mentally ill mother: relations to mother-child attachment quality. In: Solomon, J. and George, C., eds. Attachment Disorganization. Guilford Press.
74. Dwyer, S. B., Nicholson, J. M., and Battistutta, D. (2003) Population level assessment of the family risk factors related to the onset or persistence of children's mental health problems. J. Child Psychol. Psychiatry 44, 699–711.
75. Johnson, J. G., Cohen, P., Kasen, S., Smailes, E., and Brook, J. (2001) Association of maladaptive parental behavior with psychiatric disorder among parents and their offspring. Arch. Gen. Psychiatry 58(5), 453–460.
76. Mantymaa, M., Puura, K., Luoman, I., Salmelin, R. K., and Tamminen, T. (2004) Early mother-infant interaction, parental mental health and symptoms of behavioral and emotional problems in toddlers. Infant Behav. Dev. 27, 134–149.
77. Morrel, J. and Murray, L. (2001) Infant and maternal precursors of conduct disorder and hyperactive symptoms in childhood: a prospective longitudinal study from 2 months to 8 years. J. Child Psychol. Psychiatry 44, 489–508
78. Murray, L., Woolgar, M., Cooper, P., and Hipwell, A. (2001) Cognitive vulnerability to depression in 5-year-old children of depressed mothers. J. Child Psychol. Psychiatry 42, 891–899.
79. Shaw, D., Owens, E., Vondra, J., Keenan, K., and Winslow, E. (1996) Early risk factors and pathways in the development of early disruptive behavior problems. Dev. Psychopathol. 8, 679–700.
80. Hirshfeld, D. R., Biederman, J., Brody, L., Faroane, S. V., and Rosenbaum, J. F. (1997) Expressed emotion toward children with behavioral inhibition: associations with maternal anxiety disorder. J. Am. Acad. Child Adolesc. Psychiatry 36, 910–917.
81. Nelson, D. R., Hammen, C., Brennan, P. A., and Ullman, J. B. (2003) The impact of maternal depression on adolescent adjustment: the role of expressed emotion. J. Consult. Clin. Psychol. 71(5), 935–944.

82. Milgrom, J., Westley, D. T., and Gemmill, A. W. (2004) The mediating role of maternal responsiveness in some longer term effects of postnatal depression on infant development. Infant Behav. Dev. 27(4), 443–454.
83. Chaffin, M., Bonner, B. L., and Hill, R. F. (2001) Family preservation and family support programs: child maltreatment outcomes across client risk levels and program types. Child Abuse Negl. 25, 1269–1289.
84. MacMillan, H. L. (2000) Child maltreatment: What we know in the year 2000. Can. J. Psychiatry 45, 702–710.
85. Parker, S., Greer, S., and Zuckerman, B. (1988) Double jeopardy: the impact of poverty on early child development. Pediatr. Clin. North Am. 35, 1227–1240.
86. Sullivan, P. M. and Knutson, J. F. (2000) Maltreatment and disabilities: a population-based epidemiologic study. Child Abuse Negl. 24(10), 1257–1273.
87. Costello, E. J., Compton, S. N., Keeler, G., and Angold, A. (2003) Relationships between poverty and psychopathology A natural experiment. JAMA 290, 2023–2029.
88. Mason, C. A., Chapman, D. A., and Scott, K. G. (1999) The identification of early risk factors for severe emotional disturbances and emotional handicaps: an epidemiological approach. Am. J. Commun. Psychol. 27, 357–380.
89. Cogill, S. R., Caplan, H. L., Alexandra, H., Robson, K M., and Kumar, R. (1986) Impact of maternal postnatal depression on cognitive development of young children. Br. Med. J. 292, 1165–1167.
90. Du Rocher Schudlich, T. D. and Cummings, E. M. (2003) Parental dysphoria and children's internalizing symptoms: marital conflict styles as mediators of risk. Child Development 74(6), 1663–1681.
91. Keller, M. B., Beardless, W. R., Dorer, D. J., Lavori, P. W., Samuelson, H., and Klerman, G. R. (1986) Impact of severity and chronocity of parental affective illness on adaptive functioning and psychopathology in their children. Arch. Gen. Psychiatry 43, 930–937.
92. Murray, L. (1992) The impact of postnatal depression on infant development. J. Child Psychol. Psychiatry 33, 543–561.
93. Nomura, Y., Wickramaratne, P., Warner, V., Mufson, L., and Weissman, M. M. (2002) Family discord, parental depression, and psychopathology in offspring: ten year follow-up. J. Am. Acad. Child Adolesc. Psychiatry 41, 402–409.
94. Rumm, P. D., et al. (2000) Identified spouse abuse as a risk factor for child abuse. Child Abuse Negl. 24, 1375–1381.
95. Tajima, E. A. (2000) The relative importance of wife abuse as a risk factor for violence against children. Child Abuse Negl. 24, 1383–1398.
96. Kitzmann, K. M., Gaylord, N. K., Holt, A. R., and Kenny, E. D. (2003) Child witnesses to domestic violence: a meta-analytic review. J. Consult. Clin. Psychol. 71, 339–352.
97. Margolin, G. and Gordis, E. B. (2000) The effects of family and community violence on children. Annu. Rev. Psychol. 51, 445–479.
98. Johnson, J. G., Cohen, P. Smailes, E. M., Kasen, S., and Brook, J. S. (2002) Television viewing and aggressive behavior during adolescence and adulthood. Science. 295, 2468–2471.
99. Connell, A. M. and Goodman, S. H. (2002) The association between psychopathology in fathers versus mothers and children's internalizing and externalizing behavior problems: a meta-analysis. PsyB. 128, 746–773.
100. Edhborg, M., Lundh, W., Seimyr, L., and Widstrom, A. M. (2003) The parent-child relationship in the context of maternal depressive mood. Arch. Women's Ment. Health. 6, 211–216.

101. Reynolds, A. J., Temple, J. A., Robertson, D. L., and Mann, E. A. (2001) Long-term effects of an early childhood intervention on educational achievement and juvenile arrest. JAMA 285, 2339–2346.

102. Reynolds, A. J., Ou, A., and Topitzes, J. W. (2004) Paths of effects of early childhood intervention on educational attainment and delinquency: a confirmatory analysis of the Chicago Child-Parent Centers. Child Development 75, 1299–1328.

103. Brennan, P. A., Hammen, C., Katz, A. R., and LeBrocque, R. M. (2002) Maternal depression, paternal psychopathology, and adolescent diagnostic outcomes. J. Consult. Clin. Psychol. 70, 1075–1085.

104. Cicchetti, D., Rogosch, F. A., and Toth, S. L. (1998) Maternal depressive disorder and contextual risk: contributions to the development of attachment insecurity and behavior problems in toddlerhood. Dev. Psychopathol. 10, 283–300.

105. Hammen, C., Shih, J., Altman, T., and Brennan, P. A. (2003) Interpersonal impairment and the prediction of depressive symptoms in adolescent children of depressed and nondepressed mothers. J. Am. Acad. Child Adolesc. Psychiatry 42, 571–577.

106. Bowlby, J. (1988) A Secure Base: Clinical Applications of Attachment Theory. London: Routledge.

107. Beidel, D. and Turner, S. (1997) At risk for anxiety: I. Psychopathology in the offspring of anxious parents. J. Am. Acad. Child Adolesc. Psychiatry 36, 918–924.

108. Hammen, C., Adrian, C., Gordon, G., Burge, D., and Jaenicke, C. (1987) Children of depressed mothers: maternal strain and symptom predictors of dysfunction. J. Abnorm. Psychol. 96, 190–198.

109. Kurstjens, S. and Wolke, D. (2001) Effects of maternal depression on cognitive development of children over the first 7 years of life. J. Child Psychol. Psychiatry 42, 623–636.

110. Yoshida, K., Marks, M. N., Craggs, M., Smith, G. D., and Kumar, R. (1999) Sensorimotor and cognitive development of infants of mothers with schizophrenia. Br. J. Psychiatry 175, 380–387.

111. Field, T. M. (1992) Infants of depressed mothers. Dev. Psychopathol. 4, 49–66.

112. Murray, L., Fiori-Cowly, A., Hooper, R., and Cooper, P. (1997) The impact of postnatal depression and associated adversity on early mother-infant interactions and later infant outcomes. Child Development 67, 251–256.

113. Murray, L., Hipwell, A., Hooper, R., Stein, A., and Cooper, P. (1996) The cognitive development of 5-year-old children of postnatally depressed mothers. Psychiatry 37, 927–935.

114. Marlow, N. (2004) Neurocognitive outcome after very preterm birth. Arch.Dis. Child. Fetal. Neonatal. 89, F224–228.

115. Field, T. M. (1098) Interactions of preterm and term infants with their lower and middle class teenage and adult mothers. In: Field, T. M., Goldberg, S., and Stern, D., eds. High Risk Infants and Children. New York: Academic Press.

116. Lyons-Ruth, K., Easterbrooks, M. A., and Cibelli, C. D. (1997) Infant attachment strategies, infant mental lag, and maternal depressive symptoms: predictors of internalizing and externalizing problems at age 7. Dev. Psychol. 33, 681–692.

117. Kandel, E., Mednick, S. A., Kirkegaard-Sorenson, L., et al. (1988) IQ as a protective factor for subjects at high risk for antisocial behavior. J. Consult. Clin. Psychol. 56, 224–226.

118. Bugental, D. B., Blue, J., and Lewis, J. (1990) Caregiver beliefs and dysphoric affect directed to difficult children. Dev. Psychol. 26, 631–638.

119. Calkins, S. D., Hungerford, A., and Dedmon, S. E. (2004) Mother's interactions with temperamentally frustrated infants. Infant Ment. Health J. 25, 219–239.

120. Mertesacker, B., Bade, U., Haverkock, A,. and Pauli-Pott, U. (2004) Predicting maternal reactivity/sensitivity: the role of infant emotionality, maternal depressiveness/anxiety, and social support. Infant Ment. Health J. 25, 47–61.

121. Werner, E. E. (1993) Risk, resilience, and recovery: perspectives from the Kaui longitudinal study. Dev. Psychopathol. 5, 503–515.

122. Wyman, P. A., Cowen, E. L., Work, W. C., and Parker, G. R. (1991) Developmental and family milieu correlates of resilience in urban children who have experienced major life stress. Am. J. Commun. Psychol. 19, 405–426.

123. DeMulder, E. K. and Radke-Yarrow, M. (1991) Attachment with affectively ill and well-mothers: concurrent behavioral correlates. Dev. Psychopathol. 3, 227–242.

124. Van Ijzendoorn, M. H., Goldger, S., Kroonenberg, P., and Frenkal, O. (1992) The relative effects of maternal and child problems on the quality of attachment: a meta-analysis of attachment in clinical samples. Child Development 63, 840–858.

125. Barocas, R., Seifer, R., and Sameroff, A.J. (1985) Defining environmental risk: Multiple dimensions of psychological vulnerability. Am. J. Commun. Psychol. 13, 433–447.

126. Stott, F. M., Musick, J. S., Clark, R., and Cohler, B. (1983) Developmental patterns in the infants and young children of mentally ill mothers. Infant Ment. Health J. 4, 217–235.

127. Greenberg, M. T., Speltz, M. L., DeKlyen, M., and Endriga, M. C. (1991) Attachment security in preschoolers with and without externalizing problems: a replication. Dev. Psychopathol. 3, 413–430.

128. Lyons-Ruth, K., Alpern, L., and Repacholi, B. (1993) Disorganized infant attachment classification and maternal psychosocial problems as predictors of hostile-aggressive behavior in the preschool classroom. Child Development 64, 572–585.

129. Persson-Blennow, I., Binett, T. F., and McNeil, T. (1988) Offspring of women with nonorganic psychosis: antecedents of anxious attachment to the mother at one year of age. Acta Psychiatr. Scand. 78, 66–71.

130. Galler, J. R., Harrison, R. H., Ramsey, F., Forde, V., and Butler S. C. (2000) Maternal depressive symptoms affect infant cognitive development in Barbados. J. Child Psychol. Psychiatry 41, 747–757.

131. Gamer, E., Gallant, D., and Grunebaum, H. (1976) Children of psychotic mothers: an evaluation of 1-year-olds on a test of object permanence. Arch. Gen. Psychiatry 33, 311–317.

132. Ramsy, F., Forde, V., and Butler, S.C. (2000) Maternal depressive symptoms affect infant cognitive development in Barbados. J. Child Psychol. Psychiatry 41, 747–757.

133. Brennan, P. A., Hammen, C., Anderson, M. J., Bor, W., Najman, J. M., and Silliams, G. M. (2000) Chronicity, severity, and timing of maternal depressive symptoms: relationships with child outcomes at age 5. Dev. Psychol. 36, 759–766.

134. Hiscock, H. and Wake, M. (2001) Infant sleep problems and postnatal depression: a community-based study. Pediatrics 107, 1317–1322.

135. Orvaschel, H., Walsh-Allis, G., and Ye, W. (1988) Psychopathology in children of parents with recurrent depression. J. Abnorm. Psychol. 16, 17–28.

136. Oyserman, D., Mowbray, C. T., Meares, P. A., and Firminger, K. B. (2000) Parenting among mothers with a serious mental illness. Am. J. Orthopsychiatry 70, 296–314.

137. Teti, D.M. and Gelfand, D.M. (1991) Behavioral competence among mothers of infants in the first year: The mediational role of maternal self-efficacy. Child Development 62, 918-929.

138. Weissman, M. M., Warner, V., Wickramaratne, P., Moreau, D., and Olfson, M. (1997) Offspring of depressed parents: 10 years later. Arch. Gen. Psychiatry 54, 932–940.
139. Zahn-Waxler, C., McKnew, D. H., Cummings, M., Davenport, U. B., and Radke-Yarrow, M. (1984) Problem behaviors and peer interactions of young children with a manic-depressive parent. Am. J. Psychiatry 141, 236–240.
140. Caspi, A., Moffitt, T. E., Newman, D. L., and Silva, P. A. (1996) Behavioral observations at age 3 years predict adult psychiatric disorders: longitudinal evidence from a birth cohort. Arch. Gen. Psychiatry 53, 1033–1039.
141. Roza, S. J., Hofstra, M. B., vander Ende, J., and Verhulst, F. (2003) Stable prediction of mood and anxiety disorders based on behavioral and emotional problems in childhood: a 14 year follow-up during childhood, adolescence, and young adulthood. Am. J. Psychiatry 160, 2116–2121.
142. Murray, L. and Cooper, P. J. (2004) The impact of postpartum depression on child development. In: Goodyer, I., ed. Aetiological Mechanisms in Developmental Psychopathology. London: Oxford University Press.
143. Bagedahl-Strindlund, M. and Ruppert, S. (1998) Parapartum mental illness: a long-term follow-up study. Psychopathology 31, 250-259.
144. Anderson, C. A. and Hammen, C. L. (1993) Psychosocial outcomes of children of unipolar depressed, bipolar, medically ill, and normal women: a longitudinal study. J. Consult. Clin. Psychol. 61, 448–454.
145. Hammen, C. and Brennan, P. A. (2001) Depressed adolescents of depressed and nondepressed mothers: tests of an interpersonal impairment hypothesis. J. Consult. Clin. Psychol. 69, 284–294.
146. Rutter, M. and Quinton, D. (1984) Parental psychiatric disorder: effects on children. Psychol. Med. 14, 853-880.
147. Blanz, B., Schmidt, M. H., and Esser, G. (1991) Familial adversities and child psychiatric disorder. J. Child Psychol. Psychiatry 32, 939–950.
148. Hammen, C., Burge, D., and Adrian, C. (1991) Timing of mother and child depression in a longitudinal study of children at risk. J. Consult. Clin. Psychol. 59(2), 341–345.
149. Sneddon, J., Kerry, R. J., and Bant, W. P. (1981) The psychiatric mother and baby unit. A three year study. Practitioner 225, 295–1300.
150. Lyons-Ruth, K., Connell, D. B., Zoll, D., and Stahl, J. (1987) Infants at social risk: Relations among infant maltreatment, maternal behavior, and infant attachment behavior. Dev. Psychol. 23, 223–232.
151. Radke-Yarrow, M., Zahn-Waxler, C., Susman, A., and Martinez, P. (1994) Caring behavior in children of clinically depressed and well mothers. Child Development 65, 1405–1414.
152. Crittenden, P. M. and DiLalla, D. L. (1988) Compulsive compliance: the development of an inhibitory coping strategy in infancy. J. Abnorm. Child Psychol. 16, 585–599.
153. Jacobsen, T. and Miller, L. J. (1998) Compulsive compliance in a young maltreated child. J. Am. Acad. Child Adolesc. Psychiatry 37, 462–563.
154. Barnard, M. and Barlow, J. (2003) Discovering parental drug dependence: silence and disclosure. Children Soc. 17, 45–56.
155. Anthony, E. J. (1971) Folie a deux: a development failure in the process of separation-individuation. In: McDevitt, J. B. and Settlage, D. F., eds. Separation-Individuation: Essays in Honor of Margaret S. Mahler. New York: International Universities Press, pp. 253–273.

156. Rutter, M. (1966) Children of sick parents: an environmental and psychiatric study. Institute of Psychiatry Maudsley Monographs 16. London: Oxford University Press.

157. Kumpfer, K. L. (1999) Outcome measures of interventions in the study of children of substance-abusing parents. Pediatrics 10(Suppl. 5), 1128–1144.

158. Jacobsen, T. (2004) Mentally ill mothers in the parenting role: clinical management and treatment. In: Goepfert, M., Webster, J., and Seeman, M. V., eds. Parental Psychiatric Disorder: Distressed Parents and Their Families. Cambridge: Cambridge University Press, 112–122.

159. Lieberman, A. F. (1989) What is culturally sensitive intervention? Early Child Dev. Care 40, 197–294.

160. Anonymous. (2000) Children of Parents with Mental Illness. American Academy of Child and Adolescent Psychiatry.

161. Clarke, G. N., Hornbrook, M., Lynch, F., et al. (2001) A randomized trial of a group cognitive intervention for preventing depression in adolescent offspring of depressed parents. Arch. Gen. Psychiatry 58, 1127–1134.

162. Kazdin, A. E. and Weisz, J. R. (1998) Identifying and developing empirically supported child and adolescent treatments. J. Consult. Clin. Psychol. 66, 19–36.

163. Dishion, T. J. and Andrews, D. W. (1995) Preventing escalation in problem behaviors with high-risk young adolescents: immediate and 1-year outcomes. J. Consult. Clin. Psychol. 63, 538–548.

164. Kendell, R. E., Chalmers, J. C., and Platz, C. (1987) Epidemiology of puerperal psychoses. Br. J. Psychiatry 150, 662–673.

165. Kendell, R. E., Wainwright, S., Hailey, A., and Shannon, B. (1976) The influence of childbirth of psychiatric morbidity. Psychol. Med. 6, 297–302.

166. Beardslee, W. R., Salt, P., Versage, E. M., Gladstone, T. R. G., Wright E. J., and Rothberg, P. C. (1997) Sustaining change in parents receiving preventive interventions for families with depression. Am. J. Psychiatry 154, 510–515.

167. Barlow, J. and Parsons, J. (2002) Group-based parent-training programmes for improving emotional and behavioral adjustment in 0-3 year old children.. The Cochrane Database of Systematic Reviews.

168. Webster-Stratton, C. and Hammond, M. (1997) Treating children with early-onset conduct problems: a comparison of child and parent training interventions. J. Consult. Clin. Psychol. 65, 93–109.

169. Weisz, J. R., Weiss, B., Han, S. S., Granger, D. A., and Morton, T. (1995) Effects of psychotherapy with children and adolescents revisited: a meta-analysis of treatment outcome studies. PsyB 117, 450-468.

170. Eckenrode, J., Ganzel, B., Henderson, C. R., et al. (2000) Preventing child abuse and neglect with a program of nurse home visitation. JAMA 284, 1385–1391.

171. Kendrick, D., Elkan, R., Hewitt, M., et al. (2000) Does home visiting improve parenting and the quality of the home environment? A systematic review and meta analyses. Arch. Dis. Child. 82, 443–451.

172. Olds, D., Henderson, C., Cole, R., et al. (1998) Long-term effects of nurse home visitation on children's criminal and antisocial behavior. JAMA 280(14), 1238–1239.

173. Olds, D. L., Henderson, C. R., and Kitzman, H. (1994) Does prenatal and infancy nurse home visitation have enduring effects on qualities of parental caregiving and child health at 25 and 50 months of life? Pediatrics 93, 89–98.

174. Olds, D., Robinson, J., Song, N., Little, C., and Hill, P. (1999) Reducing risks for mental disorders during the first five years of life: a review of preventive interventions. Center for Mental Health Services, pp. 1–63.

175. Roberts, I., Kramer, M. S., and Suissa, S. (1996) Does home visiting prevent childhood injury? A systematic review of randomised controlled trials. Br. Med. J. 312, 29–33.
176. Bentivolgio, P. (1998) The family specialist program. Network 5, 1–2.
177. Cohler, B. J. and Musick, J. S. (1984) Interventions among psychiatrically impaired parents and their young children. In: New Dir. Ment. Health Serv. San Francisco: Jossey-Bass.
178. Lucas, L. E., Montgomery, S. H., Richardson, D. A., and Rivers, P. A. (1984) Impact project: reducing the risk of mental illness to children of distressed mothers. In: Cohler, B. J. and Musick, J. S., eds. Intervention Among Psychiatrically Impaired Parents and Their Young Children. Washington, DC: Jossey-Bass Inc., pp. 79–94.
179. University of Illinois at Chicago Women's Program. (1996) Comprehensive prenatal and postpartum psychiatric care of women with severe mental illness. Psychiatr. Serv. 47(10), 1108–1111.
180. Waldo, M C., Roath, M., Levine, W., and Freedman, R. (1987) A model program to teach parenting skills to schizophrenic mothers. Hosp. Commun. Psychiatry 38, 1110–1112.
181. Brunette, M. F., Richardson, F., White, L., et al. (2004) Integrated family treatment for parents with SMI. Psych. Rehab. J. 28, 177–180.
182. Speier, T. (1991) Final report of case management and transitional residential services for 18-40 year old dually diagnosed women with young children. In: Baton Rouge: Madre Louisiana Office of Human Services, pp. 51–53.
183. Heinicke, C. M., Fineman, N. ., Ruth, G., Recchia, S. L., Guthrie, D., and Rodning, C. (1999) Relationship-based intervention with at-risk mothers: outcome in the first year of life. Infant Ment. Health J. 20(4), 349–374.
184. Barnard, K. E., Magyary, D., Sumner, G., Booth, C. L., Mitchell, S.K., and Spieker, S. (1988) Prevention of parenting alterations for women with low social support. Psychiatry 51, 248–253.
185. Black, M. M., Prasanna, N., Kight, C., Wachtel, R., Roby, P., and Schuler, M. (1994) Parenting and early development among children of drug-abusing women: effects of home intervention. Pediatrics 94, 440–448.
186. Gelfand, D. M., Teti, D. M., Seiner, S. A., and Jameson, P. B. (1996) Helping mothers fight depression: evaluation of a home-based intervention program for depressed mothers and their infants. J. Clin. Child Psychol. 25, 406–422.
187. Wasik, B. H. and Bryant, D. M. (2001) Home Visiting. Thousand Oaks: Sage Publications.
188. McNaughton, D. B. (2004) Nurse home visits to maternal-child clients: a review of intervention research. Public Health Nurs. 21, 207–219.
189. Sweet, M. A. and Appelbaum, M. I. (2004) Is home visiting an effective strategy? A meta-analytic review of home visiting programs for families with young children. Child Development 75, 1435–1456.
190. Kitzman, H., Olds, D. L., Sidora, K., Henderson, C. R., Hanks, C., Cole., R., Luckey, D. W., Bondy, J., Cole, K., and Glazner, J. (2000) Enduring effects of nurse home visitation of maternal life course: a three year follow-up of a randomized trial. JAMA 283, 1983–1989.
191. Macleod, J. and Nelson, G. (2000) Programs for the promotion of family wellness and the prevention of child maltreatment: a meta-analytic review. Child Abuse Negl. 24, 1127–1149.

192. Horowitz, J. A., Bell, M., Trybulski, M., Munro, B. H., Moser, D., Hartz, S. A., McCordic, L., and Sokol, E. S. (2001) Promoting responsiveness between mothers with depressive symptoms and their infants. J. Nurs. Scholarship 33, 323–329.

193. Fraser, J. A., Armstrong, K. L., Morris, J. P., and Dadds, M. R. (2000) Home visiting intervention for vulnerable families with newborns: follow-up results of a randomized controlled trial. Child Abuse Negl. 24, 1399–1429.

194. Marcenko, M. O. and Spence, M. (1994) Home visitation services for at-risk pregnant and postpartum women: a randomized trial. Am. J. Orthopsychiatry 64, 468–478.

195. Lyons-Ruth, K. and Melnick, S. (2004) Dose-response effect of mother-infant clinical home visiting on aggressive behavior problems in kindergarten. J. Am. Acad. Child Adolesc. Psychiatry 43, 699–707.

196. Hinden, B., Biebel, K., Nicholson, J., et al. (2002) Steps toward evidence-based practice for parents with mental illness and their families. Mental Health Services, Substance Abuse and Mental Health Services Administration.

197. Straus, M. A. (1992) Children as witnesses to marital violence: a risk factor for lifelong problems among a nationally representative sample of American men and women. Report of the Twenty-Third Ross Roundtable, pp. 98–109.

198. Thompson-Cooper, I., Fugere, R., and Cormier, B. (1993) The child abuse reporting laws: an ethical dilemma for professionals. Can. J. Psychiatry 38, 557–561.

199. Weinstein, B., Levine, M., Kogan, N., Harkavy-Friedman, J., and Miller, J. M. (2000) Mental health professionals experiences reporting suspected child abuse and maltreatment. Child Abuse Negl. 24, 1317–1328.

200. Nicholson, J., Sweeney, E. M., and Geller, J. L. (1998) Mothers with mental illness: II. Family relationships and the context of parenting. Psychiatr. Serv. 49, 643–649.

201. Herman, S. P. (1997) Practice parameters for child custody evaluation. American Academy of Child and Adolescent Psychiatry. J. Am. Acad. Child Adolesc. Psychiatry 36(10 Suppl.), 57s–68s.

202. Budd, K. S. and Holdsworth, M. J. (1996) Methodological issues in assembling minimal parenting competence. J. Clin.Child Psychol. 25, 2–14.

203. Jacobsen, T. and Hofmann, V. (1997) Children's attachment representations: Longitudinal relations to behavior and competence in middle childhood and adolescence. Dev. Psychol. 33, 703-710.

204. Rudolph, B., Larson, G. L., Sweeny, S., Hough, E. E. and Arorian, K. (1990) Hospitalized pregnant psychotic women: characteristics and treatment issues. Hosp. Commun. Psychiatry 41, 159–163.

205. Stewart, D. and Gangbar, R. (1984) Psychiatric assessment of competency to care for a new-born. Can. J. Psychiatry 29, 583–589.

206. Gruenbaum, L. and Gammeltoft, M. (1993) Young children of schizophrenic mothers: Difficulties of intervention. Am. J. Orthopsychiatry 63, 16–27.

207. Simms, M. D. and Horwitz, S. M. (1996) Foster home environments: a preliminary report. Dev. Behav. Pediatr. 17, 170–175.

Index

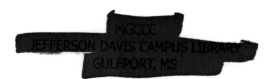